Lecture Notes in Computer Science 9545

Commenced Publication in 1973
Founding and Former Series Editors:
Gerhard Goos, Juris Hartmanis, and Jan van Leeuwen

More information about this series at http://www.springer.com/series/7409

Xiaolong Zheng · Daniel Dajun Zeng
Hsinchun Chen · Scott J. Leischow (Eds.)

Smart Health

International Conference, ICSH 2015
Phoenix, AZ, USA, November 17–18, 2015
Revised Selected Papers

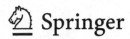 Springer

Editors
Xiaolong Zheng
Institute of Automation, Chinese Academy
  of Sciences
Beijing
China

Daniel Dajun Zeng
Department of MIS
University of Arizona
Tucson, AZ
USA

Hsinchun Chen
University of Arizona
Phoenix, AZ
USA

Scott J. Leischow
Mayo Clinic
Scottsdale, AZ
USA

ISSN 0302-9743   ISSN 1611-3349   (electronic)
Lecture Notes in Computer Science
ISBN 978-3-319-29174-1   ISBN 978-3-319-29175-8   (eBook)
DOI 10.1007/978-3-319-29175-8

Library of Congress Control Number: 2015960232

LNCS Sublibrary: SL3 – Information Systems and Applications, incl. Internet/Web, and HCI

Printed on acid-free paper

This Springer imprint is published by SpringerNature
The registered company is Springer International Publishing AG Switzerland

Preface

Advancing informatics for health care and health-care applications has become an international research priority. There is increased effort to transform reactive care to proactive and preventive care, clinic-centric to patient-centered practice, training-based interventions to globally aggregated evidence, and episodic response to continuous well-being monitoring and maintenance. The annual International Conference for Smart Health (ICSH) began in 2013. This first conference, held in Beijing, China, attracted over 50 contributors and participants from all over the world, providing a forum for meaningful multidisciplinary interactions. In the following year (2014), the conference was also held in Beijing, China. This year (2015), the International Conference for Smart Health (ICSH 2015) was held in Phoenix, Arizona, USA.

ICSH 2015 was organized to develop a platform for authors to discuss fundamental principles, algorithms, or applications of intelligent data acquisition, processing, and analysis of health-care information. Specifically, this conference mainly focused on topics and issues including medical monitoring and information extraction, clinical and medical data mining, health data analysis and management, big data and smart health, and health-care intelligent systems and clinical practice. We are pleased that many high-quality technical papers were submitted, accompanied by evaluation with real-world data or application contexts. The work presented at the conference encompassed a healthy mix of computer science, medical informatics, and information systems approaches.

The 1.5-day event encompassed presentations of 33 papers. The organizers of ICSH 2015 would like to thank the conference sponsors for their support and sponsorship, including the University of Arizona, Mayo Clinic, the Chinese Academy of Sciences, and National Natural Science Foundation of China. We also greatly appreciate the following technical co-sponsors, IEEE SMC Technical Committee on Homeland Security, and Institute for Operations Research and the Management Sciences (INFORMS). We further wish to express our sincere gratitude to all Program Committee members of ICSH 2015, who provided valuable and constructive review comments.

November 2015

Xiaolong Zheng
Daniel Dajun Zeng
Hsinchun Chen
Scott J. Leischow

Organization

Program Committee

Muhammad Amith	University of Texas Health Science Center, USA
Mohd Anwar	North Carolina A&T State University, USA
Yigal Arens	The University of Southern California, USA
Ian Brooks	University of Illinois at Urbana-Champaign, USA
David Buckeridge	McGill University, Canada
Zhidong Cao	Chinese Academy of Sciences, China
Nitesh V. Chawla	University of Notre Dame, USA
Guanling Chen	University of Massachusetts Lowell, USA
Amar Das	Geisel School of Medicine at Dartmouth, USA
Ahmed Gomaa	Marywood University, USA
Natalia Grabar	University of Lille, France
Hung-Hsuan Huang	Ritsumeikan University, Japan
Kun Huang	Ohio State University, USA
Ernesto Jimenez-Ruiz	University of Oxford, UK
Hung-Yu Kao	National Cheng Kung University, Taiwan
Kyoji Kawagoe	Ritsumeikan University, Japan
Kenneth Komatsu	Arizona Department of Health Services, USA
Qingchao Kong	Chinese Academy of Sciences, USA
Erhun Kundakçioğlu	Ozyegin University, Turkey
Dingcheng Li	Mayo Clinic, USA
Jiao Li	Chinese Academy of Medical Sciences, China
Qiudan Li	Chinese Academy of Sciences, China
Xiaoli Li	Institute for Infocomm Research, Singapore
Xin Li	City University of Hong Kong, SAR China
Yunji Liang	The University of Arizona, USA
Jiaqi Liu	Chinese Academy of Sciences, China
Jian Ma	University of Colorado, USA
Deepti Mehrotra	Amity University, India
Mevludin Memedi	Dalarna University, Sweden
Riccardo Miotto	Columbia University, USA
Hamed Monkaresi	University of Sydney, Australia
Jin-Cheon Na	Nanyang Technological University, Singapore
Radhakrishnan Nagarajan	University of Kentucky, USA
Michael O'Grady	University College Dublin, Ireland
Xiaoming Sheng	University of Utah, USA
William Song	Dalarna University, Sweden
Xiaolong Song	Harbin Institute of Technology, China

W. Nick Street	The University of Iowa, USA
Cui Tao	University of Texas Health Science Center at Houston, USA
Jason Wang	New Jersey Institute of Technology, USA
Jiaojiao Wang	Chinese Academy of Sciences, USA
May D. Wang	Georgia Institute of Technology and Emory University, USA
Chunhua Weng	Columbia University, USA
Hui Yang	University of South Florida, USA
Chaogui Zhang	Marywood University, USA
Mi Zhang	Michigan State University, USA
Qingpeng Zhang	City University of Hong Kong, SAR China
Yong Zhang	Tsinghua University, China
Zhu Zhang	Chinese Academy of Sciences, USA
Kang Zhao	University of Iowa, USA

Organizing Committee

Conference Co-chairs

Hsinchun Chen	University of Arizona, USA
Daniel Dajun Zeng	University of Arizona, USA; Chinese Academy of Sciences, China
Scott J. Leischow	Mayo Clinic, USA

Program Co-chairs

Daniel Neill	Carnegie Mellon University, USA
Raghu Santanam	Arizona State University, USA
Yanchun Zhang	Victoria University, Australia

Workshop Co-chairs

John Brownstein	Harvard Medical School, USA
Chunxiao Xing	Tsinghua University, China
Hsin-Min Lu	National Taiwan University, Taiwan

Publication Co-chairs

Xiaolong Zheng	Chinese Academy of Sciences, China
Wendy Chapman	University of Utah, USA

Finance Co-chairs

Ahmed Abbasi	University of Virginia, USA
Donald Adjeroh	West Virginia University, USA

Publicity Co-chairs

Kwok Tsui	City University of Hong Kong, SAR China
Cathy Larson	University of Arizona, USA

Additional Reviewers

Carr, Dominic
Li, Yumei
Myneni, Sahiti
Song, Dezhao
Wang, Xi
Zhang, Shaozhong
Zhou, Jiaqi
Zuo, Zhiya

Contents

Health Data Analysis and Management

Medical Monitoring and Information Extraction

SilverLink: Smart Home Health Monitoring for Senior Care

Joshua Chuang[1], Lubaina Maimoon[1(✉)], Shuo Yu[2], Hongyi Zhu[2],
Casper Nybroe[2], Owen Hsiao[3], Shu-Hsing Li[3], Hsinmin Lu[3],
and Hsinchun Chen[2]

[1] Caduceus Intelligence Corporation, Tucson, AZ, USA
{joshua.chuang,lubainamaimoon}@gmail.com
[2] Artificial Intelligence Lab, University of Arizona, Tucson, AZ, USA
{shuoyu,zhuhy}@email.arizona.edu, casper@nybroe.com,
hchen@eller.arizona.edu
[3] Health Information Research, National Taiwan University, Taipei, Taiwan
owen.w.hsiao@gmail.com, shli@management.ntu.edu.tw,
luim@ntu.edu.tw

Abstract. Senior care has become one of the pressing societal challenges faced by many developed and emerging countries, including the US (the aging baby boomer) and China (the reverse 4-2-1 family pyramid due to one child policy). Despite failing health, most senior citizens prefer to live independently at home and hence the focus of current healthcare technologies have shifted from traditional clinical care to "at-home" care for the senior citizens. We propose to develop SilverLink, a system that is unique in its smart and connected technologies and will offer: (1) affordable and non-invasive home-based mobile health technologies for monitoring health-related motion and daily activities; (2) advanced mobile health analytics algorithms for fall detection, health status progression monitoring, and patient health anomaly detection and alert; and (3) a comprehensive patient health activity portal for reporting user activity and health status and for engaging with family members. This system will initially be launched in the US, in China and in Taiwan and will aim to overcome the limitations of existing home-care solutions.

Keywords: Health big data · Home health monitoring · Health progression monitoring · Senior care · Gait analysis

1 Introduction

Senior citizens face many challenges to their independence, including a decline in mobility or cognition or chronic physical health conditions that compromise their ability to maintain their independence. For example, according to data from the National Safety Council, there were 12,900 deaths from falls in 2003 among those over the age of 65; with 7,500 of those deaths occurring in homes [1].

Presently, friends or family members provide care for most senior citizens. Family caregiving is both emotionally and physically demanding and is generally unpaid. According to a study, the estimated value of this unpaid care is $257M dollars annually [2].

© Springer International Publishing Switzerland 2016
X. Zheng et al. (Eds.): ICSH 2015, LNCS 9545, pp. 3–14, 2016.
DOI: 10.1007/978-3-319-29175-8_1

As most senior citizens prefer to "age in place," the number of older adults living alone continues to increase with at least one out of three non-institutionalized senior citizens living alone [3]. Independent living (e.g., private households) will be an important housing option for the future, particularly for the newly aged [4]. The applications of in-home monitoring technologies will have enormous potential for assuaging the burdens of caregivers and family members.

There are several potential technologies under development for remote health monitoring. These technologies range from in-house lifestyle monitoring to fall detection and monitoring of health vitals such as blood pressure, etc. [5]. The major limitations of existing products in this category include the high cost of technology, lack of flexibility in use, and limited one-dimensional data collection and analytics to "intelligently" monitor health status of senior citizens at-home. Even with recent developments, there is a need for an affordable but smart and non-invasive health monitoring system. Hence, we are motivated to develop, evaluate, and commercialize an easy to use, all encompassing smart and connected home health monitoring system, called SilverLink. SilverLink combines personal emergency response, lifestyle monitoring, and advanced analytics for providing more effective remote care to senior citizens at an affordable price. The significance of the innovation lies in the system's unique ability to combine unobtrusive assistance with real time data monitoring and emergency alerts, and preventive care including health progression analysis and fall risk prediction on an easy-to-use platform.

2 Literature Review and Related Systems

2.1 Mobile Health Monitoring Techniques

Remote monitoring devices gather data about patients' status and relay it to healthcare providers/caregivers on a regular basis. They have not only helped patients to manage a variety of chronic diseases, but also paved a path for communicating with patients beyond the acute care setting. Lifestyle monitoring is crucial to health management for the elderly, who often forget to perform everyday tasks such as taking medications, etc. Mobile health monitoring techniques often use environmental sensors, video recording tools, and/or other surveillance equipment (either alone or in combination) to monitor patients at home. These techniques are often used in conjunction with cloud computing and are often limited in their functionality. Lack of privacy is also a major issue with most monitoring techniques.

Another application of mobile health monitoring is monitoring human motion. The way a physical activity is performed by a human is highly indicative of their health and quality of life. Quantification and reliable measurement of daily physical activity can allow an effective assessment of a person's daily activities as well as the effects of numerous medical conditions and treatments, especially in people suffering from chronic diseases such as arthritis, cardiovascular or neurodegenerative diseases that can often affect gait and mobility [6]. There are several studies in the fields of activity identification, motion tracking, and exercise monitoring including gait monitoring and fall detection. Most products developed in labs use more than one sensor to gather data for analysis of gait pattern. The greater the number of sensors attached to the users, the more accurate the gait that can be modeled from this data. This research is promising but has been mainly conducted within a lab environment and may not be applicable to real life situations: a drawback of existing gait monitoring devices.

2.2   Health Activity Portals and Support

Due to health and mobility issues, an elderly person's world is often smaller — both physically and socially. Digital technology has an obvious role to play here by connecting people virtually when being together is difficult or impossible. Research shows that "persuasive technology" [7] such as in the form of personal messages, frequent communication via photos, videos, and other means can often help motivate people to change their attitudes, and in turn better manage their health. For example, portals such as DiabeticLink provide a platform for diabetics to track and easily visualize health data on the portal and improve health outcomes by monitoring how one health factor can affect another [8].

2.3   Advanced Mobile Analytics

Due to the progress in mobile and sensor technology, it is now possible to collect healthcare information about any patient in a home-based environment. Data collected can range from movement of objects (e.g., displacement of a pillbox) to human motion (e.g., walking, jogging, sitting). This collected data can be used to document medical trends and further analysis of the collected data and patterns can prove useful in predicting health outcomes, thus reducing costs associated with treatment.

Today, healthcare analytics is moving toward a model that will incorporate predictive analytics and enable creation of more personalized healthcare, by predicting patient behavior [9]. Falls are among the most common and serious problems facing older adults and are associated with considerable mortality, morbidity and reduced functioning. Presently a combination of accelerometers and gyroscopes are used to collect data for predicting risk of falls. Electrocardiogram (ECG) data is commonly used to monitor arrhythmias that cause syncope resulting in falls. Capillary finder stick glucose readings are also used to signal hypoglycemia, a condition that contributes to falls. The common algorithms used for pre-processing the signal data include low-pass filtering and wavelet filtering. Variables that can be drawn from such signals to predict the risk of falls include angular velocity, linear acceleration, etc. One limitation of existing tools is that they lack monitoring capabilities for progression of Frailty (slow and natural health deterioration) in older adults.

The existing solutions to home health monitoring are divided into two main categories: (1) Personalized Emergency Response Systems for fall detection and signaling for help and (2) Home-Use Monitoring with Sensors for mobile health.

Personalized Emergency Response Systems (PERS). This is one of the most widely used technology-based home care solutions today. PERS provides an easy way to summon assistance, with the push of a button, in case of an emergency. Advanced PERS also possess fall detection capabilities; however, they do not provide all the components of home health monitoring, e.g., activity monitoring, medicine reminders, etc. Some examples of these devices include Alert 1, Phillips Medical Alert System, Bay Medical Systems and Medical Guardian. None of these systems can actively monitor user at-home activity or health status or provide any "intelligent" or proactive assistance. In addition, Internet-connected fitness wristbands (e.g., FitBit) and health-monitoring smart watches (e.g., Apple Watch) are gaining traction with the youth. These devices use accelerometers for activity level tracking and calorie counting, sensors for heart rate and temperature measurement, and GPS for location tracking. Despite their emerging popularity, such devices do not target home care or activity monitoring for the aging population.

Home-Use Monitoring with Sensors. Some of the more basic and mature home monitoring systems such as home security systems (e.g., ADT home security) and home video surveillance (e.g., Nest Cam, ADT Pulse) do not adopt or leverage advanced multi-sensor technologies or cloud-based intelligent analytics services. Some Smart Home researchers used object sensors with pressure sensors on the floor to recognize users' daily activities, which is not easily applicable in real home settings [10]. Among the emerging technology leaders in this space, MyLively has shown the most promise. Despite its initial validation, MyLively lacks several critical function-alities such as gait analysis; health progression monitoring; health tracking and a proactive analytics algorithm to generate automated alerts upon detection of health anomalies.

3 System Design

3.1 SilverLink Architecture

The SilverLink system consists of both hardware and software components for various types of home monitoring and analytics services. The hardware components include multiple sensors; a home gateway and an SOS alarm pendant/wristband. The software components consist of data collection API, a database, an analytics engine and a web portal. The overall service architecture is shown in Fig. 1. The SilverLink system will use object and human sensors placed inside a user's home for the purpose of remote monitoring. The object sensors will be attached to relevant household objects that can help indicate user activity or health status based on users' preference and lifestyle, e.g., pillbox (indicating medication compliance), refrigerator (indicating regular food intake), shower or bathroom door (indicating personal hygiene routines), front/garage door (indicating exiting/entering a home), etc. The human sensor (one for each user) attached on the user's body at all times will continuously record any motion performed (walking, sitting, falling) by the user. The user will also be provided with an SOS alarm pendant/wristband for emergencies. A pre-configured gateway will use BLE and 3G communication techniques to receive and transmit data collected from the sensors to the Datacenter where the advanced analytics engine will then process this data and check for any abnormalities in the movement patterns.

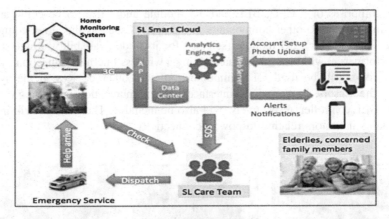

Fig. 1. SilverLink architecture: hardware (sensors/gateway), software (analytics/portal), and services

The SilverLink web portal will provide a platform (on devices such as laptops, tablets, mobile phones, etc.) to visualize the health information collected by the sensors. The analytics engine will process the data to make deductions based on pattern recognition and these deductions will in turn stimulate notifications/alerts when a shift in pattern in detected. The personalized response system with the SOS alarm button can be activated (by the user) to alert the emergency response team, who will confirm the emergency via a telephonic call and check for false alarms. Upon receiving a confirmation (or in the event that no contact is established) the emergency response team will be sent out to the user's residence to provide the necessary help.

3.2 Hardware Design for Home Activity Sensors and Gateway

SilverLink has three types of activity sensors: (1) object sensors, (2) human sensors, and (3) SOS alarm pendant/wristband (Fig. 2a and b). The object and human sensors are comprised of high-sensitivity tri-axis acceleration chips. Each sensor further includes a wireless communication system, such as Bluetooth (e.g., BLE 4.0) and will periodically emit signals to indicate the sensor status and to synchronize the sensor with other components of the monitoring system. A coin cell battery will power the sensor enclosed in a lightweight and durable casing with an attachment mechanism that allows the sensor to be attached to a variety of different objects. For human motion monitoring, the sensor will have an additional hook or loop for users to easily attach the sensor to their belt/keychain.

The SOS alarm (Fig. 2b) will comprise of an easy-to-use push button alarm sensor that will be used to send a distress signal. LEDs on the body of the alarm will indicate the status of the signal (i.e. sent to/received by the datacenter) to the user.

The home gateway (Fig. 2c) will typically be located inside the residence of a user and will be configured to receive signals and data transmitted from one or more sensors placed inside the house (object sensors) or on the user (human sensor). The home gateway comprises of a CPU, BLE and 3G module and will also be configured to transmit information to other components in the system such as the cloud-computing network. The gateway's 3G module (selected for its wide availability, low cost, and stable performance) will be used for maintaining a wireless Internet connection, while a BLE controller will be used for communication with other devices in the system, including the sensors. Programming interfaces, in communication with the gateway's CPU and BLE controller, respectively, will also be included. The gateway will include typical status indicators relating to power, connectivity, etc.

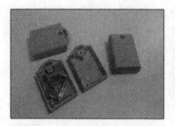 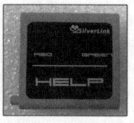 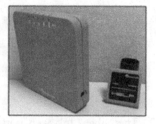

Fig. 2. a. (left) Customizable object and human sensors prototype; **b.** (center) The SOS alarm prototype; **c.** (right) The Home Gateway prototype.

3.3   Data Collection API and Activity Database

The data collection API will be used to collect data from the different sensors placed in a user's home. A datacenter will be configured to store raw data collected from activity sensors and send it to the datacenter via the gateway using a 3G-communication protocol. Examples of the types of data stored in the tables include gateway, sensor and system information; raw sensor log data; sanitized data for analysis; processed data representing user activities; and web portal management data such as user login and profile, links, notifications, etc.

3.4   Process Design for Advanced Analytics Engine

SilverLink's novel analytics engine is configured to process and analyze data obtained by other components of the system. Accordingly, the analytics engine employs an algorithm (e.g., an abnormal pattern detection algorithm) to perform such tasks as advanced pattern recognition. Figure 3 shows the flow of data through the monitoring system and the analytics engine. Data is sourced from the remote sensors and transmitted through the monitoring system to the data collection API such that a set of raw sensor data is generated and is subjected to data transformation and integration steps for noise reduction and sanitization. Various analytics approaches including pattern recognition and signal detection to generate user activity data and define signal patterns are then performed on the data. These signals will then either be recorded and stored in user activity tables or used to send out notifications to family members/caregivers.

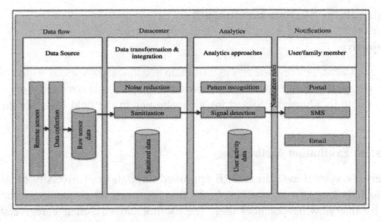

Fig. 3. SilverLink software design: data flow, datacenter, analytics, and notifications

3.5 Design for SilverLink Web Portal

The SilverLink web portal is an online monitoring and data visualization tool designed to allow family members/caregivers to remotely monitor their loved ones.

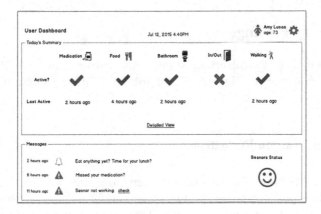

Fig. 4. SilverLink's user dashboard displaying a user's activity summary for the day

The SilverLink web portal offers utilities such as user sign in or registration (sign up), user dashboard to view monitoring data (Fig. 4), sensor configuration (sensor status and location of the sensor), notifications, notification settings (selection of the threshold for notification/alert generation) and administrative options (adding or editing a new user profile). It provides a passage for communication between the user and their family member through a feature called SilverMail, a video and photo-sharing interface. The web portal provides password-protected access to registered users and will be accessible from, or transmit information to computers, tablets or smartphones.

4   Preliminary System Evaluation

4.1   Objective

The aim of evaluating the system was to obtain feedback on various aspects of SilverLink's design and usage for system improvement and to uncover areas of potential research to help in advancing SilverLink's capabilities in the field of senior care.

4.2   System Evaluation Methodology

The SilverLink system evaluation (IRB approved through the University of Arizona) was conducted using two approaches. In the first approach we conducted introductory research by interviewing potential users (i.e., senior citizens, their caregivers/family members and physicians) to gauge user need and obtain preliminary feedback on the current version of the SilverLink prototype. The second approach was to test the prototype in a laboratory setting (or mock home environments) to evaluate factors such as the operating distance between the Gateway and the sensors (range), battery life, data transmission rate, data loss rate, system errors, stability of the website and the capabilities of the analytics engine. The preliminary interviews were conducted in the US, whereas the laboratory tests were conducted in the US and in Taiwan.

5   Preliminary Findings

The alpha prototype of the SilverLink system was developed in April 2015. Results from the preliminary evaluation (April–August 2015) of the alpha prototype are summarized below.

5.1   SilverLink Taiwan Evaluation

Internal System Testing. The internal tests were conducted in three different home settings. The floor plan and house structures were carefully selected to bring diversity to the test scenarios. There were five separate tests that were conducted on each of the sensors (1 human sensor and 4 object sensors) and their signal activity was measured at distances of 1 M through to 10 M. During the tests, the subject wore the human sensor at all times, i.e. while walking, sitting and sleeping. The object sensors were placed on objects such as pillboxes, refrigerator door, front door, and the bathroom door while a subject was asked to displace each object in predefined test cases with 5 repetitions. It was found that the pass rate (the number of times the system recorded the event divided by the actual number of events) was 70–80 % for object sensors while it was less than 60 % for the human sensors. The average range of the object and human sensors was found to be approximately 7.3 m.

5.2   SilverLink US Evaluation

Preliminary Interviews. The preliminary evaluation of the SilverLink prototype included introductory interviews conducted with several potential users. The 9 interviewees included a 72-year-old patient with Parkinson's and his wife, an 85-year-old man afflicted with Spinal Stenosis and his caregiver, a couple (female aged 68 and male aged 75) who had recently experienced a fall, two physicians, and an expert working with a local center on aging. These interviews were very useful in determining the need for a system like SilverLink. The wife of the Parkinson's patient commented, "This system will put me at ease whenever I am away from my husband." while others provided feedback on the size of the SOS wristband. One interviewee said, "It is too big and I would not like to wear it on my wrist." Another observation during these interviews was that the elderly people often have trouble wearing watches due to conditions such as arthritis and hence it was determined that a wrist band may not be the most suitable form for an SOS alarm. A domain expert also provided research findings from previously conducted form factor studies and this information was critical to the redesigning of the SOS alarm.

Internal System Testing. To estimate the signal loss rate, one internal subject (male, age 23, of average height and weight) was fitted with two sensors, then asked to perform a series of actions including sitting, standing, and walking, at locations of varying distances from the gateway. Three locations were selected to test whether the sensor-gateway distance will affect the signal loss rate. At Locations 1 and 2, all actions were performed within 5 meters from the gateway. At Location 3, the sensor was around 10 meters from the gateway, and there existed a wall between them. The signal loss rate varied between 30 to 70 % at Locations 1 and 2, but increased to 90 % at Location 3. In one instance at Location 3, the gateway did not receive any signals at all. Based on the initial test results, a future improvement will be enhancing the stability of signal transmission.

6   Preliminary Mobile Sensor Research

6.1   Research Design

While living alone, a senior person may encounter different scenarios that are worth attention from his/her caregivers. For instance, (1) walking at a normal speed around the house performing daily chores; (2) walking at a drastically decreased speed on a certain day; (3) sitting on a chair for most part of the day and seldom standing or walking; or (4) lying on a bed for 24 h. Such situations are often indicative of a person's health condition (such as healthy, improving, deteriorating or even in a state of emergency). Inferences drawn from such data can help a senior citizen's caregiver and/or doctor to formulate focused health plans. The human sensor used for activity/motion detection contains a tri-axial accelerometer, which tracks the user's actions and sends acceleration signals to the gateway. Analytic algorithms are needed to aggregate the signals to high-level parameters (e.g., walking speed and step count) and make meaningful inferences. Najafi et al. [11] proposed activity recognition algorithms based on a single tri-axial accelerometer, much similar to our setting. However, the location for the accelerometer is restricted to the center of the chest, and its orientation has to be determined beforehand, i.e., the sensor cannot be set upside-down or be tilted in an arbitrary angle. Furthermore, high sampling frequencies (40 to 120 Hz) are preferred in such studies, which, lead to a limited battery life for the sensors (15 days at maximum).

The first part of our research is focused on developing an algorithm (for the human sensor) to deliver the walking speed of a user, using a sampling rate of 10 Hz with extended battery life, 30–50 % physical data loss, arbitrary location for sensor attachment (firm and not dangling) to the user, and an arbitrary orientation of the sensor. Solving the motion detection problem in this real setting has been a challenge for researchers. We aim to solve this problem by reconstructing the inertial reference system based on the tri-axial acceleration signals. Further inferences (e.g., posture/activity recognition) will also rely on this algorithm.

The second part of our research is Activity of Daily Living (ADL) Recognition. Activity of Daily Living refers to the basic self-care activities performed by a person each day. Analysis of activity data can reveal patterns that are indicative of a person's lifestyle and can be used to improve health outcomes, especially for senior citizens. Current research is based on using only object sensors, e.g. pressure sensors for ADL recognition. However, in a real home setting, using object sensors or human sensor alone is not sufficient for ADL recognition as the activity performer's information is not included in the object sensor data. For example, in the case of a caregiver preparing lunch for a user, the activity of opening the fridge detected by object sensor (attached to the fridge door) can be associated with either the caregiver or the user in the room. The object sensor fails to distinguish between the user and the caregiver. Similarly, the human sensor alone does not provide sufficient data on the kind of activity a user performs. Our preliminary research is focused on evaluating how the use of object sensors with a human sensor (with the advanced algorithm) can give us a better understanding of a user's ADL and help in ADL recognition.

6.2 Preliminary Research Findings

As part of our preliminary research, we used our sensors to collect data patterns for different user motions such as running, walking, standing, sitting and falling down. These patterns will be instrumental in developing the algorithm for pattern recognition and health prediction for senior citizens. Figure 5a and b show a graphical representation of the patterns obtained while a person is walking, running or falling down respectively. These patterns are far more complex and varied in real life and identifying them to make meaningful inferences is an integral part of our research.

For preliminary research on ADL, we used both an object sensor and a human sensor together to determine their combined effectiveness in ADL recognition. Several experimental scenarios were set up in a home environment to understand the interaction between a user and the object. In every scenario, the human sensor was attached to the user's left shirt pocket. Object sensors were placed on a fridge door, a chair in the kitchen, a pillbox, and a bathroom door. Each pair of scenarios compared interactions

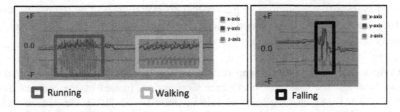

Fig. 5. a. (left) Represents running and walking motion; **b.** (right) Represents a person falling

between user performing the activities and others performing the activities while the user is simply moving. For example, scenario pair 1&2 involved (1) user walking to the fridge and opening the fridge door (2) Finding and grabbing items (3) Closing the fridge door and (4) Walking away. In the plots (Fig. 6a and b), the x-axis denotes the time and y-axis denotes the acceleration level. The shaded area depicts the time period when the fridge was open (from the first triggered signal to the last triggered signal). In Scenario 1, we noticed that user's interactions with the fridge resulted in a difference between motion data collected inside and outside the shaded time period. In contrast, movements captured by the human sensor in Scenario 2 were consistent throughout all time periods. We can infer that the user's movement and "using the fridge" activity has less relevance compared with Scenario 1. This observation result introduced an efficient way to extract human-object interaction that could be a helpful feature or criterion in user's ADL recognition.

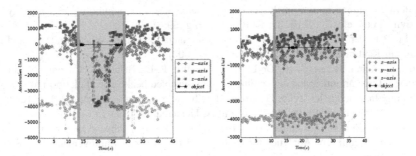

Fig. 6. a. (left) Scenario 1: User used the fridge. **b.** (right) Scenario 2: Others used the fridge while the user was walking.

7   System Improvement and Future Development Plans

Presently, the team is focusing on improving hardware and software functionalities such as operating range, battery life, SOS design, stability of data transmission, and data visualization on the SilverLink web portal. Further research into utilizing both object sensors and human sensors for the ADL recognition will be conducted and will be accompanied by detailed gait analysis (using human sensors) and algorithm enhancement (for determining the walking speed in users) to better understand cases with arbitrary sensor orientations (e.g., vertical to horizontal). The team will also be conducting an extensive 100-person interactive user study (in the US, China and Taiwan) to obtain further feedback on updated versions of the system.

Acknowledgements. This work is supported in part by the University of Arizona Artificial Intelligence Lab and the Caduceus Intelligence Corporation, funded by the National Science Foundation (IIP-1417181) and the National Taiwan University (NTUH). We wish to acknowledge our collaborators in the U.S. and Taiwan for their research support. We would also like to extend our gratitude to Miss Xiao Liu for her contributions.

References

1. National Safety Council. Report On Injuries in America, (2003, 2004). http://www.nsc.org/library/report_injury_usa.htm
2. Toseland, R.W., Smith, G., McCallion, P.: Family caregivers of the frail elderly. In: Gitterman, A. (ed.) Handbook of Social Work Practice with Vulnerable and Resilient Populations. Columbia University, New York (2001)
3. Cannuscio, C., Block, J., Kawachi, I.: Social capital and successful aging: the role of senior housing. Ann. Intern. Med. **139**(5 pt. 2), 395–399 (2003)
4. Mann, W.C., Marchant, T., Tomita, M., Fraas, L., Stanton, K., Care, M. J.: Elder acceptance of health monitoring devices in the home. Winter **3**(2), 91–98 (2001–2002)
5. Brownsell, S.J., Bradley, D.A., Bragg, R., Catlin, P., Carlier, J.: Do community alarm users want telecare? J. Telemed. Telecare. **6**(4), 199–204 (2000)
6. Najafi, B., Aminian K., Paraschiv-Ionescu, A., Loew, F., Büla C.J., Robert, P.: Ambulatory system for human motion analysis using a kinematic sensor: monitoring of daily physical activity in the elderly. IEEE Trans. Biomed. Eng. **50**(6) 2003
7. Fogg, B.J.: Persuasive Technology: Using Computers to Change What We Think and Do. Morgan Kaufmann Publishers, San Francisco (2002)
8. Chen, J., Chen, H., Li, S.-H., De La Cruz, H., Wu, P.-L., Hsiao, O., Chuang, J., Liu, X.: DiabeticLink: an integrated and intelligent cyber-enabled health social platform for diabetic patients. In: Zheng, X., Zeng, D., Chen, H., Zhang, Y., Xing, C., Neill, D.B. (eds.) ICSH 2014. LNCS, vol. 8549, pp. 63–74. Springer, Heidelberg (2014)
9. Cortada, J., Gordon, D., Lenihan, B.: Advanced analytics in healthcare. In: Strome, T.L. (ed.) Healthcare Healthcare Analytics for Quality and Performance Improvement, pp. 183–203 (2013). Web
10. Krishnan, N.C., Cook, D.J.: Activity recognition on streaming sensor data. Pervasive Mobile Comput. **10**, 138–154 (2014)
11. Najafi, B., Armstrong, D.G., Mohler, J.: Novel wearable technology for assessing spontaneous daily physical activity and risk of falling in older adults with diabetes. J. Diab. Sci. Technol. **7**(5), 1147–1160 (2013)

Real-Time Models to Predict the Use of Vasopressors in Monitored Patients

André Braga[1], Filipe Portela[1,2(✉)], Manuel Filipe Santos[1],
António Abelha[1], José Machado[1], Álvaro Silva[3], and Fernando Rua[3]

[1] Algoritmi Research Centre, University of Minho, Guimaraes, Portugal
cfp@dsi.uminho.pt
[2] ESEIG, Porto Polytechnic, Vila do Conde, Portugal
[3] Intensive Care Unit, Centro Hospitalar do Porto, Porto, Portugal

Abstract. The needs of reducing human error has been growing in every field of study, and medicine is one of those. Through the implementation of technologies is possible to help in the decision making process of clinics, therefore to reduce the difficulties that are typically faced. This study focuses on easing some of those difficulties by presenting real-time data mining models capable of predicting if a monitored patient, typically admitted in intensive care, will need to take vasopressors. Data Mining models were induced using clinical variables such as vital signs, laboratory analysis, among others. The best model presented a sensitivity of 94.94 %. With this model it is possible reducing the misuse of vasopressors acting as prevention. At same time it is offered a better care to patients by anticipating their treatment with vasopressors.

Keywords: Vasopressors · INTCare · Intensive medicine · Real-time · Data mining · Vital signs · Laboratory results

1 Introduction

There is an ongoing effort to implement Information Technologies (IT) in medical facilities, since they can ease various developed activities. In Intensive Medicine (IM) there are numerous devices and technologies helping intensivist to develop their job more precisely, in order to take care of critically ill patients.

The use of Data Mining (DM) is one of such technologies becoming more common in Intensive Care Units (ICU) where the patient is continuous monitored and it is possible collecting data in real-time. Objectively, it seeks to use data produced by many devices and transform it into new knowledge helping the decision making process.

In ICUs the use of vasopressors is very common in order to improve patient condition, however sometimes the therapy is not applied in the correct time. In order to provide a better patient care this study was conducted. The aim of this study is to use DM in order to predict if a patient will need to take a vasopressor or not. If the prediction is verified, the intent is to alert the intensivists. So that they can act before that necessity materializes itself. Otherwise these models are useful to avoid wrong prescriptions.

Data Mining models were induced using real data provided by Hospital Santo António, Centro Hospitalar do Porto, Porto, Portugal. The data were collected from

© Springer International Publishing Switzerland 2016
X. Zheng et al. (Eds.): ICSH 2015, LNCS 9545, pp. 15–25, 2016.
DOI: 10.1007/978-3-319-29175-8_2

vital sings monitors presented in the ICU, laboratory analysis and Electronic Health Record (EHR).

Analysing the developed DM models, very good results were achieved. The best model reached a sensitivity of 94.94 %.

Apart from the introduction, this article is composed by other four chapters. Background is the Sect. 2 where it presents information relative to related work. The Sect. 3 - Study Description - enunciates the methods and tools used in the development of the study and it is presented through the CRISP-DM phases. In the Sect. 4 is presented and discussed the results of the study. Lastly, in the Sect. 5 is drawn the conclusion regarding to the study.

2   Background

Information Systems and Technologies are very important nowadays and allowed progress and success beyond imagined in many diverse areas. The area of Intensive Medicine (IM) belongs to the medical sciences and it seeks to help critically ill patients [1]. Through prevention, diagnosis and treatment, intensivists try to recover the patient's to prior state of health [2]. These activities take place in Intensive Care Units (ICU) which are facilities specifically designed for these types of patients, where the existence of life-support devices that monitor patients' vital sings is abundant. Along with the use of drugs these represent a strong ally to help patients [3].

The use of vasopressors is on focus here. This is a type of drug normally used to increase blood pressure (BP) in patients where BP is minimal and patient's life is at risk [4]. Adrenaline, Noradrenaline and Dopamine are three developed vasopressors that mimic the effects of neurotransmitter substances of the sympathetic nervous system. They act as agonists in α_1 and α_2 adrenergic receptors being responsible for vaso-constriction, which in turn increases blood pressure [5]. The use of vasopressors need to be very carefully planned when a patient is with arrhythmias [6, 7].

The interest in study the use of vasopressors comes from the realization of INTCare [8], a research project being developed in Centro Hospitalar do Porto (CHP). This project implemented an information system in the hospital where the acquisition process was modified. The data acquisition changed from a manual, on paper way to an automatic, electronic and real-time process [9, 10]. The interactions within the system are done through intelligent agents. These agents act autonomously and belong to four different subsystems: Data Acquisition, Knowledge Management, Inference and Interface [11]. Due to an iterative process, it is now a Pervasive Intelligent Decision Support System (PIDSS) which using Data Mining (DM) supports the decision making process in ICU. This PIDSS is able to predict patient's outcome [12, 13], organ failure [14], readmission [15, 16], discharge and length of stay [17, 18], among others [19]. Data Mining can be define as a process of looking for patterns in great amounts of data, with the intent of describing the data or use it to predict future events. It is the conversion of data into useful information [20].

Being DM an integral part of the INTCare system [21] this study seeks to improve on a prior study [22] which had the objective of developing data mining models capable of predicting the use of vasopressors in monitored patients of intensive care units. DM models used variables from vital sings monitors, laboratory analysis and Electronic Health Record (EHR) to make predictions upon the future necessity of vasopressor intake. The variables were selected based on possible causes for various health conditions that require vasopressors as treatment. In total six different scenarios combining the variables and four different algorithms – Naïve Bayes, Support Vector Machines, Decision Tree and Generalized Linear Model – where induced. In this first phase only were used raw data without classes. The results achieved were very satisfactory having the best model reached the 90.72 % in the sensitivity metric.

Despite the results being very good there was still the intent to try and improve upon those results. This time some changes were made to the dataset and to the percentage of test/training of the models, in order to see how the results would cope with that. While before the vital sings and laboratory analysis variables used raw values, this time the values were aggregated into classes, with clinical meaning.

This work represents an ongoing effort of trying to innovate and augment the conditions offered by intensive care facilities of CHP, so that the treatment given to patients is always improving and the intensivists can make more precise decisions.

3 Study Description

3.1 Method and Tools

This study was developed according to the guidelines provided by the Cross Industry Standard Process for Data Mining (CRISP-DM), a methodology often used in solving data mining related problems. This methodology is composed by six phases, which are Business Understanding, Data Understanding, Data Preparation, Modeling, Evaluation and Deployment. The possibility of moving backwards and forward is one of the characteristics that makes CRISP-DM a very versatile methodology.

Oracle SQL Developer was the tool used to perform the Extract Transforming and Loading Process (ETL) and induce data mining models. It is an Integrated Development Environment (IDE) used for development and management of Oracle Databases. The modeling part of CRISP-DM in which data mining models were developed was done recurring to the Oracle Data Miner extension available in Oracle SQL Developer.

3.2 Business and Data Understanding

Based on patient's clinical data, the goal of this study is to improve the results of previous developed data mining models to predict if a patient will need vasopressors or not. This way it is possible to provide patients a higher quality of care, by allowing intensivists to make more precise decisions. Also this study differentiates from the previous study because it seeks to aggregate the various variables in classes (using clinical knowledge) and realize if that will increase the quality of the results.

CHP is the provider of the data being used in this study, which concerns vital signs, laboratory analysis and Electronic Health Record (EHR) of patients admitted to the

Intensive Care Unit (ICU). The data being used ranges from January 6th, 2015 to May 18th, 2015 and holds 1259 rows of data concerning 56 distinct patients.

In total seventeen variables were used: SPO2, ECG_HR, ART_SYS, TEMP_T1, PH, Erythrocytes, Potassium, Glucose, Leucocytes, Lactate, PCO2, Hemoglobin, Age, Sex, Provenience, Type_Hospitalization and Hospitalization_Surgery. The target variable is VSPGeral which represents if the patient did take a vasopressor or not. Below in Table 1, it is possible to overview the variables used, their type and source.

Table 1. Variables overview

Variable	Type	Source
Saturation of oxygen (SPO2)	String	Vital signs
Hearth rate (ECG_HR)	String	Vital signs
Blood pressure (ART_SYS)	String	Vital signs
Temperature (TEMP_T1)	String	Vital signs
Leucocytes and erythrocytes	String	Lab analysis
Potassium and potential hydrogen (PH)	String	Lab analysis
Glucose and hemoglobin	String	Lab analysis
Pressure of carbone dioxide (PCO2) and lactate	String	Lab analysis
Dopamine, noradrenaline and adrenaline	String	Lab analysis
Age	Number	EHR
Sex	String	EHR
Provenience	String	EHR
Type_Hospitalization	String	EHR
Hospitalization_Surgery	String	EHR
VSPGeral	String	–

3.3 Data Preparation

In this phase the Extract, Transform and Loading (ETL) process was executed. Since great part of the issues concerning the data used in the previous study, the only iterations done this time was the transformation of the values from string type to number type through the use of a function and the aggregation of the variables' results into classes with clinical meaning. The reason for this change is centered on the fact that a normal distribution could hold results in the wrong class. Therefore the results were divided in three classes: Critical Low, Normal and Critical High. Critical Low represents values below the reference values, Normal represents value within the reference values and Critical High represents values above the reference values.

In Table 2 it is presented the variables and values' range for each of the classes.

Table 2. Variables and values' range per class

	Variable	Units	Critic low	Normal	Critic high
Vital signs	Temperature (TEMP)	°C	34–36	36–38	38–45
	Blood pressure (ART SYS)	mmHg	0–90	90–180	180–500
	Heart rate (ECG_HR)	BPM	0–60	60–120	120–250
	SPO2	%	0–90	90–100	100–500
Laboratory analysis	Hemoglobin	g/dL	<12.00	12.0–18.0	>18.00
	PH		<7.35	7.35–7.45	>7.45
	Leukocytes	$10^3/\mu L$	<4.00	4.00–11.00	>11.00
	Potassium	mmol/L	<3.50	3.50–5.30	>5.50
	Lactate	mmol/L	<0.50	0.50–2.20	>2.20
	Glucose	mg/dl	<70.00	70.00–105.00	>105.00
	PCO2	mmHg	<32.00	32.00–45.00	>45.00
	Erythrocytes	$10^6/\mu L$	<4.10	4.10–5.50	>5.50

To change each attribute's field to a class an update to the attributes table was made. This operation changed the field of the attribute to a class name according to the value in the attribute's field. To calculate these classes an algorithm to track patient condition [23] able to calculate critical events [24] was adopted. This method was also repeated for every single one of the variables belonging to vital signs and laboratory analysis. As example it is the updated of Leucocytes attribute:

```
UPDATE PATIENT_DMCLASSES
   SET LEUCOCYTES = CASE
   WHEN LEUCOCYTES < 4.0 then "Critical Low"
   WHEN LEUCOCYTES >= 4.0 AND LEUCOCITOS <=11.0 then
   "Normal"
   WHEN LEUCOCYTES > 11.0 then "Critical High"
END.
```

The creation of the target variable VSPGeral resulted from the combination of the three vasopressor variables: Dopamine, Adrenaline and Noradrenaline. When a row had at least one of these three variables with value "1", the VSPGeral value for that row was 1. Otherwise the patient did not receive a vasopressor and VSPGeral value was 0.

3.4   Modeling

Data mining models were built according to the objective of the study in this phase. Since the objective is to predict a discrete result, i.e., if a patient will need to take a vasopressor or not, the data mining function to be used is Classification.

The structure of the data mining models was maintained the same as in the previous study, resulting in a distribution of the target variable (VSPGeral) with 37.81 % of patients having taken vasopressors while 62.19 % of patients did not take any vasopressor. The variables were aggregated into groups in order to understand how they could influence the results of the data mining models. In Table 3 it is possible to see which group each variables belong.

Table 3. Variables aggregated in groups

Group	Variables
Vital Signs (VS)	SPO2, ECG_HR, ART_SYS, TEMP_T1
Lab Analysis (LA)	PH, Erythrocytes, Potassium, Glucose, Leucocytes, Lactate, PCO2, Hemoglobin
Patient Admission (PA)	Provenience, Type_Admission, Admission_Surgery
Case Mix (CM)	Age, Sex

After the formation of the groups, six new scenarios were modeled. At first the same distribution was used for test and training, respectively, 40 % and 60 %, but afterwards Cross Validation (all data for training and test) was used for test in order to see the effects on the results. Table 4 displays the modeled scenarios and the groups that compose them.

Table 4. Scenarios and their group of variables

Scenarios	Groups
S1	VS + LA + PA + CM
S2	VS + LA + PA
S3	VS + LA + CM
S4	LA + CM
S5	VS + CM
S6	PA + CM

Each one of the scenarios were executed using four data mining algorithms: Support Vector Machine (SVM), Decision Tree (DT), Naïve Bayes (NB) and Generalized Linear Model (GLM), which are all the algorithms available in the software being used.

The combination of scenarios and algorithms results in a total of 48 models (6 scenarios * 4 algorithms * 2 validation techniques). The following expression can represent a general model:

$$M_n = A_x + S_i + T_z + V_t$$

In the expression M_n is the model with a classification approach (A_x), a scenario (S_i), an algorithm (T_z) and a validation technique (V_t):

In Table 5 is presented the settings used for each one of the data mining algorithms.

Table 5. Data mining algorithm's settings

Support Vector Machine	
Kernel Function	Gaussian
Tolerance Value	0,001
Active Learning	Yes
Decision Tree	
Homogeneity Metric	Gini
Maximum Depth	7
Minimum Records in a Node	10
Minimum Percent of Records in a Node	0,05
Minimum Records for a Split	20
Minimum Percent of Records for a Split	0,1
Naive Bayes	
Pairwise and Singleton Threshold	0
Generalized Linear Model	
Reference Class name	1
Missing Value Treatment	Mean Mode
Ridge Regression	Disable
Approximate Computation	Disable

3.5   Evaluation

When the evaluation phases of CRISP-DM is reached, the results given by each one of the data mining model, each scenario should be analyzed in order to conclude which scenario has the best results. In this study the results were analyzed based on a confusion matrix and Receiver Operating Characteristic (ROC) curves. The analysis of the confusion matrix resulted on the production of results based on three different metrics: sensitivity, specificity and accuracy.

Being the main goal the prediction of the necessity to take a vasopressor, the main metric selected was sensitivity, because it focuses in predicting true positive values, i.e. patients that will have to take a vasopressor. These analyzes were done over two attempts: the first attempt (CL1) differentiates from the previous study because it has vital signs and analysis' values aggregated in classes. The second attempt (CL2) is equal to CL1, except instead of using a distribution of 40/60 (%) for test/training. CL2 used Cross Validation for test and training. The intent is to understand how the clinical classes and the percentage of test/training of data can affect the final results.

4   Discussion

As in the previous study, the focus was to have very sensitive models. In this case the objective was to see if the results got better results based on the aggregation of the variables' values into classes and later by evaluating using CV. The general results were better not only for sensitivity, but also for specificity and accuracy. It was used the same threshold: 85 % for sensitivity, 70 % for accuracy and 60 % for specificity.

The first attempt using the aggregation in classes and a distribution of test/training of 40/60 (%) resulted in better results than in the previous study without classes.

In Table 6 are presented the scenarios (Sc), algorithms (Al) and values of the best three models for metric, belonging to each attempt.

Table 6. Top 3 models per metric

Previous study			CL1			CL2		
Sensitivity			Sensitivity			Sensitivity		
Sc	Al	Value	Sc	Al	Value	Sc	Al	Value
S1	SVM	90.72 %	S6	SVM	94.18 %	S6	SVM	94.94 %
S1	NB	89.22 %	S1	DT	93.18 %	S3	SVM	94.44 %
S3	NB	88,68 %	S3/S4	DT	92.89 %	S1	SVM	94.01 %
Specificity			Specificity			Specificity		
Sc	Al	Value	Sc	Al	Value	Sc	Al	Value
S3	SVM	82.72 %	S1	SVM	85.14 %	S1	SVM	87.57 %
S4	SVM	76.00 %	S3	SVM	79.17 %	S4	SVM	85.51 %
S1	NB	70.44 %	S2	SVM	75.94 %	S3	SVM	83.49 %
Accuracy			Accuracy			Accuracy		
Sc	Al	Value	Sc	Al	Value	Sc	Al	Value
S3	SVM	86.02 %	S1	SVM	89.61 %	S1	SVM	91.50 %
S4	SVM	82.84 %	S3	SVM	87.29 %	S4	SVM	90.23 %
S1	SVM	81.14 %	S6	SVM	84.75 %	S3	SVM	89.91 %

Through the observation of Table 6 we can infer that the use of classes in CL1 resulted in an increase of the metrics values, when compared to the Previous Study in which were used the variable values, instead of classes. On the other hand, CL2 which used cross validation (CV) also proved to increase results for all measures when to compare to the first attempt, and even more so when compared to the previous study.

In parallel with the models of the previous study, all of the metrics increased. In CL1, sensitivity increased in average 3.88 %, specificity 3.69 % and accuracy 3.87 %.

On the other hand, CL2 which also used classes but used CV for test and training showed even better results than the first attempt. This time the increase relative to the previous study was much more substantial, having the sensitivity increased in average 4.92 %, specificity 9.14 % and accuracy 7.21 %.

The best model is now belonging to CL2, where scenario 6 and algorithm SVM surpassed the both best models from Previous Study and CL1 with 94.94 %.

Concerning the ROC curves, it is possible to observe in Figs. 1 and 2 that the use of classes increased marginally the area under the curve of the most sensitive models belonging to CL1 and CL2. While in the previous study the ROC curve of the most sensitive model had a value of 83.06 %, now CL1 has a value of 84.75 % and CL2 has a value of 83.80 %.

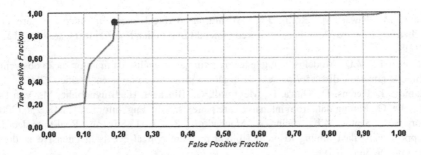

Fig. 1. CL1 – S6/SVM – ROC curve

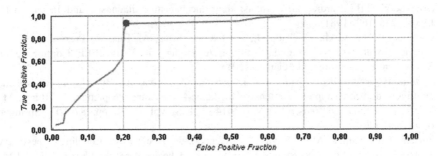

Fig. 2. CL2 – S6/SVM – ROC curve

5 Conclusion

The results obtained in this study represent the success of the objectives defined - the improvement of the results attained in the previous study. Prediction results increased on all metrics, but more importantly on sensitivity, which it is the metric that predicts if the patient will need to take a vasopressor. This improvement will increase the strength that previous models already had. At first it benefits the patients by avoiding the side effects that vasopressors might have. In second this models seeking to improve their health condition. In fact intensivists will have less stressful and uncertain decisions and the hospital will reducing costs and waste of resources by avoiding wrong therapeutics associated to the use of vasopressors.

Overall the correct implementation of data mining models that can predict a relevant aspect concerning patient's health is always very important and welcome.

Acknowledgments. This work has been supported by FCT - Fundação para a Ciência e Tecnologia within the Project Scope UID/CEC/00319/2013 and the contract PTDC/EEI-SII/1302/2012 (INTCare II).

References

1. Kaur, M., Pawar, M., Kohli, J.K., Mishra, S.: Critical events in intensive care unit. Indian J. Crit. Care Med.: Peer-reviewed Official Publ. Indian Soc. Critical Care Med. **12**, 28 (2008)
2. Silva, Á.J.B.M.D.: Modelos de intelegência artificial na análise da monitorização de eventos clínicos adversos, disfusão/falência de orgãos e prognóstico do doente crítico (2007)
3. Ramon, J., Fierens, D., Güiza, F., Meyfroidt, G., Blockeel, H., Bruynooghe, M., Van Den Berghe, G.: Mining data from intensive care patients. Adv. Eng. Inform. **21**, 243–256 (2007)
4. Portela, F., Santos, M.F., Abelha, A., Machado, J., Rua, F.M., Silva, Á.: Real-time decision support using data mining to predict blood pressure critical events in intensive medicine patients, 9456 (2015)
5. Elliott, J.: Alpha-adrenoceptors in equine digital veins: evidence for the presence of both alpha~1 and alpha~2-receptors mediating vasoconstriction. J. Vet. Pharmacol. Ther. **20**, 308–317 (1997)
6. Greenberg, H.B.: Cardiac arrhythmias: their mechanisms, diagnosis, and management. JAMA **246**, 169 (1981)
7. Portela, F., Santos, M., Machado, J., Abelha, A., Silva, Á., Rua, F.: Preventing patient cardiac arrhythmias by using data mining techniques. In: 2014 IEEE Conference on Biomedical Engineering and Sciences (2014)
8. Portela, F., Santos, M.F., Machado, J., Abelha, A., Silva, Á., Rua, F.: Pervasive and intelligent decision support in intensive medicine – the complete picture. In: Bursa, M., Khuri, S., Renda, M. (eds.) ITBAM 2014. LNCS, vol. 8649, pp. 87–102. Springer, Heidelberg (2014)
9. Portela, C.F., Santos, M.F., Silva, Á., Machado, J., Abelha, A.: Enabling a pervasive approach for intelligent decision support in critical health care. In: Cruz-Cunha, M.M., Varajão, J., Powell, P., Martinho, R. (eds.) CENTERIS 2011, Part III. CCIS, vol. 221, pp. 233–243. Springer, Heidelberg (2011)
10. Portela, C.F., Santos, M.F., Silva, Á., Machado, J., Abelha, A., Rua, F.: Data mining for real-time intelligent decision support system in intensive care medicine (2013)
11. Santos, M.F., Portela, C.F., Vilas-Boas, M.: Intcare: multi-agent approach for real-time intelligent decision support in intensive medicine (2011)
12. Santos, M.F., Mathew, W., Portela, C.F.: Grid data mining for outcome prediction in intensive care medicine. In: Cruz-Cunha, M.M., Varajão, J., Powell, P., Martinho, R. (eds.) CENTERIS 2011, Part III. CCIS, vol. 221, pp. 244–253. Springer, Heidelberg (2011)
13. Boas, M.V., Santos, M.F., Portela, C.F., Silva, A., Rua, F.: Hourly prediction of organ failure and outcome in real time in Intensive Care Medicine (2010)
14. Portela, C.F., Santos, M.F., Silva, Á., Machado, J., Abelha, A.: Pervasive and intelligent decision support in critical health care using ensembles. In: Bursa, M., Khuri, S., Renda, M. (eds.) ITBAM 2013. LNCS, vol. 8060, pp. 1–16. Springer, Heidelberg (2013)
15. Braga, P., Portela, C.F., Santos, M.F.: Data mining models to predict patient's readmission in Intensive care units. In: ICAART - International Conference on Agents and Artificial Intelligence (2014)

16. Veloso, R., Portela, C.F., Santos, M.F., Silva, Á., Rua, F., Abelha, A., Machado, J.: Categorize readmitted patients in intensive medicine by means of clustering data mining. Int. J. E-Health Med. Commun. (IJEHMC) (2015). (accepted for publication)
17. Veloso, R., Portela, C.F., Santos, M., Machado, J.M.F., Abelha, A., Silva, Á., Rua, F.: Real-time data mining models for predicting length of stay in intensive care units (2014)
18. Portela, C.F., Oliveira, S., Veloso, R., Santos, M.F., Abelha, A., Machado, J., Silva, Á., Rua, F.: Predict hourly patient discharge probability in intensive care units using data mining. ScienceAsia J. (ICCSCM 2014) (2014)
19. Oliveira, S., Portela, C.F., Santos, M.F.: Pervasive universal gateway for medical devices. In: Recent Advances in Electrical Engineering and Education Technologies (SCI 2014), pp. 205–210 (2014)
20. Hardin, J.M., Chhieng, D.C.: Data mining and clinical decision support systems. In: Berner, E.S., Facmi, F. (eds.) Clinical Decision Support Systems. Springer, New York (2007)
21. Portela, C.F., Pinto, F., Santos, M.F.: Data mining predictive models for pervasive intelligent decision support in intensive care medicine. In: INSTICC (ed.) KMIS 2012, Barcelona (2012)
22. Braga, A., Portela, C.F., Santos, M.F., Machado, J., Abelha, A., Silva, Á., Rua, F.: Data mining to predict the use of vasopressors in intensive medicine patients. Jurnal Teknolog, Penerbit UTM Press (2016). (accepted for publication)
23. Portela, C.F., Oliveira, S., Santos, M., Machado, J., Abelha, A.: A real-time intelligent system for tracking patient condition. In: Bravo, J., Hervás, R., Villarreal, V., Caro, L., Silva, C., Peralta, B., Herrera, O., Barrientos, S., et al. (eds.) AmIHEALTH 2015. LNCS, vol. 9456, pp. 91–97. Springer, Heidelberg (2015). doi:10.1007/978-3-319-26508-7_9
24. Portela, C.F., Gago, P., Santos, M.F., Machado, J., Abelha, A., Silva, Á., Rua, F.: Pervasive real-time intelligent system for tracking critical events in intensive care patients (2013)

An Approach to Automate Health Monitoring in Compliance with Personal Privacy

Nikolay Kazantsev[1], Daniil Korolev[1], Dmitry Torshin[2], and Anna Mikhailova[1(✉)]

[1] Higher School of Economics, National Research University, ul. Myasnitskaya, 20,
Moscow, Russia
{nkazantsev,agmikhaylova}@hse.ru,denbrubeck@gmail.com
[2] CJSC «АйТи», ul. Leninskaya Sloboda, 19, Moscow 115280, Russia
dmitry@torsh.in

Abstract. The main goal of this study is to build a secure information ecosystem that connects patients, doctors, medical and insurance companies, sports organizations, fitness centers, manufacturers of telemedicine devices and medical systems for constant monitoring, long-term analysis and quick alerting over sensitive patient's data. This paper provides the extended literature analysis on topic and summarizes state-of-the-art in development of Personal Medical Wearable Device for Distance Healthcare Monitoring X73-PHD (mHealth).

Keywords: E-health · Medical information systems · Information privacy · Reliability · Experimentation · Security · Human factors · Theory

1 Research Motivation

In recent years, the healthcare industry has acknowledged the benefits of efficient service systems. Software-as-a-Medical Device (SaMD) was recognized as one of emerging parts of XaaS ("everything as a service").

In our research we aim to develop a personal health monitoring device to allow an early detection of patient's cardiovascular and endocrine diseases (hypertension, diabetes) to lower death and disability rates in distant rural areas in Russia. We keen on increasing this technology diffusion and adoption due to fair information privacy policies over patient's sensitive data.

In this short paper we expand the overview of medical device in Russia and describe the functional characteristics of created medical product.

2 Overview of Medical Portable Devices in Russia

A number of studies [1, 2, 5] show that the adoption of electronic medical devices assisting ageing societies in everyday life contain huge potential and "*encourage better doctor-patient interaction*" regarding patient symptoms and quality-of-life monitoring. For instance, in Taiwan where the elder population is expected to reach 20 % of the total population by the end of 2025 a group of scholars [6] integrated the health control

© Springer International Publishing Switzerland 2016
X. Zheng et al. (Eds.): ICSH 2015, LNCS 9545, pp. 26–30, 2016.
DOI: 10.1007/978-3-319-29175-8_3

monitor with iPhone device. Their paper contained review on 17 immobile and mobile long-distance health monitoring systems available on the world market. We extend this work by a short reviewing the same attempts in Russia.

Medical information systems' (MIS) market in Russia contains several promising products and the market itself is emerging: Medesk cloud platform[1], Eureka[2], Patient[3], qMS[4] monitoring services provide remote diagnostics storing personal patients health cards and making appointments scheduling. Their advantages vary from multi-server data storage (Medesk), modularity (Eureka), duplicated data storage mechanism (qMS) and free database system (Patient).

The abovementioned products are facing today a number of patient's information privacy and information security concerns. Prospective users perceive aspects of privacy policy differently ("right to privacy") and proposed medical monitoring benefits (after the privacy loss) could look vague [3, 7]. Moreover sensitive private data imposes high risks for insurance companies that (in the era of Big Data) expect to build their patients-handling and pricing models according to the electronic medical records collected.

We acknowledge that the demand of accumulating the best functionalities in a holistic, easy-to-use, functional and secure MIS at affordable price still exist. But the mentioned risks show how easily the acceptance of a new product might fail without handling information privacy and security.

3 Our Attempt – Health Monitor

That is why one of our primary concerns developing Remote Health MIS were: protected full patient recovery life-cycle information storage (automated gathering, transfer and storage) (1); and full patient control over data possession by signing a Commission sharing agreement (CSA) prior to device usage (2) (Fig. 1).

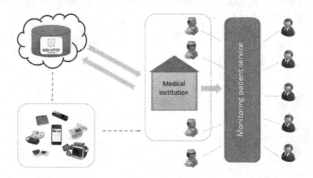

Fig. 1. Model of mHealth information environment

---
[1] http://www.medesk.md/ru/.
[2] http://www.eureca.ru/index.php?id=220.
[3] http://medotrade.ru/MIS-Patsiyent.
[4] http://www.sparm.com/products/qms.

To reach this goal specific software was developed to automate the gathering, transfer and storage of medical information processes, information consolidation and analysis, prognosis and risk detection of person's health indicators, organization of rapid response in cases of emergency, maintenance and correction of patient's treatment plan. Table 1 summarizes the benefits of developed solution for three stakeholder groups.

Table 1. List of benefits of proposed solution

Medical organization	Doctors	Patients
Rise of patients loyalty due to the increased QoS	Controlling the assigned patients' prescriptions	Personalized service inc. CSA according to **patient privacy understanding**
Remote functional diagnostics in cases of qualified medical personal absence	Case management of the clinically supervises patients	Easy to use way of monitoring health status and Remote medical advisement
Management of the quantity of in-person patients' attendance	Work hour's management rationalization	**Encrypted channels of data transmission**
Costs optimization	Remote advisement due to the videoconferencing, chatting and email	Recovery hour's management rationalization

To the current moment we developed a Web-portal with personal account of the patient, doctor and administrator of the health facility and a number of electronic devices that now are being verified in target groups [4], (Fig. 2).

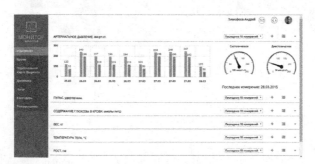

Fig. 2. Health indicators displayed realtime on the web portal

The solution provides vast functionality for adding, reading and analyzing patients' health indicators. Statistics of the selected indicators can be seen over time, so that conslusions about the possibility of the diseases can be drawn based on the collected data. Health indicators' data can be added either manually or via integration with other services or devices. The solution also provides functionality for the communication with the current patient's doctors. Due to the concerns of patient's confidentiality, the communication is encrypted and can bee seen only by the participants, in this case the doctor and the patient (Fig. 3).

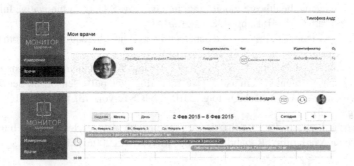

Fig. 3. View over personal patient's schedules

The solution also provides functionality for the personal patient's schedules, that has all the scheduled appointments, procedures and prescriptions.

4 Conclusion

Developed mobile application provides following functionality:

- Secure health indicators transfer (from phones and tablets of the patient)
- Encrypted storage of information (health indicators data and self-observation diary, doctor's prescription, medical tests results, etc.)
- Remote medical consultation: videoconferencing, chatting and e-mail
- Integration with external systems (medical information systems and insurance companies' systems)
- Encrypted personal data storage and obligatory data disclosures for dealing with information privacy

Acknowledgments. The developers of «Health monitor» system thank the CJSC «АйТи» and National Research University Higher School of Economics for a tight and productive cooperation and the support of the Ministry of Education and Science of Russian Federation (the contract No. 02. G 25.31.0033) without which it would be impossible to complete the research.

References

1. Almashaqbeh, G., Hayajneh, T., Vasilakos, A.V.: A cloud-based interference-aware remote health monitoring system for non-hospitalized patients. In: Global Communications Conference (GLOBECOM), 2014 IEEE, pp. 2436–2441, 8–12 December 2014

2. Bielli, E., et al.: A wireless health outcomes monitoring system (WHOMS): development and field testing with cancer patients using mobile phones. BMC Med. Inform. Decis. Mak. **4**(1), 7 (2004)
3. Laudon, K.C.: Markets and privacy. Commun. ACM **39**(9), 92–104 (1996)
4. Raznometov, D.A., Korsakov, I.N.: Algorithms for gathering wireless wearavle sensors information in remote healthcare monitoring. In: Uvaysov, S.U. (ed.) Innovative Information Technologies. Part 2. M.: HSE, pp. 438–442 (2014)
5. Wilkowska, W., Ziefle, M.: Privacy and data security in E-health: requirements from the user's perspective. Health Inform. J. **18**(3), 191–201 (2012)
6. Wu, Y.-C., Hsu, W.-H., Chang, C.-S., Yu, W.-C., Huang, W.-L., Chen, M.-J.: A smart-phone-based health management system using a wearable ring-type pulse sensor. In: Sénac, P., Ott, M., Seneviratne, A. (eds.) MobiQuitous 2010. LNICST, vol. 73, pp. 409–416. Springer, Heidelberg (2012)
7. Yee, G., Korba, L., Song, R.: Ensuring privacy for e-health services. In: The First International Conference on Availability, Reliability and Security, ARES 2006. IEEE (2006)

Mobile Cloud Computing as an Alternative for Monitoring Child Mental Disorders

Shavely S. Pusey[1], Jorge E. Camargo[1(✉)], and Gloria M. Díaz[2]

[1] Laboratory for Advanced Computational Science and Engineering Research,
Antonio Nariño University, Bogotá, Colombia
{chsinisterra,jorgecamargo}@uan.edu.co
[2] Grupo de Investigación en Automática, Electrónica y Ciencias Computacionales,
Instituto Tecnológico Metropolitano, Medellín, Colombia
gloriadiaz@itm.edu.co

Abstract. Smartphones have opened a new world of opportunities in the context of health care. Particularly, they can be used in behavioral monitoring scenarios. This paper presents a system based on mobile and cloud computing technologies for managing multimodal and unstructured data in an ubiquitous and pervasive platform. The proposed system allows parents, teachers and tutors to collect information of children behavior. The proposed system aims to provide a technological tool for aiding psychologists and psychiatrists to perform evidence-based diagnosis and therapy as a strategy to improve the management of mental disorders in children and adolescents.

Keywords: Mental disorders · Cloud computing · mHealth · Behavior tracking

1 Introduction

Mental disorders are syndromes characterized by clinically significant alterations from expected cognitive, social and emotional development becoming a pathological phenomenon [1]. These disorders have been considered as an important public health. It is estimated that a total of 13 % − 20 % of children around the world experience a mental disorder in one year, but only a small portion of them receive treatment; especially in low and middle income countries [20].

Cognitive Behavioral Therapy (CT) has shown encouraging results for the treatment of mental disorders in children, still above pharmacological treatments. This type of therapy refers to a class of interventions that share the basic premise that mental and psychological disorders are generated and maintained because of cognitive factors [11]. It is based on functional analysis of conduct, which focuses on identifying variables that influence the occurrence of behavior problems. CBT allows to establish cause-effect relationships between the child behavior and her/his environment [9].

The first step to initiate a CBT intervention is to identify and separate the behaviors, which vary from what is considered as normal from those considered

© Springer International Publishing Switzerland 2016
X. Zheng et al. (Eds.): ICSH 2015, LNCS 9545, pp. 31–42, 2016.
DOI: 10.1007/978-3-319-29175-8_4

as pathological. It is important to take into account the social factors of child environment and the levels of frequency and intensity. It is also relevant to assess characteristic behaviors manifested by children in various environments such as school, home, or any other place in which children remain. Due to the impossibility of performing continuous specialized observation of all possible child environments, psychologists and psychiatrists turn to the appreciation of child relatives, teachers and tutors.

Observations are commonly captured with evaluation instruments such as paper-based questionnaires [2]. These instruments have been criticized due to aspects such as memory lapses, attention problems, and emotional reasons, which could change adult testimony when they meet psychologist. Moreover, credibility of child testimony is even more complex because the confusion between what is considered reality and fiction by children, as it is revealed by a psychoanalytic study [18]. Therefore, it is recommended to follow an observation process and track child behavior by people involved in development of the infant in a systematic way [2].

Paper-based diagnostic tests are being widely used by psychologists nowadays, however, they present several disadvantages related to subjectivity and availability. Subjectivity because traditional evaluation measures of paper-based test strongly depends on the psychologist criteria. Availability because relatives do not have at hand a mechanism to record data when children behavior events happens [8]. Figure 1 shows a real paper-based instrument used to assess anxiety symptoms.

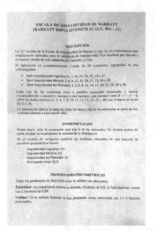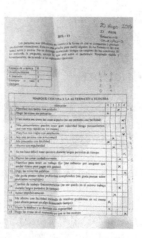

Fig. 1. Paper-based test using the Barrat scale.

The development of mobile applications that support clinical processes is a growing field that promises to be useful in behavioral health care. Specifically for improving the evidence of characteristics of behavior that are out of clinic environments [3–5]. Recently, some works have been developed for providing support to observational processes in cognitive behavioral therapy. The system presented in [8] involves a mobile system and a web component for the monitoring of bipolar patients. In [6], authors present a system for self-managing of schizophrenia symptoms. In [12] authors integrate a mobile application, a web component, SMS messages and email for the tracking eating disorders in adolescents.

These applications are high storage demanding due the need of constant observational records and to the complexity of multimodal and unstructured data that should be managed (images, audio and video) [21]. Thus, the need of accessing all patient information at the right time is critical. Medical records must be available and accessible to all the involved people in the diagnosis and therapy processes [21].

This paper proposes the use of cloud computing as a strategy for developing behavioral registration technologies that requires large storage and access to unstructured data. The proposed platform provides tools that allows to access to evidence of behavior characteristics at different environments in which children remain. Consequently, it is expected that the proposed system improves therapy and diagnosis processes in children and adolescents with mental disorders.

The paper is structured as follows: Sect. 2 presents the proposed cloud computing architecture as well as opportunities and reasons for choosing this alternative; Sect. 3 describes system requirements for building the proposed system; Sect. 4 presents details of the developed system; Sect. 5 provides an overview of a first system validation; and finally, Sect. 6 concludes the paper and presents some ideas for future work.

2 Cloud Computing and Mobile Health

Mobile Cloud Computing (MCC) is a paradigm in which mobile applications use infrastructure for storing and processing data in the cloud. This architecture uses cloud platforms that are dynamically scalable [16] and follows a pay-per-use premise. One of the biggest MCC service providers is Amazon Web Services (AWS), which provides a set of services accessible through Internet [19].

Cloud computing is considered as an unlimited resource that is accessible in anytime and anywhere (while internet service are available), which offers the possibility of maintain ubiquity and pervasiveness in applications [15]. Cloud computing also brings an easy and fast access to computing resources [10].

The increasing use of smartphones in health care scenarios [17] makes data grows exponentially [21]. Therefore, larger storage capacities are typically needed by mobile devices to efficiently operate. Additionally, energy limitations on mobile devices [15] make it necessary an environment that allows storage, search, share and analyze patient information [21].

The combination of cloud computing architectures, wireless networks, and mobile computing, allows to minimize technological constraints of mobile devices. A mobile cloud computing architecture solves problems such as low capacity, security and privacy [7,15].

An MCC architecture follows one of the following paradigms: (1) Platform as a service (PaaS), allowing customers to develop, run, and manage Web applications; (2) Infrastructure as a service (IaaS), which provides virtualized computing resources over the Internet; (3) Software as a service (SaaS), which is a software licensing and delivery model in which software is licensed on a subscription hosted solution; and (4) Back-end as a Service (BaaS), which is a new cloud computing model that provides web and mobile developers with a way to connect their applications to backend cloud storage and APIs exposed by back end applications while also providing features such as user management, push notifications, and integration with social networking services [7,21].

The Baas paradigm is one of the most attractive options nowadays because mobile app developers do not have to do complex tasks such as installation, configuration, administration and integration between mobile and server, typical of the other three paradigms. There are available in the market some Baas implementations. One of the most popular is *Parse*[1], which provides the following features:

- It allows to manage everything about system back-end: application users, sending and reception of notifications, and data analysis.
- It offers high availability to access patient information every time.
- It provides interoperability and sharing information with all professionals involved into the diagnosis and therapy processes [21].
- It implements Non-SQL databases (Cassandra, MongoDB, Redis), which allows to efficiently store and manage multimodal data such as audio, video, and images.
- It uses Amazon EC2 (elastic computing) that allows automatically scale the system on demand.

3 System Description

This section presents characteristics of the developed system in terms of clinical and technical factors.

3.1 Clinical Characteristics

The following clinical features were implemented in the application:

- Collaborative environment that involves child relatives and health professionals in diagnosis and therapy processes.
- Data protection due to the sensitivity of clinical and personal child information.
- Setting of predominant behaviors for each type of mental disorder, with possibility of adding specific behaviors.

---

[1] https://www.parse.com/.

- Pervasive and ubiquitous behavior tracking to record information about *with whom the child was* and *where the child was*.
- Functional behavioral assessment tool.
- Graphical visualization of behavioral observation records that allows to identify predominant behaviors and its environments.
These characteristics are mainly related with user needs, which correspond to functional requirements.

3.2 Technical Characteristics

The following technical features were implemented in the application:

- Capture of multimodal data such as images, audio and video.
- Scalable storage to support massive volumes of captured data.
- User authentication based on login and password.

These three aspects were very important to define the architecture of the system, which correspond to non-functional requirements.

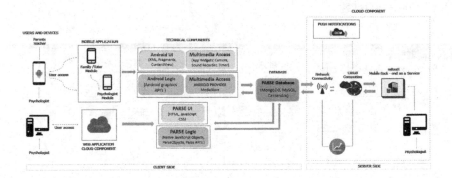

Fig. 2. System architecture composed of two parts: client-side and server-side components.

4   The BehAppy System

The *BehAppy* system consists of two main components: a mobile application and a back-end component. As shown in Fig. 2, the mobile component was developed as an Android application that provides functionality of signing in/login in to the system, and recording data of child behavior events. The web component is part of the back-end, which provides to health professionals access to user information (parents, teachers, grandparents, etc.), analyze behavioral records, and configure system parameters.

4.1 Mobile Application

Mobile application was built following the well-known model-view-controller software design pattern, which establishes a three layer architecture: view or user interface (GUI), controller or business logic and, model or data layers. The GUI was built using XML (Extensible Markup Language), and Java language. The application access to multimedia devices (camera, audio, timer) for recording behavioral events, using an **App Widgets** implementation. The application logic was managed through Android Application Programming Interfaces (APIs), which manage the answers to requests generated by the GUI. The data layer is managed by Parse, which provides a set of functions to store, access, modify and delete data in an efficient way.

The main objective of the *BehAppy* application is to support diagnosis and therapy processes through a tool that also to acquire multimodal data of children behavior in order to improve the observation in all environments in which a child remain. As illustrated in the Fig. 2, the mobile application has two submodules: the first one is focused on roles that participate in the child development environment (parents, teachers, tutors, and other relatives), and the second one focuses on professionals (psychologist, therapist) that participate in the diagnosis or therapy processes.

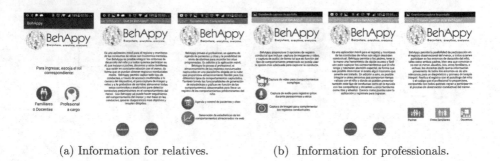

(a) Information for relatives.   (b) Information for professionals.

Fig. 3. Information module.

Relatives Module. This module allows the integration of relatives in the behavior recording process. The main idea is to allow to register important child behavior events. This information will be useful for finding correlations between events, people, environment, etc., in posterior analysis phase. This module is composed of three submodules described below:

1. *Information module:* It describes through three screens the main objective of the application and other key information such as what is *BehAppy*, who can use the application, how to use it and a brief description of the provided functionality. This module is illustrated in Fig. 3a.

2. *Registration process:* The registration form and application login establishes three "roles" to make the register in *Behappy.* As it was mentioned before, it is important to integrate information of the different environments in which the infant develops, home, school or other activities that the child performs. But also it is important register the people who share these activities with the child, by which each relative must be registered independently. By default, three register options were included: parent, teacher, tutor or family/guardian. Each role has access to different information concerning the infant, because the information that parents know about the child is not the same as the teacher must know. Among the data requested for registering on the application, name, username, email, and account password were established. In addition, an unique infant registration code is provided by the professionals module when It makes the registry of the infant as new patient. This code must be entered by parents and teachers or other relatives, and this is the way as the behavioral records catched by the application will be identified.

3. *Conductual recording:* This module allows to perform the recording of each characteristic behavior. For each register user must select the type of behavior that will be registered and the data modality, i.e. image, video or audio. Behavior types must be previously defined by the health professional in the patient register process. Each captured record is sent to the server for doing it accessible to the health professional.

Health Professional Module. Because not all mental disorders present the same characteristics behavior, this module provides mental health professional to register children that will be tracked and to configure the specific behavior that must be recorded for each. This module includes three submodules: an information module, a health professional registration module and a patient registration and management.

1. *Information module:* similar to he relatives module, the information module presents general information about the application features and functionality, as it is shown in Fig. 3b. Specifically, this module informs about the application description at clinical level, functionality of both relatives and professional modules, and explains how to use the application.

2. *Registration module:* personal data for creating a system account such as name, username, email, ID number, professional card number and password, are required. This type of account enable user to register patients, to manage the recording registers and to visualize information reports.

3. *Patient registration and management module:* this module provides to health professionals functions for handling patients that require to be tracked. The behavior tracking process starts with a registration, which requires some personal and clinical information of the child such as name, age, parent's names, school age, reason for the consult, mental health history, among others. Once the child is registered, the application generates a code, which should be provided to the child relatives for allowing to register new behavior events.

Through this module, a health professional has access to a set of patients with his/her associated records. In addition, the professional can record appointments and configure reminder alarms of meeting therapies of each patient.

Some application screenshots are shown in Fig. 4.

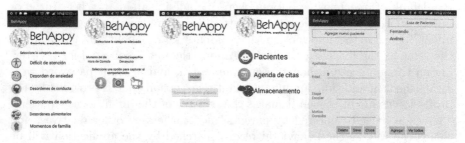

    (a) Relative's module.   (b) Professional's module.

Fig. 4. Main functionality of *BehAppy* mobile application

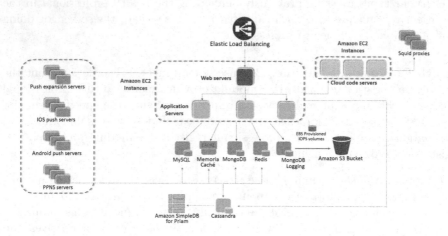

Fig. 5. Server-side architecture (adapted from a AWS case study: Parse [13])

4.2 The Back-End Component

As illustrated in Fig. 5, the back-end service provides a comprehensive set of architectural components for display, storing and processing data. In our case we implement two of them: (1) A web component designed for providing health professional access to recorded data, as an additional option to mobile application, which allows another visualization possibilities, and (2) A server that allows the management of large unstructured and multimodal data. Web interfaces were designed using HTML, CSS and JavaScript, whilst storing and processing features were implemented with the Parse cloud services.

Web component involves two menus: The main menu located at the top center (horizontally) and a sub-menu in the upper left corner (vertically). The first one provides data visualization functions, data analytics, push-up notifications and system configuration options. The second one changes according to the selected main menu option. Below, some functionality of the web component is described.

Notifications. The web component managed in the cloud provides the functionality for sending and receiving push-up notifications through the use of Google Cloud Messaging (GCM). Thus, when a new behavioral record is registered, a notification is sent to a professional.

Data Analytics. One of the main features of the web component is to provide statistical analysis of the stored data. Figure 6 shows the amount users that participate in the recording process and the influence of each user in the quantity of registered data. This tool allows to identify in which environment there exist more characteristic behaviors related to a mental disorder. The amount of stored behavioral records can be also viewed via graphs that indicate the highest peaks or times where the child has more anomalous behaviors.

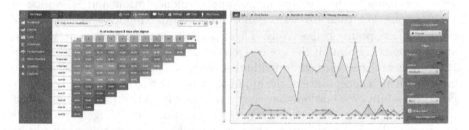

Fig. 6. System audience analysis and statistics module

Data Storing and Processing Component. The server component that manages all stored data (users, notifications, behavioral records, etc.) is managed in the cloud. Incoming data traffic is automatically distributed by making use of Amazon Web Services and Amazon Elastic Cloud Computing (Amazon EC2), which provide re-sizable compute capacity in the cloud.

Since the system server component must handle a high amount of multimodal and unstructured data, Parse uses the MongoDB Non SQL database, Redis and Cassandra. The first one provides flexible storage schemes required by the system; the second one allows to manage send/receive notifications (push-ups); and the third one, provides a stronger service to increase data storage.

Finally, because the importance of behavioral records for diagnosis and therapy processes, Amazon Elastic Block Store (Amazon EBS) is used to create snapshots frequently for each piece of stored data, increasing the security of stored data. Each Amazon EBS volume is automatically replicated to protect data in case of component failures, providing high availability and durability of the stored information.

5 Preliminary System Evaluation

The proposed system was developed with the support of a team of mental health professionals, who determined the basic set of clinical and functional requirements, and supply continuous feedback in the development process. System evaluation was carried out through a qualitative survey that was composed of three kinds of assessment categories: functional, usability and needs satisfaction. Items were evaluated through four approval criteria using the Likert's Scale [14], where 4 indicates totally agree, 3 indicates agree, 2 indicates disagree and 1 indicates totally disagree.

Five psychologists participated in this evaluation, all of them belonging to cognitive-conductual perspective and are specialized on children. One psychologist had not postgraduate studies, two had specialization degree and two doctorate degree. Results are discussed below:

- For the functionality evaluation, seven criteria were considered including application clarity, information provided, ease of recording functionality, characteristic behavior fitting, usefulness appointment option and relevance of notifications. For each survey the minimum and maximum score was in the range of 7–28 points respectively. Thus, participants could score between 28 and 140 points. From all the applied surveys, it was obtained a total score of 129 points and the average individual score was 25.8. These results allow to interpret a high acceptance of the application by the participant psychologists.
- For the usability evaluation they were evaluated five criteria including colors combination, letter size, ease of use of registration, recording and appointments modules. For each survey the maximum and minimum scores could be 20 and 5 points respectively, which means a maximum of 100 and minimum of 25 for the summarized result. From all applied surveys, it was obtained a total score of 95 points, with an individual average score of 19, which allows to infer that the application is highly usable.
- For the user needs satisfaction point of view, three criteria were used: contribution on the diagnosis and therapy processes, interest on acquiring and using the application in his/her daily consult, and usability for other mental health professionals. This evaluation just considered YES/NO answers, where YES scores 1 point and NO scores 0 points. All surveys obtained 3 points in this part, which allows to establish that the proposed system is a feasible tool for demanding needs in mental health care area.

6 Conclusions and Future Work

Mobile technologies have shown to be useful for aiding the diagnosis process of children mental disorders. Recent mobile capturing technologies have generated an exponential growing of multimodal and non-structured data that require to be stored and analyzed to infer behavioral patterns in order to enable health specialist to obtain more accurate diagnosis and effective therapeutic interventions.

The cloud computing approach and its integration with mobile technology is a very successful combination for supporting health activities and specifically to support mental health care. Based on an applied survey, we conclude that the proposed system is very necessary for mental health professionals and its contribution to diagnosis and therapy is of high relevance. As future work we will perform a validation of the proposed system in a real patient environment, which will involve parent referents, tutors and teachers. Likewise, we plan to implement data mining techniques to analyze collected data for future platform versions.

Acknowledgments. This work was funded by Universidad Antonio Nariño through the project 20131088 "Desarrollo de herramientas diagnósticas basadas en annalisis de neuroimágenes para la identificación de pacientes con enfermedades neuropsiquiátricas". This work was partially funded by BIGDATA SOLUTIONS SAS.

References

1. American Psychiatric Association. Diagnostic and Statistical Manual of Mental Disorders (2013)
2. Amorós, M.O., Carrillo, X.M., Alcázar, A.I.R., Saura, C.J.I., Saura, C.J.I., Carrillo, F.J.M., Alcázar, A.I.R., Amorós, M.O., Carrillo, X.M., Alcázar, I.A.R.: La terapia cognitivo-conductual en problemas de ansiedad generalizada y ansiedad por separación : Un análisis de su eficacia. Anales de Psicol. **19**(2), 193–204 (2003)
3. Apps4SpecialEducation. Behavior tracking (2015)
4. AutismApps. Behavior management, ef and data tools (2015)
5. BehaviorTrackerPro. Skill tracker pro (2015)
6. Kaiser, S.M., Brenner, C.J., Begale, M., Duffccy, J., David, C.M., Ben-Zeev, D.: Development and usability testing of focus: a smartphone system for self-management of schizophrenia. Psychiatric Rehabil. J. **36**(4), 289–296 (2013)
7. Cloud Standards Customer Council. Impact of Cloud Computing on Healthcare, November 2012
8. Frost, M., Marcu, G., Hansen, R., Szaanto, K., Bardram, J.E.: The MONARCA Self-assessment System: Persuasive Personal Monitoring for Bipolar Patients. IEEE, New York (2011)
9. Hanely, G.P., Iwata, B.A., McCord, B.E.: Functional analysis of problem behavior: a review. J. Appl. Behav. Anal. **36**(2), 147–185 (2003)
10. Hoang, D.B., Chen, L.: Mobile cloud for assistive healthcare (MoCAsH). In: Proceedings - 2010 IEEE Asia-Pacific Services Computing Conference, APSCC 2010, pp. 325–332 (2010)
11. Hofmann, S.G., Asnaani, A., Vonk, I.J.J., Sawyer, A.T., Fang, A.: The efficacy of cognitive behavioral therapy: a review of meta-analyses. Cogn. Ther. Res. **36**(5), 427–440 (2012)
12. Bauman, A., Hebden, L., Balestracci, K., McGeechan, K., Denney-Wilson, E., Harris, M., Allman-Farinelli, M.: 'TXT2BFiT' a mobile phone-based healthy lifestyle program forpreventing unhealthy weight gain in young adults: study protocol for arandomized controlled trial. Trials J. **14**, 75 (2013)

13. Charity Majors. AWS case study: Parse. http://aws.amazon.com/solutions/case-studies/parse/. Accessed 24 Dec 2015
14. McLeod, S.A.: Likert scale - simply psychology (2008). http://www.simplypsychology.org/likert-scale.html. Accessed 24 Dec 2015
15. Parameswari, R., Prabakaran, N.: An enhanced Mobile HealthCare Monitoring System in mobile cloud computing. Int. J. Adv. **1**(10), 804–807 (2012)
16. Prasad, M.R., Gyani, J., Murti, P.R.K.: Mobile cloud computing: implications and challenges. J. Inf. Eng. Appl. **2**(7), 7–16 (2012)
17. Rahimi, M.R., Ren, J., Liu, C.H., Vasilakos, A.V., Venkatasubramanian, N.: Mobile cloud computing: a survey, state of art and future directions. Mob. Netw. Appl. **19**, 1–11 (2013)
18. Ajuriaguerra, J.: Manual de Psiquiatria Infantil, 5th edn. Toray-Masson, Barcelona (1976)
19. Varia, J.: Architecting for the cloud: best practices. Compute **1**, 1–23 (2010)
20. World-Health-Organization. Mental health: a state of well-being (2014)
21. Youssef, A.E.: A framework for secure healthcare systems based on big data analytics in mobile cloud computing environments. Int. J. Ambient Syst. Appl. **2**(2), 1–11 (2014)

Network Analysis of Ecological Momentary Assessment Data for Monitoring and Understanding Eating Behavior

Gerasimos Spanakis[1]([⊠]), Gerhard Weiss[1], Bastiaan Boh[2], and Anne Roefs[2]

[1] Department of Knowledge Engineering, Maastricht University,
6200 Maastricht, MD, The Netherlands
{jerry.spanakis,gerhard.weiss}@maastrichtuniversity.nl
[2] Faculty of Psychology and Neuroscience, Maastricht University,
6200 Maastricht, MD, The Netherlands
{bastiaan.boh,a.roefs}@maastrichtuniversity.nl

Abstract. Ecological Momentary Assessment (EMA) techniques have been blooming during the last years due to the emergence of smart devices (like PDAs and smartphones) that allow the collection of repeated assessments of several measures (predictors) that affect a target variable. Eating behavior studies can benefit from EMA techniques by analysing almost real-time information regarding food intake and the related conditions and circumstances. In this paper, an EMA method protocol to study eating behavior is presented along with the mobile application developed for this purpose. Mixed effects and vector autoregression are utilized for conducting a network analysis of the data collected and lead to inferring knowledge for the connectivity between different conditions and their effect on eating behavior.

Keywords: Ecological momentary assessment · Mixed effects · Vector autoregression · Network analysis

1   Introduction

Nowadays, rapid technological advancement has allowed the introduction of modern devices (PDAs, mobile devices, electronic diaries, smartphones, etc.) into the collection and study of -almost- real-time data from real-world environments. These processes provide researchers with a harness of data that need to be analysed in an effective way. Ecological Momentary Assessment (EMA) [16] is an umbrella term for all methods used to repeatedly assess individual subjects in daily life. Reports can be created either randomly (e.g. selecting some time moments per day) or can even be event triggered. EMA has a number of advantages over more traditional methods [14] for the assessment of different measured values and a broad field of applications [13] (such as substance abuse, psychopathology, levels of pain, levels of physical activity, emotional states).

© Springer International Publishing Switzerland 2016
X. Zheng et al. (Eds.): ICSH 2015, LNCS 9545, pp. 43–54, 2016.
DOI: 10.1007/978-3-319-29175-8_5

Another field that EMA can provide more insight is the predictors of unhealthy eating behavior, and thereby can contribute to a better understanding of the mechanisms of eating behavior. The insights gained using this method can be used for developing ecological momentary interventions (EMI) [7], which consists of intervening in real-time, right in the situations in which it is most important, and most likely to have an effect. Furthermore, an open problem is the analysis of these predictors: How the different predictors (e.g. emotions, cognitions) are interrelated, change over time and are related to eating behavior.

In this paper, we present a method for analysing data collected using EMA utilizing a smartphone application and how mixed effects models (ME) with vector autoregression (VAR) can help reveal the network dynamics of how predictors like emotions affect each other but also eating behavior.

2   Related Work

2.1   Mixed Effects Models (ME) and Vector AutoRegression (VAR)

Mixed effects models refer to a variety of models which have as a key feature both fixed and random effects [5]. Fixed effects are ones in which the possible values of the variable are fixed across all samples (e.g. age) whereas random effects refer to variables in which the set of potential values can change (according to the individual). Mixed effects models are utilized in looking into research data where users are organized at more than one level. More specifically, a level-1 submodel describes how individuals change over time (fixed effects) and a level-2 submodel describes how these changes vary across individuals (random effects). The main advantage of mixed effects models is that they take into consideration variation across individuals that is not generalizable to the independent variables.

Mixed effects (ME) models can capture the multiple levels of organisation of EMA data but are not able to show evolution over time or how variables affect each other from one time point to the next. Vector autoregression (VAR) is an econometric model used to capture these interdependencies among multiple time series [18]. VAR models extend the univariate autoregression (AR) models by allowing for more than one evolving variable. Each variable is represented by an equation explaining its evolution based on its own lags and the lags of all the other model variables.

2.2   Studies on EMA Data and ME-VAR Models

EMA research methods use mobile technology (diaries, PDAs, smartphones etc.) in order to collect repeated measurements on the same unit (i.e. humans, plants, samples depending on the study) over time. Variables measured depend on the kind of study (agriculture, medical health, physical sciences, engineering) and can hold continuous, binary or ordinal values. An EMA framework allows the researcher to ask subjects to answer questions or to perform certain actions when predetermined conditions are met. These conditions can be anything from a certain time of day to the occurrence of events of interest, such as being about to eat or being tempted to eat.

Some of the main advantages of EMA methods are: (a) real-time assessments increase ecological validity and minimize retrospective bias, (b) repeated assessments can reveal dynamic processes, (c) multimodal assessments can integrate psychological, physiological, and behavioral data, (d) setting- or context-specific relationships of variables or events can be identified, (e) interactive feedback can be provided in real time and (f) assessments in real-life situations enhance generalizability.

During the last years EMA studies have been conducted in several fields like Tobacco use and relapse [15], social anxiety [9], mood disorders and mood dysregulation [4] and many more. There is also a great variety of EMA studies regarding eating behavior [3,8,12]. These studies demonstrated that by capturing eating behavior in everyday life, it is possible to reveal the factors affecting eating events like hunger experiencing, sorts of (non-)leisure activities undertaken, social circumstances and states of affective arousal (positive or negative emotions).

Combination of mixed effects models and vector autoregression is a technique which gains ground in analysing data (not only EMA). Brain connectivity has been investigated using ME-VAR techniques [6] from a functional MRI dataset. Besides graphical approaches, researchers are able to translate complex relations to tangible networks. For example, in psychopathology, symptom networks (created by interplay between symptoms) [1] can be used to extract useful information. Such network structures reveal that patterns of temporal influence allow symptoms to directly or indirectly connect and interact [2].

3   Description of the EMA Method

An iPhone application was developed in-house that allows people to report potential obesity-promoting factors in real time (see Table 1 for these factors), by filling in brief questionnaires. Such relatively unobtrusive on-line self-monitoring can yield more accurate results than retrospective (questionnaire) assessment. Ecological momentary assessment was performed in two ways: (a) *Event sampling*: participants were instructed to use the application immediately prior to eating something and (b) *Random sampling*: Limited input was requested at pseudo-random time points throughout the day (pseudo-random means that day is divided in 8 boxes and samples occur at random times in each of the boxes aiming at covering all day intervals).

In detail, the application is a logbook, which is used every time the user eats something and when the user is prompted (randomly) to report his/her status. The latter data points are used to generate a baseline by assessing user's status at random moments throughout the day. When an eating moment is about to happen, the user is required to provide short feedback about the emotional state, the food product, the thought that preceded food intake, and the circumstances. In addition, the user is also asked to add a picture of the food intake.

Table 1. Data collection using iPhone application

Variable	Format
Date saved *	date-month-year hour-min-sec
Craving *	VAS item (0–10)
Emotion worried *	VAS item (0–10)
Emotion angry/annoyed *	VAS item (0–10)
Emotion stressed/tense *	VAS item (0–10)
Emotion relaxed/at ease *	VAS item (0–10)
Emotion cheerful/happy *	VAS item (0–10)
Emotion sad/depressed *	VAS item (0–10)
Emotion bored *	VAS item (0–10)
Specific craving *	Selection from a table of 19 images
Location	Free text
Circumstances	Free text
Specific eating *, +	Selection from a table of 19 images
Thoughts regarding to eating +	Free text
Food intake image +	Image file in .png format

(*) denotes variables used in current paper analysis
(+) denotes variables present only in event-contingent samples

The ESM study followed 100 participants (equally divided to healthy-weight and obese, as defined by objective Body Mass Index (BMI) measurements) over the course of 14 days. Every day subjects were randomly notified by a beeper (random sampling) between 0730 and 2230 with an interval of two hours. Besides that, when they are about to eat something they fill out a similar questionnaire but containing the food information. This process resulted in an average of 10 responses (including random samples and eating events) per user per day. The dataset is multi-level and complex containing information about users and their eating events, emotions, circumstances, locations for several time moments during the days they participated in the study. In detail, the information collected using the application are presented in Table 1.

For the purpose of the analysis presented in the next Section, we selected a number of items that captured the mood state of users and the items that captured their eating behavior (they are denoted by (*) in Table 1). Mood states are measured using seven emotions using Visual Analogue Scale (VAS). Regarding eating behavior, the assessment of user's craving (on VAS) was measured in each time point. Also, cravings for specific items have been included by allowing users to select an image (out of 19 possible choices) which is most similar to the craving they experience. There is also the option that users did not have a specific craving. The same idea is applied for specific eating: Whenever an eating event occurs, user selects an image (out the 19 possible) that is most similar to the food consumed. For random sampling events, users are considered to eat nothing at that moment. This broad selection (19 possible choices) allows us to categorize each specific item either to healthy or unhealthy food (where *unhealthy* refers mostly to high caloric food items and *healthy* to all other itmes). This categorization allows specific craving and eating to take three different values: healthy, unhealthy or nothing. So in total there are 10 variables: 8 continuous (emotions and craving) and 2 categorical (craving for healthy/unhealthy/nothing and eating healthy/unhealthy/nothing).

4   Description of the Model

Combination of mixed effects and vector autoregression leads to representations of the model variables based on all other variables' lags (itself included) and each lagged variable has both a fixed and a random effect. An exact description of the mixed effects vector autoregression model of order p (ME-VAR(p)) that captures the data described with (*) in Table 1 is the following:

$$\mathbf{Y}^i(t) = \left[\sum_{k=1}^{p} \mathbf{A}_k^i \cdot \mathbf{Y}^i(t-k)\right] + + \left[\sum_{k=1}^{p}\left\{(\mathbf{b}_k^i + \mathbf{c}_k^t) \cdot \mathbf{Y}^i(t-k)\right\} + \mathbf{e}^i(t)\right] \quad (1)$$

The explanation of the elements in this Equation is as follows.

1. $\mathbf{Y}^i(t)$ is the vector of variables for individual i at time t. Dimension of vector is R, where R is the number of different variables measured and used in this model, i.e. the variables referred at the end of previous Section.
2. $\mathbf{A}_k^i$ is the person-specific (i) direct connectivity matrix at lag k. This $R \times R$ matrix quantifies how $\mathbf{Y}^i(t-k)$ directly predicts $\mathbf{Y}^i(t)$. The first part of the Equation in the brackets represents the fixed effect part of the model.
3. $\mathbf{b}_k^i$ is the individual-specific random effect which describes the variability in the connectivity among different participants and that is defined by the superscript i.
4. $\mathbf{c}_k^t$ is the time-specific random effect which describes the variability in the connectivity in different time periods of data collection which are defined by superscript t.
   $\mathbf{e}^i(t)$ describes the per-person vector of error terms as Gaussian variables ($e_t \sim N(0, \sigma_\omega^2)$) and also satisfying the non-correlation condition over time.

Equation 1 demonstrates the importance of mixed effects models and how the connectivity matrix can be decomposed into fixed and random components:

$$\mathbf{A}_k^i = \mathbf{A}_k + \mathbf{b}_k^i + \mathbf{c}_k^t \quad (2)$$

where: $\mathbf{A}_k$ is the fixed effect connectivity matrix common in population from which persons are sampled, $\mathbf{b}_k^i$ is the random effect deviation of individual i from the common population connectivity matrix associated to lag k and $\mathbf{c}_k^t$

is the random effect deviation of time period t from the common population connectivity matrix associated to lag k. The elements of matrices $\mathbf{b}_k^i$ and $\mathbf{c}_k^t$ are modelled as mutually independent Gaussian random variables (like $\mathbf{e}^i(t)$).

For the purpose of this study, a ME-VAR(1) model was introduced with the variables presented with (*) in Table 1. Because specific_craving and specific_eating are categorical variables, they need to be introduced as dummy variables in the ME-VAR model, by leaving one out as the reference level. Nothing was selected as reference level for both cases, allowing to compare healthy and unhealthy to this. By this coding, R is 12, thus there are 12 Equations (8 for the continuous variables and 4 for craving healthy/unhealthy and eating healthy/unhealthy).

Testing for Significance Among Obese and Healthy-Weight People and Further Remarks. One of our primary goals is to investigate differences in behavior between healthy-weight and obese people. Under the proposed model, this can be achieved by introducing two indicator factors for the two groups (obese and healthy-weight) and replacing connectivity matrix $\mathbf{A}_k^i$ with a formula $\left[\mathbf{A}_{k,ob}^i W_{ob}^i + \mathbf{A}_{k,hw}^i W_{hw}^i\right]$ where W_c^i are used to differentiate between the two groups ($c = \{hc, ob\}$) and $\mathbf{A}_{k,c}^i$ denote the connectivity matrices of each group. Equation 1 is now rewritten as follows:

$$\mathbf{Y}^i(t) = \left\{\sum_{k=1}^{p} \left(\mathbf{A}_{k,ob}^i + \boldsymbol{\Delta}_k W_{hw}^i + \mathbf{b}_k^i + \mathbf{c}_k^t\right) \cdot \mathbf{Y}^i(t-k)\right\} + \mathbf{e}^i(t) \qquad (3)$$

This way the parameter matrix $\boldsymbol{\Delta}_k$ (dimension $R \times R$) is directly tested via $H_0 : \boldsymbol{\Delta}_k = 0$ for $k = 1, ..., P$. Note that when $\boldsymbol{\Delta}_k \neq 0$ then the effective connectivity for the two groups is different at lag k. Using a similar formulation, one can also test for differences in effective connectivity across any other group or parameter than we want to include.

Regarding lagging the data, it should be noted that clock starts again at the beginning of the day, meaning that the last measurement of a day does not affect (or predict) the first measurement of the next day, something which is in accordance with literature (e.g. [11]). Regarding time, it is assumed that the time intervals between two consecutive measurements are approximately equal, but even without this assumption the introduction of time as a random factor (see the next Section for more) overcomes this issue. Stationarity was checked using the Kwiatkowski-Phillips-Schmidt-Shin (KPSS) test [10] confirming that the data have a (weekly) constant mean and variance and no trend for every subject and every variable. Moreover, despite we present here results for lag=1 (ME-VAR(1) model), we also fitted models for lag=2 and lag=3, as well as a day-aggregated model (i.e. average of variables for one day) where 24 h was the lag. Space limitations do now allow the presentation of these results but since eating unhealthy can be very spontaneous, ME-VAR(1) model is considered to be the best choice for detecting the micro-level changes in people status.

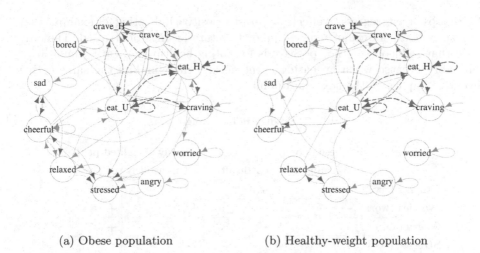

(a) Obese population   (b) Healthy-weight population

Fig. 1. Fixed effects networks for lag=1: predicting time (t) from time (t−1) (crave_H= craving healthy, crave_U=craving unhealthy, eat_H=eating healthy, eat_U=eating unhealthy). Green solid line implies that originating item's value at time (t−1) positively predicts endpoint item's value at time (t). Red dashed line implies that originating item's value at time (t−1) negatively predicts endpoint item's value at time (t). Only significant connections are shown, thicker arrows imply stronger relations (Color figure online)

5   Experimental Analysis

5.1   The Population Network

We construct two networks based on the population of obese and healthy-weight people and the ME-VAR(1) model described before. The networks are based on the connectivity matrix $\mathbf{A}_1$ of Eq. 1 as modified by Eq. 3 for the two groups (index 1 will be skipped from now on when referring to ME-VAR(1)). Each network is represented by a graph G comprising a set of $V = 12$ nodes (one for each variable) together with a set of E edges, which are 2-element subsets of V. More specifically, an edge is related with two nodes i and j and its weight is a direct reflection of the coefficient $A(i,j)$, which expresses the strength of the relation between item i at time $t-1$ and item j at time t. To clearly demonstrate positive and negative effects respectively, edges are drawn green when $A(i,j) > 0$ and red when $A(i,j) < 0$. Also, the thickness of edges is relative to the value of $A(i,j)$, meaning that the thicker the edge between two nodes, the stronger the relation between these nodes. These networks (based on connectivity matrices $\mathbf{A}_{ob}$ and $\mathbf{A}_{hw}$) are depicted in Fig. 1. Only significant connections are depicted (i.e. p-value of the t-statistic is smaller than 0.05).

A few general conclusions on the dynamical network structure between the twelve variables can be derived. Obese people have a more dense structure (which implies more complex relations between emotions and eating related events).

Self-loops or autoregressive effects are mostly positive indicating for example that the current experience of stressed predicts future feelings of stressed. The only case that self-loops are not positive is for eating healthy and eating unhealthy, probably because when an eating event occurs, that inhibits the same eating event to happen at the next data point.

Table 2. Predictors for eating events

Predictor	Obese people		Healthy Weighted people	
	eat_unhealthy	eat_healthy	eat_unhealthy	eat_healthy
Craving (crv)	++	++	++	++
Worried (worr)	-	-	+	+
Angry (ang)	-	-	+	+
Stressed (stsd)	-	-	- -	-
Relaxed (rlx)	++	-	+	- -
Cheerful (chrf)	++	- -	++	-
Sad (sad)	+	- -	-	+
Bored (brd)	+	-	-	+
crave_H (crvH)	- -	++	- -	++
crave_U (crvU)	++	- -	++	- -
eat_H (eatH)	- -	- -	- -	- -
eat_U (eatU)	- -	- -	- -	- -

(+) shows positive relation, (++) shows positive significant relation
(-) shows negative relation, (- -) shows negative significant relation

Table 2 demonstrates all (regardless their significance) positive and negative predictors for eating healthy and unhealthy for the two groups (obese and healthy weighted). Some remarks given this Table are:

- Craving positively affects eating either healthy or unhealthy.
- Craving for something healthy (or unhealthy respectively) positively predicts eating healthy (or unhealthy respectively).
- Positive emotions (relaxed and cheerful) positively predict eating unhealthy with relaxed being more significant for obese people.
- Stressed appears to inhibit eating for both groups.
- Sad, bored, worried and angry have an opposite effect on eating for both groups, demonstrating the differences in the two groups.

5.2   The Random Effects Networks

This individual variability can also be immediately observed in the networks of individual subjects. For this purpose, the matrices $\mathbf{A}_1^i$ and $\mathbf{b}_1^i$ of Eq. 2 are utilized. Figure 2 illustrates the individual networks for two persons randomly selected from the obese people sample.

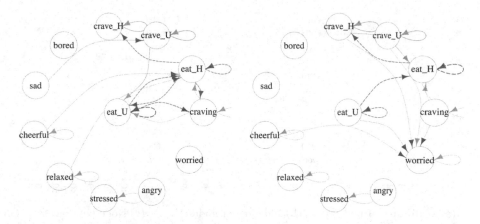

Fig. 2. Individual networks of two different (random, obese) users

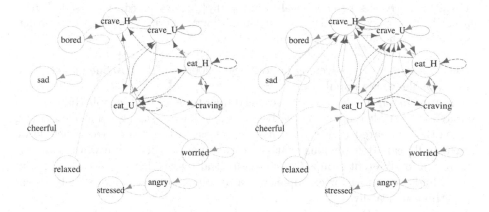

(a) Baseline network for 10:00-12:00 block (b) Baseline network for 18:00-20:00 block

Fig. 3. Networks for specific time periods of day

The network on the left has a quite strong self-loop for craving unhealthy and a strong connection to eating unhealthy, which means that this person has often unhealthy cravings (self-loop) but also tends to give in by eating something unhealthy. Also, the positive emotions have a negative affect on eating healthy. On the other hand, the network of the participant on the right implies that eating in general (healthy or unhealthy) has a negative affect on worried and also craving unhealthy predicts worried. Obviously, worried is an emotion which can be further monitored for this specific user.

Another target of the current approach was to investigate the effect of time of day in the networks but also to eating behavior. This can be achieved by taking into account the c_1^t of Eq. 2. Figure 3 illustrates networks for a morning period

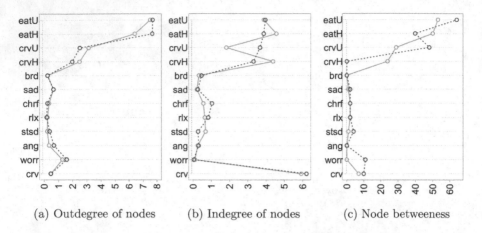

(a) Outdegree of nodes   (b) Indegree of nodes   (c) Node betweeness

Fig. 4. Centrality analysis of networks of obese and healthy-weight people blue dashed line = obese people, cyan solid line = healthy-weight people (eat{H,U} = eat{healthy, unhealthy}, crv{H,U} = crave{healthy,unhealthy}, brd = bored, sad = sad, chrf = cheerful, rlx = relaxed, stsd = stressed, ang = angry, worr = worried, crv = craving) (Color figure online)

(1000–1200) and for an evening period (1800–2000) for the baseline model (fixed effects of the whole population).

Figure 3b is more dense (because it is dinner time for most people that participated in the study) and also positive emotions have a stronger affect on eating unhealthy compared to Fig. 3a which represents a time block when people do not usually eat. It is obvious that these time-period-specific networks can also be drawn for different groups (obese versus healthy-weight) but also for different individuals, assessing for example, when an obese person is more likely to eat something unhealthy.

5.3 Graph Analysis Measures

By treating these networks as graphs, it is possible to perform a graph-based analysis in order to reveal which nodes (i.e. variables) have stronger effect on the network. Figure 4 illustrates three centrality analysis measures (outdegree, indegree and betweeness values) for the networks of obese and healthy-weight people (see Fig. 1) but taking into account all connections (regardless of significance).

The outdegree is a measure of how a node connects to other nodes (thus it takes into account edges that originated from this node to all others) and shows how this node influences and affects other nodes. Figure 4a suggests that eating (either healthy or unhealthy) severely affects all other nodes (emotions) in the next time point. Outdegree value (for eating healthy or unhealthy) is larger for obese people which is in contrast to craving (for healthy or unhealthy) which takes larger values healthy people.

The indegree is a measure of how other nodes connect to a specific node (thus, it takes into account edges that end up at a specific node from all others) and shows how this node is influenced or affected by other nodes. Figure 4b suggests that craving (numeric value) is severely affected by other nodes. Healthy weighted people also have higher indegree for eating healthy than unhealthy, in contrast to obese people where the relation is slightly inverse. The same pattern applies for craving (either for healthy or unhealthy). Also, positive emotions (cheerful and relaxed) have higher indegrees for obese people, also meaning that they are expected to receive greater effect from other nodes.

Finally, the betweeness value is a measure which is indicative of which nodes are more central in the network, so they are important for defining the status of people at each time point (for more information see [17]). Figure 4c suggests that eating unhealthy is the node with the largest betweeness value (with eating healthy being second largest) and the difference between eating healthy and unhealthy is even larger for obese people, suggesting that unhealthy eating is much more important in defining obese people's situation and status. Other interesting findings are that craving (the numeric value) has larger betweeness value for obese people, suggesting that they eventually experience more craving (and possibly satisfy them more often). Finally, negative emotions (like worried and stressed) also have large betweeness values for obese people, which is also an indication that could reveal interesting dynamic relations between emotions and unhealthy eating.

6   Conclusion and Further Work

In this paper we proposed a mixed effects vector autoregression (ME-VAR) model to analyse EMA data related to eating behavior and emotions. Data were collected using an iPhone application developed specifically for this study and they represent almost real-time information about predictors of eating behavior. The ME-VAR model allows the combination of mixed effects (fixed and random) along with time lagging leading to insightful findings. Results presented suggest that there is a complex network affecting multiple variables and events which can vary not only according to groups of people (like obese or healthy-weight) but also to individual persons and to the time block of day.

Further analysis will involve finding ways to include more complex variables (like location, circumstances or thoughts) which will enhance the ability to monitor persons' behavior (through measuring their data) in order to (early) detect moments that each person will be more prone to eating unhealthy. Ultimate goal would be to utilize knowledge acquired from current analysis in order to accurately predict (person-specific) unhealthy eating moments.

References

1. Borsboom, D., Cramer, A.O.J.: Network analysis: an integrative approach to the structure of psychopathology. Ann. Rev. Clin. Psychol. **9**(1), 91–121 (2013). PMID: 23537483
2. Bringmann, L.F., Lemmens, L.H.J.M., Huibers, M.J.H., Borsboom, D., Tuerlinckx, F.: Revealing the dynamic network structure of the beck depressioninventory-II. Psychol. Med. **45**, 747–757, 3 (2015)

3. Carels, R.A., Douglass, O.M., Cacciapaglia, H.M., O'Brien, W.H.: An ecological momentary assessment of relapse crises in dieting. J. Consult. Clin. Psychol. **72**(2), 341–348 (2004)
4. Ebner-Priemer, U.W., Trull, T.J.: Ecological momentary assessment of mood disorders and mooddys regulation. Psychol. Assess. **21**(4), 463 (2009)
5. Gelman, A.: Analysis of variance - why it is more important than ever. Ann. Statist. **33**(1), 1–53, 02 (2005)
6. Gorrostieta, C., Ombao, H., Bdard, P., Sanes, J.N.: Investigating brain connectivity using mixed effects vector autoregressive models. NeuroImage **59**(4), 3347–3355 (2012)
7. Heron, K.E., Smyth, J.M.: Ecological momentary interventions: incorporating mobile technology into psychosocial and health behaviour treatments. Br. J. Health Psychol. **15**(1), 1–39 (2010)
8. Hofmann, W., Adriaanse, M., Vohs, K.D., Baumeister, R.F.: Dieting and the self-control of eating in everyday environments: an experience sampling study. Br. J. Health Psychol. **19**(3), 523–539 (2014)
9. Kashdan, T.B., Lorraine, R.: Collins. Social anxiety and the experience of positive emotion and anger ineveryday life: an ecological momentary assessment approach. Anxiety Stress Coping **23**(3), 259–272 (2010). PMID: 19326272
10. Kwiatkowski, D., Phillips, P.C.B., Schmidt, P., Shin, Y.: Testing the null hypothesis of stationarity against the alternative of a unit root: how sure are we that economic time series have a unit root? J. Econometrics **54**(13), 159–178 (1992)
11. Lavie, P.: Sleep-wake as a biological rhythm. Ann. Rev. Psychol. **52**(1), 277–303 (2001)
12. McKee, H.C., Ntoumanis, N., Taylor, I.M.: An ecological momentary assessment of lapse occurrences in dieters. Ann. Behav. Med. **48**(3), 300–310 (2014)
13. Moskowitz, D.S., Young, S.N.: Ecological momentary assessment: what it is and why it is a method of the future in clinical psychopharmacology. J. Psychiatry Neurosci. **31**, 13–20 (2006)
14. Shiffman, S.: Conceptualizing analyses of ecological momentary assessment data. Nicotine and Tob. Res. (2013)
15. Shiffman, S., Stone, A.A., Hufford, M.R.: Ecological momentary assessment. Ann. Rev. Clin. Psychol. **4**(1), 1–32 (2008)
16. Stone, A.A., Shiffman, S.: Ecological momentary assessment (EMA) in behavorial medicine. Ann. Behav. Med. **16**(3), 199–202 (1994)
17. White, D.R., Borgatti, S.P.: Betweenness centrality measures for directed graphs. Soc. Netw. **16**(4), 335–346 (1994)
18. Zellner, A.: An efficient method of estimating seemingly unrelated regressions and tests for aggregation bias. J. Am. Stat. Assoc. **57**(298), 348–368 (1962)

Chronic Disease Related Entity Extraction in Online Chinese Question and Answer Services

Yan Zhang[1(✉)], Yong Zhang[1], Yanshen Yin[1], Jennifer Xu[2],
Chunxiao Xing[1], and Hsinchun Chen[1,3]

[1] Research Institute of Information Technology, Tsinghua National Laboratory
for Information Science and Technology, Department of Computer Science
and Technology, Tsinghua University, Beijing, China
zhang-yan14@mails.tsinghua.edu.cn,
hchen@eller.arizona.edu
[2] Computer Information Systems, Bentley University, Waltham, USA
jxu@bentley.edu
[3] MIS Department, University of Arizona, Tucson, USA

Abstract. Chinese chronic disease entity extraction aims to extract health
related entities from online questions and answers (QA). Our research tackles
challenges in Chinese chronic disease entity extraction from three aspects:
Chinese health lexicons construction, feature development, and equivalence
conjunctions tagging. We construct large scale Chinese health lexicons based on
expert knowledge and the Web resources; develop a feature extraction approach
that draws out character, part-of-speech, and lexical features from QA data; and
improve the performance of answer entity extraction by leveraging equivalence
conjunctions (punctuation marks and conjunctional words) in Chinese to capture
dependencies between tags of entities. Experiments on question and answer
entity extraction demonstrate that the Precision, Recall and F-1 score are
improved using our proposed features, and the Precision and F-1 score can be
further improved by considering equivalence conjunctions.

Keywords: Entity extraction · QA · Health lexicon

1 Introduction

Aging population has become a serious problem in many countries around the world.
In China, the number of seniors aged 60 and above had risen to 212 million (15.5 %)
by the end of 2014 [9]. These seniors have a pressing need for high quality medical
services for treating their chronic diseases, which greatly worsen their quality of life. In
China, about 86.6 % of total deaths in 2012 were caused by chronic diseases, such as
diabetes, hypertension, etc. [9]. Unfortunately, high quality healthcare resources have
long been in short supply in China. In large cities such as Beijing, an average physician
may have to see around a hundred patients every day, and literally has no time to
answer patients' questions in detail or to provide personalized medical advice.

© Springer International Publishing Switzerland 2016
X. Zheng et al. (Eds.): ICSH 2015, LNCS 9545, pp. 55–67, 2016.
DOI: 10.1007/978-3-319-29175-8_6

This situation has been mitigated to some extent by online medical and healthcare services such as health portals, blogs, Questions and Answers (QAs), and discussion forums. For instance, QA services, whether they are community-based or expert-based, encompass a large amount of user generated content (UGC) and have become an alternative channel through which patients seek health-related information. How to leverage UGC and provide quality QA services is a nontrivial problem.

In this research, we propose a named entity extraction approach to help improve health-related QA services in China using UGC data. Entity extraction, or entity recognition (ER), aims to recognize and identify entities out of unstructured texts. A named entity is a contiguous sequence of textual tokens for representing the name of an object in a certain class (e.g., person or organization). The entity can be general (e.g., organization names) or domain specific (e.g., medicine names). The extracted entities are used to measure the similarity between questions and answers. Generally speaking, if an answer and a question have more common entities, it is more likely that the answer is for addressing the question. Therefore, entity extraction can help identify and construct answers to patient questions with higher relevance and quality.

Entity extraction is essentially a multi-class classification task, which assigns an entity label to each word in a sentence. One of the biggest challenges for Chinese entity extraction is the lack of standard domain lexicons. In techniques and applications for extracting entities out of English texts, there often are a number of domain lexicons available for text processing. For example, the Unified Medical Language System (UMLS [10]) has been widely used in text mining applications in the medical domain. Unfortunately, there has not been a standard Chinese lexicon available for the medical and health domain. Another challenge is the processing of Chinese UGC data. UGCs are usually not formal writing and tend to have a lot of "noises," such as incorrect syntax, misspellings, lay-person terms, or missing punctuations. Furthermore, some unique Chinese punctuation marks, such as the enumeration comma "、", which is used to separate items in a series, need special treatment. For example, in the sentence "治疗糖尿病的方法有药物疗法、运动疗法、饮食疗法。(Treatments for diabetes include medication therapy, physical therapy, and diet therapy.)", the enumeration comma can be leveraged to help identify entities of the same types.

The main contribution of our study is two-fold. First, we construct Chinese chronic disease lexicons to facilitate chronic disease entity extraction in online Chinese QA services. Second, we propose a CRF-based entity extraction approach for Chinese chronic disease entity extraction. In this approach, we define QA entity types based on analysis of large amounts of QA data, extend the tags to leverage unique punctuation marks (i.e., enumeration comma) and conjunctions in Chinese to capture dependencies between tags of entities, and propose a feature extraction approach to extracting character, part-of-speech, and lexical features from online QA. Experiments on health related QA entity extraction show promising performance of our approach.

The remainder of the paper is organized as follows. Section 2 introduces the related work. Section 3 presents our research design. We report on our experiments and results in Sect. 4. The last section concludes this paper.

2 Related Work

Entity extraction in our study aims to extract entities related to chronic diseases from the UGC in online QA services. The extracted entities are used to measure the similarity between the questions and answers by identifying the common entities. In this section, we review the literature on QA systems and entity extraction methods.

QA Systems. There are two types of QA systems: domain-independent and domain-specific. Here we focus on the domain-specific QA systems. In the medical domain, two QA systems, MedQA [6] and AskHERMES [2], are well-known. MedQA was developed in 2006 and is the first QA system for physicians. MedQA uses the records from MEDLINE and Internet. AskHERMES was released in 2011 and employs the UMLS in question analysis. It relies on a dynamic hierarchical categorization model to select answer sentences, and uses question-oriented keywords to assemble the final answers. It not only provides the answers to a user question, but also suggests related questions. Few studies can be found for Chinese QA systems. Peng et al. [13] developed a Chinese QA system based on an enterprise knowledge base. Zhang et al. [15] designed a document retrieval method for a Chinese QA system using professional documents.

Entity Extraction. Feature extraction and entity classification are two major components in entity extraction techniques. Feature extraction is to extract a set of relevant features for building robust learning models. In machine learning approaches, feature extraction is very critical and can significantly affect the performance of entity classification. Prior entity extraction studies have adopted various types of features, including word and contextual features [3], structural features and denotation features, which consider the coherence or appropriateness of the selected entity strings [12]. [14] groups features into different dimensions: word-level features, list lookup features, contextual features, and language-specific features.

Entity classification is to classify extracted entities (terms or words) into predefined target classes, i.e., to assign a class label to each entity. Three types of entity classification methods have been proposed in the literature, namely, supervised learning, semi-supervised learning, and unsupervised learning [8]. Supervised learning includes a training stage and testing stage. During the training, records with class labels are used to construct the classification model (a.k.a. classifier). The classifier is then tested using the test data (i.e., records with their known class labels removed). Among the many supervised methods, Hidden Markov Model (HMM), Maximum Entropy, Support Vector Machine (SVM), and Conditional Random Field (CRF) are the most widely used. Unsupervised learning does not require model training. The most widely used approach is clustering. Other unsupervised techniques employ lexicon, words' pattern, and unlabeled corpus. Semi-supervised learning [11] uses two kinds of samples in the training set: one set with labeled records and the other with no labels. The semi-supervised learning combines the supervised learning with unsupervised learning to reduce the effort to label samples and achieve high accuracy at the same time. In our experiments we choose a supervised learning method: CRF [7]. CRF is one of the most effective methods for sequence labeling such as part-of-speech tagging and entity extraction. Entity extraction is different from general classification in that labels of neighboring items are dependent. For example, while "heart" is an organ, "heart disease" is a disease. Unlike traditional classification methods that classify each word separately, CRF considers the interdependency between labels by incorporating graphical models.

Although entity extraction has been included in medical QA systems in English, little research has been done for systems in Chinese due to the lack of standard domain lexicons and the unique characteristics of Chinese. In our research, we build Chinese lexicons for chronic diseases, design entity tags and extract features considering the QA and Chinese characteristics, and apply a CRF-based machine-learning approach to classifying the entities when processing questions and constructing answers.

3   Research Design

Figure 1 presents the system architecture for our chronic disease related entity extraction approach. It contains two components: Chinese Chronic Disease Lexicons and Question and Answer Entity Extraction. There are two main steps in our CRF-based QA entity extraction approach: Entity Tag Design and Feature Extraction.

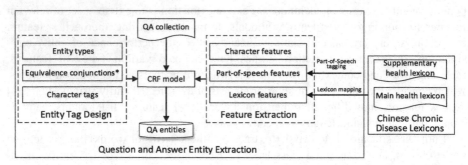

* for answer entity extraction only.

Fig. 1. System Architecture

3.1   Chinese Chronic Disease Lexicons

The extraction of Chinese medical and health-related entities relies on a high quality Chinese chronic condition lexicon. We create two lexicons in our study: an expert-based main lexicon, and a Web-based supplementary lexicon.

Main Health Lexicon. We collaborated with domain experts to create our main lexicon based on professional dictionaries and medical textbooks. The lexicon consists of terms and phrases for diseases, symptoms, diagnosis, medicines, and their relationships. The lexicon is organized in a database, whose metadata are presented in Table 1.

Table 1. The schema of the main health lexicon

Table name (attributes)	#Records
Disease (Name, Subject, System, Department (>=1), Body Part (>=1))	512
Symptom (Name)	2,162
Diagnosis (Name, Abbreviation)	1,080
Medicine (Name, Manufacturers(>=1), URL, Alias)	3,200
Disease-Symptom (Disease, Symptom)	4,738
Disease-Diagnosis (Disease, Diagnosis)	3,049
Disease-Medicine (Disease, Medicine)	6,673

Supplementary Health Lexicon. Manually constructing a domain lexicon is labor-intensive and time-consuming as experts must identify not only concepts but also their relationships. As a result, this manual construction approach is only applicable for small-sized lexicons and can hardly scale up. To construct a more complete, large-scale health lexicon, we collected entries from existing health lexicons on the Web (pinyin. sogou.com, dict.bioon.com, zzk.xywy.com, jib.xywy.com, and yao.xywy.com), and created a supplementary lexicon. Although entities contained in these online resources are concepts without associated metadata and relationships, they greatly reduced the time and effort required by the manual approach. We categorized the concepts into nine classes and placed them in eight tables, as shown in Table 2.

Table 2. Supplementary health lexicon

Table name	Examples	#Records
Disease and symptom	Diabetes mellitus, gingival bleeding	31,452
Medicine	Melbine	38,726
Food	Banana, rice, coffee	26,893
Organ	Lymph gland, heart	6,089
Sign	Urine, sweat	149
Index	Temperature, blood-sugar, lymphokine	3,314
Diagnosis	NMR, CT, pregnancy test	3,473
Treatment	Nasal fistula excision, bone transplantation	8,493

3.2 Question and Answer Entity Extraction

Entity extraction is essentially a sequence labeling task that assigns words and phrases in a sentence sequence to their proper entity types. We use the Conditional Random Field model (CRF) [5], which is based on the Maximum Entropy model (MaxEnt) and the Hidden-Markov model (HMM). The formula is shown as follows:

$$p(\mathbf{y}|\mathbf{x}) = \frac{1}{Z(\mathbf{x})} \exp\{\sum_{k=1}^{K} \lambda_k f_k(y_t, y_{t-1}, \mathbf{x}_t)\}, \tag{1}$$

where **x** is the input/observed data sequence; **y** is the output/hidden label sequence; $\mathbf{x_t}$ is the input feature for word at position t; y_t is the output label of word at position t; K is the number of feature function; f_k is the k_{th} feature function; λ_k is the weight of the k_{th} feature function; and Z is a normalization factor of the form

$$\sum_y \exp\{\sum_{k=1}^{K} \lambda_k f_k(y_t, y_{t-1}, \mathbf{x_t})\}.$$

The feature function $f_k(y_t, y_{t-1}, \mathbf{x_t})$ is the key component of CRF model. It captures the co-occurrence between y_t and $\mathbf{x_t}$, which reflects the dependency between the output entity tag and the input feature of current word, and between y_t and y_{t-1}, which reflects the dependency between entity tags of two adjacent words. Note that $\mathbf{x_t}$ is a vector that can be a data sequence rather than a single value. Hence, by applying such feature function, it catches not only a large amount of observable knowledge from the input data sequence, but also the Markov chain dependency relationships between hidden entity tags that need to be inferred.

As λ_k is the parameter to be estimated, what we need to provide for the model is the alternative output entity tags for each word y_t, and the input features for each word $\mathbf{x_t}$. Hence, the CRF-based entity extraction requires two preceding steps: Entity Tag Design and Feature Extraction.

Entity Tag Design

Entity Types. Entity extraction is a multi-class classification task which assigns a label to each word in a sentence. In our study, entities are the words in questions and answers on QA websites. To identify the targeted classes to be extracted, we analyzed the QA data on three major Chinese QA services (39.net, xywy.com, and 120ask.com) and categorized the entities into the types shown in Table 3. Note that entity types frequently used in questions and answers are different, hence we need to extract them separately.

Table 3. Entity types in questions and answers

	Type	Tag	Examples
Question	Disease and symptom	d	Diabetes mellitus, renal failure
	Medicine and food	m	Plantago seed, melbine
	Diagnosis	c	Electrocardiogram, NMR
	Treatment	t	Laser therapy, cystectomy
	Organ	o	Kidney, heart
	Index	i	Body temperature, glucose
	Organ symptom	os	Pain, erythema
	Index description	is	A little high, normal
Answer	Disease and symptom	d	Diabetes mellitus, renal failure
	Medicine	m	Traditional Chinese or western medicine
	Food	f	Watermelon, millet porridge
	Diagnosis	c	Electrocardiogram, NMR
	Treatment	t	Laser therapy, cystectomy
	Organ	o	Kidney, heart
	Index	i	Body temperature, glucose

Equivalence Conjunctions. There exist some dependencies between entity tags of certain words. For example, entities around conjunction words such as "和 (and)", "或 (or)" and "及 (as well as)" are very likely to have the same tags. Similarly, the enumeration comma (" 、 "), a special Chinese punctuation, separates a series of terms of the same type. We call these words "equivalence conjunctions." While conjunction words in English also join two sentences, the above mentioned Chinese equivalence conjunctions usually join terms, which makes it appropriate for identifying entities with same tags. Equivalence conjunctions are frequently found in answer text where a list of symptoms, conditions, and medicines are named. The problem is that it is difficult to capture such information using a Markov model. According to the Markov property, the latter tag (y_t) is only influenced by the preceding tag (y_{t-1}), which is the tag of equivalence conjunctions instead of the tag of the preceding entity. To leverage such dependencies between entity tags, we design some tags for equivalence conjunctions in answer texts.

- Tag enumeration comma as "*dn?*", where "?" is determined by the tag of the preceding word.
- Tag equivalence conjunction words (e.g., "和", "或", "及") as "*l?*", where "?" is determined by the tag of the preceding word.

The following is an example of an answer containing enumerated Chinese medicine names, which are tagged correctly following the two rules.

- 建议在医生当面指导下服用颈复康颗粒\m 、\dnm 芬必得\m 、\dnm 舒筋活血片\m 进行治疗。
- Translation: I recommend you take <u>Jingfukang Granules\m</u> 、\dnm <u>Fenbid\m</u> 、\dnm <u>Shujinhuoxue tablets\m</u> under the direction of your physician.

Character Tags. A Chinese word may consist of several characters, e.g., "糖尿病" for "diabetes". One way for entity tagging is to perform Chinese word segmentation first, and then assign a tag for each word. However, the overall performance may be influenced by the segmentation accuracy because only words included in the dictionary in the segmentation tool can be identified and assigned a tag. Character tagging, which tags every character instead of words, is a common technique for addressing this problem [16]. Hence, we extend the existing tags by adding two prefixes *B* and *I* to each tag. For example, *d* is extended as *Bd* and *Id*. If a character is tagged as *Bd*, it is the beginning of some disease entity. If a character is tagged as *Id*, it is in the middle or at the end of one entity. As tags listed in Table 3 are for health related entities only, we need four extra tags for words that don't fall into this category:

- *Bf, If* – negation words (e.g., no, not, without, etc.).
- *D* – the comma sign (,).
- *J* – the period sign (.).
- *O* – characters not included in any entity.

The major difference between our approach and previous studies in entity tag design is that, rather than only tagging terms, we also design tags for Chinese equivalence conjunctions, which help identify neighboring words that share same entity types. Furthermore, not only words but also characters found in Chinese health QA contents are tagged, which helps extract more entities from the informal and noisy UGC texts.

Feature Extraction. Feature extraction is to extract feature values from the input data. Three types of features are used in our study: character features, lexical features, and part-of-speech features. *Character feature* is the character in a sentence. Take "心脏病" ("heart disease") for example: when the character "病" ("disease") appears in a word, it usually indicates a disease entity. *Lexical feature* is the class label (tag) assigned to each character based on the health lexicons. It is derived by mapping each word in a sentence to the lexicons, and then assigning a symbol to each character in the words by extending the class label with two prefixes *B* and *I*. For example, as "心脏病" is included in the disease table of the lexicon, the lexical features (i.e., tags) of these three characters are "Bd, Id, Id". Intuitively, if a word is included in a health lexicon, it probably belongs to a given entity type. *Part-of-speech feature* is the part-of-speech tags derived from NLPIR, a Chinese NLP toolkit [1]. For example, as "苹果" ("apple") is tagged as a noun by NLPIR, the part-of-speech features of these characters are then "Bn, In". Generally, nouns are more likely to be the disease entities than adjectives or verbs.

We do not use the feature of current position as input directly. Still take "heart disease" for example, if we use the lexicon symbol of "heart", it will probably be labeled as an organ. But if we take into account "disease," which is the following word of it, it should be labeled as part of a disease entity. The idea behind it is that the entity type of current word y_t is not only determined by the feature tag of current word, but also influenced by the feature around the word. Hence, by varying the observation range, we can derive various input features. We define following x_t based on our analysis:

Character Feature. We denote C_0 as the current character, C_{-i} as the i_{th} character before the current character, C_i as the i_{th} character after the current character. Hence, x_t that considers character feature can be:

- C_0. This is the most common feature template. For example, "糖Bd尿Id病Id" ("sugar Bd urine Id disease Id").
- C_{-2} and C_{-1}. For example, in "服O用O二Bm甲Im双Im胍Im片Im" ("taking metformin tablets"), "二" (the first Chinese character of metformin) is tagged as "Bm" because "服用" ("taking") usually appears before medicine Bm.
- C_1 and C_2. For example, "格Bm列Im齐Im特Im胶Im囊Im" ("Gliclazide capsule"), "特" (the last Chinese character of Gliclazide) is tagged as "Im" because "胶囊" ("capsule") usually appears after medicine Im.
- Similar unigram features also used in our study are: C_{-2}, C_{-1}, C_1, C_2.
- Similar bigram features also used in our study are: C_{-1} and C_0, C_0 and C_1.

Lexical Feature. We denote L as the lexicon-based tag. Hence, x_t that considers lexical feature can be:

- L_0. For example, "hand" is tagged as "organ" as it is included in the organ table of the lexicons.
- L_{-1} and L_0, L_0 and L_1.

Part-of-Speech Feature. We denote P as the part-of-speech tag. Hence, $\mathbf{x_t}$ that considers part-of-speech feature can be:

- P_{-1}, P_0, P_1. For example, an adjective is often followed by a noun.
- P_{-1} and P_0, P_0 and P_1.

We use CRF++ [4] as our CRF implementation.

4 Experiments

Our research aims to improve the performance of CRF-based entity extraction approach from two aspects: extracting large sets of features considering characteristics of both Chinese and health related QA, and leveraging equivalence conjunctions to identify entity of the same types. To validate the effectiveness of proposed approach, we first compare the performance of question entity extraction using different features, and then the performance of answer entity extraction including equivalence conjunctions or not. Both experiments reflect the performance and design rationality of our approach.

4.1 Data

We collected medical and health related QA data from three major Chinese QA service websites: 39.net, xywy.com, and 120ask.com. On these websites, users can ask questions and get answers and advice from real physicians and healthcare professionals. One service, 39.net, also allows other users to answer questions. 1.27 million questions and 2.26 million answers were collected in total. The date range was between July 2007 and May 2015. We then randomly sampled 1,112 questions and 1,266 answers from the dataset and manually tagged each sentence with predefined entity types. Ten-fold cross validation was conducted based on these labeled data.

4.2 Evaluation Metrics

For a N classification problem, we build a $N \times N$ confusion matrix C, where $C(i,j)$ is the number of label j predicted as i. Based on this matrix, we calculate the precision, recall, F-Measure for each class.

- Precision of i: $P = \dfrac{C(i,i)}{\sum_j C(i,j)}$
- Recall of i: $R = \dfrac{C(i,i)}{\sum_j C(j,i)}$
- F-Measure of i: $F = \dfrac{(a^2+1)PR}{a^2(P+R)}$, (when a = 1, it degrades to F1-Score - $F_1 = \dfrac{2PR}{P+R}$)

We use the average values of all indexes as performance metrics of the classifier.

4.3   Question Entity Extraction

In the question entity extraction process, we used three types of features: character features, lexical features, and part-of-speech features. As character features are the most common feature and are usually included in entity extraction, we designed four experiments by combining features on the condition that character features are used:

- Experiment (1): character features only;
- Experiment (2): character features and part-of-speech features combined;
- Experiment (3): character features and lexical features combined;
- Experiment (4): all three types of features combined.

The performance of the above combinations is evaluated as shown in Table 4. We first explore the effectiveness of using the three features. From the most commonly used character feature (experiment 1) to the combination of the three (experiment 4), performance of all types of entity extraction is improved except index description and precision of treatment. We then explore the effects of different features. The comparison between experiment (2) and (4) suggests that the inclusion of lexical features significantly improves certain performance (precision, recall, or F1-score) for entity extraction of disease, medicine, diagnosis, organ, index, and the average. The comparison between experiment (3) and (4) suggests that the inclusion of POS features significantly improves certain performance for entity extraction of diagnosis, organ, index, and organ symptom. Overall, the inclusion of character, lexicon and POS feature significantly improve the average performance of question entity extraction. From pure character feature to the combination of three features, F1-score increased from 0.79 to 0.82.

Table 4. The performance of different feature combinations

Entity Type	Metric	(1) Char.	(2) Char. + POS	(3) Char. + Lex.	(4) Char. + POS + Lex.
Disease	Precision	0.936	0.936	0.956	**0.955**$^{** \&\&}$
	Recall	0.899	0.908	0.939	**0.944**$^{**\&\&}$
	F1-score	0.917	0.922	0.947	**0.949**$^{**\&\&}$
Medicine	Precision	0.914	0.894	0.935	0.923
	Recall	0.796	0.838	0.801	**0.815**$^{\&}$
	F1-score	0.849	0.863	0.862	**0.864***
Diagnosis	Precision	0.870	0.894	0.858	0.912
	Recall	0.619	0.615	0.580	**0.635**$^{\#}$
	F1-score	0.707	0.715	0.675	**0.739**$^{\&\#}$
Treatment	Precision	0.833	0.821	0.817	0.816
	Recall	0.614	0.633	0.627	0.634
	F1-score	0.702	0.712	0.702	0.709
Organ	Precision	0.870	0.859	0.869	0.880
	Recall	0.621	0.685	0.786	**0.814**$^{**\&\&\#\#}$
	F1-score	0.721	0.759	0.823	**0.844**$^{**\&\&\#}$

(Continued)

Table 4. (*Continued*)

Entity Type	Metric	(1) Char.	(2) Char. + POS	(3) Char. + Lex.	(4) Char. + POS + Lex.
Index	Precision	0.936	0.932	0.952	**0.944**$^{*\ \&\&\ \#\#}$
	Recall	0.929	0.933	0.926	0.930
	F1-score	0.932	0.932	0.938	0.937
Organ symptom	Precision	0.765	0.784	0.785	0.786
	Recall	0.529	0.584	0.547	**0.601**$^{**\#\#}$
	F1-score	0.622	0.668	0.641	**0.678**$^{**\#\#}$
Index description	Precision	0.843	0.807	0.827	**0.803***
	Recall	0.698	0.688	0.680	**0.676***
	F1-score	0.759	0.738	0.742	0.730
Average	Precision	0.875	0.872	0.880	**0.883**$^{**\ \&\&}$
	Recall	0.742	0.762	0.763	**0.781**$^{**\&\&\#\#}$
	F1-score	0.794	0.806	0.809	**0.823**$^{**\&\&\#\#}$

Note: Comparison between experiment (1) and (4): * $p < 0.05$; ** $p < 0.01$; comparison between (2) and (4): $^{\&}$ $p < 0.05$; $^{\&\&}$ $p < 0.01$; comparison between (3) and (4): $^{\#}$ $p < 0.05$; $^{\#\#}$ $p < 0.01$.

4.4 Answer Entity Extraction

For answer entity extraction, we add a new tag - equivalence conjunction. As shown in Table 5, equivalence conjunction improves the performance of all types of the entity extractions except the recall of diagnosis, treatment, and organ, and significantly improves certain performance (Precision, Recall, or F1-score) of disease, medicine, organ, index, and the average. The reason for the decrease is that in the test set, the equivalence conjunctions are seldom used for these three entities, and, when equivalence conjunctions are considered, characters with no equivalence conjunction around them are less likely to be tagged as entities. Overall, the use of equivalence conjunction can significantly improve the precision and F1-score of answer entity extraction.

Table 5. The performance of equivalence conjunction

Entity type	Metric	No equivalence conjunction	With equivalence conjunction
Disease	Precision	0.913	**0.920****
	Recall	0.866	0.867
	F1-score	0.888	**0.892***
Medicine	Precision	0.896	0.906
	Recall	0.846	0.849
	F1-score	0.869	**0.876***
Food	Precision	0.869	0.872
	Recall	0.771	0.781
	F1-score	0.813	0.821

(*Continued*)

Table 5. (*Continued*)

Entity type	Metric	No equivalence conjunction	With equivalence conjunction
Diagnosis	Precision	0.887	0.888
	Recall	0.808	0.803
	F1-score	0.842	0.842
Treatment	Precision	0.828	0.833
	Recall	0.726	0.718
	F1-score	0.771	0.769
Organ	Precision	0.682	**0.709***
	Recall	0.587	0.584
	F1-score	0.623	0.636
Index	Precision	0.923	**0.932****
	Recall	0.891	0.895
	F1-score	0.906	**0.913***
Average	Precision	0.869	**0.877***
	Recall	0.809	0.809
	F1-score	0.835	**0.839****

* $p < 0.05$;. ** $p < 0.01$.

5 Conclusion and Future Work

It is important to build automatic health QA systems to help people get high-quality answers to their concerns. This paper presents an entity extraction approach based on CRF, which considers both QA and Chinese characteristics by entity tag design and feature extraction. To recognize the entities, we create Chinese Chronic Disease lexicons based on expert knowledge and Web resources. Our experiments demonstrate the effectiveness of our approach. In the future, we plan to increase the size of Chinese chronic condition lexicon, add more training and test samples, and refine our entity extraction approach using different classification models and more feature types.

Acknowledgments. This work was supported by the National High-tech R&D Program of China (Grant No. SS2015AA020102), National Basic Research Program of China (Grant No. 2011CB302302), the 1000-Talent program, and the Tsinghua University Initiative Scientific Research Program. We thank the research assistance provided by Qingbo Cao at Tsinghua University.

References

1. Big Data Search and Mining Lab, BIT.: Natural Language Processing and Information Retrieval Sharing Platform. http://www.nlpir.org/
2. Cao, Y., Liu, F., Simpson, P., Antieau, L., Bennett, A., Cimino, J.J., Ely, J., Yu, H.: Askhermes: an online question answering system for complex clinical questions. J. Biomed. Inform. **44**(2), 277–288 (2011)

3. Keretna, S., Lim, C.P., Creighton, D.C., Shaban, K.B.: Enhancing medical named entity recognition with an extended segment representation technique. Comput. Methods Programs Biomed. **119**(2), 88–100 (2015)
4. Kudo, T.: CRF++: Yet Another CRF toolkit. http://taku910.github.io/crfpp/
5. Lafferty, J., McCallum, A., Pereira, F.C.: Conditional random fields: Probabilistic models for segmenting and labeling sequence data (2001)
6. Lee, M., Cimino, J., Zhu, H.R., Sable, C., Shanker, V., Ely, J., Yu, H.: Beyond information retrieval—medical question answering. In: AMIA Annual Symposium Proceedings, vol. 2006, p. 469. American Medical Informatics Association (2006)
7. McCallum, A., Li, W.: Early results for named entity recognition with conditional random fields, feature induction and web-enhanced lexicons. In: Proceedings of the seventh conference on Natural language learning at HLT-NAACL 2003, vol. 4, pp. 188–191. Association for Computational Linguistics (2003)
8. Nadeau, D., Sekine, S.: A survey of named entity recognition and classification. Lingvisticae Investigationes **30**(1), 3–26 (2007)
9. National health and family planning commission of the people's republic of China (2015). http://www.nhfpc.gov.cn/
10. Nlm.nih.gov: Unified Medical Language System (UMLS). http://www.nlm.nih.gov/research/umls/
11. Pasca, M., Lin, D., Bigham, J., Lifchits, A., Jain, A.: Organizing and searching the world wide web of facts-step one: the one-million fact extraction challenge. In: AAAI, vol. 6, pp. 1400–1405 (2006)
12. Pasupat, P., Liang, P.: Zero-shot entity extraction from web pages. In: Proceedings of the 52nd Annual Meeting of the Association for Computational Linguistics, ACL 2014. Long Papers, Baltimore, MD, USA, 22–27 June 2014, vol. 1, pp. 391–401 (2014)
13. Peng, X.Y., Chen, Y., Huang, Z.W.: A Chinese question answering system using web service on restricted domain. In: 2010 International Conference on Artificial Intelligence and Computational Intelligence (AICI), vol. 1, pp. 350–353. IEEE (2010)
14. Shaalan, K.: A survey of arabic named entity recognition and classification. Comput. Linguis. **40**(2), 469–510 (2014). http://dx.doi.org/10.1162/COLI_a_00178
15. Zhang, H., Xu, S., Li, W., Zhu, L.: XML-based document retrieval in Chinese diseases question answering system. In: (Jong Hyuk) Park, J.J., Adeli, H., Park, N., Woungang, I. (eds.) Mobile, Ubiquitous, and Intelligent Computing. LNEE, vol. 274, pp. 211–217. Springer, Heidelberg (2014)
16. Zhao, H., Kit, C.: Unsupervised segmentation helps supervised learning of character tagging for word segmentation and named entity recognition. In: IJCNLP, pp. 106–111. Citeseer (2008)

Sentiment Analysis on Chinese Health Forums: A Preliminary Study of Different Language Models

Yan Zhang[1(✉)], Yong Zhang[1], Jennifer Xu[2], Chunxiao Xing[1],
and Hsinchun Chen[1,3]

[1] Research Institute of Information Technology, Tsinghua National Laboratory
for Information Science and Technology, Department of Computer Science
and Technology, Tsinghua University, Beijing, China
zhang-yan14@mails.tsinghua.edu.cn,
hchen@eller.arizona.edu
[2] Computer Information Systems, Bentley University, Waltham, USA
jxu@bentley.edu
[3] MIS Department, University of Arizona, Tucson, USA

Abstract. Sentiment analysis on Chinese health forums is challenging because of the language, platform, and domain characteristics. Our research investigates the impact of three factors on sentiment analysis: sentiment polarity distribution, language models, and model settings. We manually labeled a large sample of Chinese health forum posts, which showed an extremely unbalanced distribution with a very small percentage of negative posts, and found that the balanced training set could produce higher accuracy than the unbalanced one. We also found that the hybrid approaches combining multiple language model based approaches for sentiment analysis performed better than individual approaches. Finally we evaluated the effects of different model settings and improved the overall accuracy using the hybrid approaches in their optimal settings. Findings from this preliminary study provide deeper insights into the problem of sentiment analysis on Chinese health forums and will inform future sentiment analysis studies.

Keywords: Sentiment analysis · Chinese health forum · Language model

1 Introduction

Chronic diseases have become more common in many countries. In China, the number and percentage of patients diagnosed with chronic diseases continue to increase rapidly in recent years. For example, a recent study estimates that there are 113.9 million Chinese people with diabetes and 493 million with pre-diabetes [17]. To better manage their health, more and more people use the Internet to seek health-related information such as the symptoms, causes, and treatments of chronic diseases. Among many types of online services, discussion forums have become increasingly popular. According to a study by the Pew Research Center [3], 80 % of American Internet users have looked for health-related information online, among whom 34 % have read about health-related

© Springer International Publishing Switzerland 2016
X. Zheng et al. (Eds.): ICSH 2015, LNCS 9545, pp. 68–81, 2016.
DOI: 10.1007/978-3-319-29175-8_7

personal stories from other users; and 5 % have posted health-related comments, questions, or information in online forums. Many health forums have also emerged in China to offer a platform for patients to communicate with other users.

These health forums can help alleviate the demand pressure on healthcare resources. Meanwhile, forum users may form communities, and give and receive psychological and social support, which is crucial to their recovery. Hence, analyzing the sentiment polarity (i.e., positive or negative) that users express in their posts offers a great opportunity to understand the opinions, feelings, and emotions associated with their health conditions. It may also have a practical impact on online healthcare services by helping moderators of online health communities more efficiently prioritize their responses to users [5], identify influential members, provide better social support to their members, and get innovative ideas for designing new forums.

Although many new approaches have been proposed, sentiment analysis remains a challenging task because of the language, platform, and domain characteristics. First, automatically extracting sentiment from texts is difficult as people's expressions of their feelings may be obscure, ambiguous, and hard to understand for both humans and computers. Second, analyzing sentiment in user generated contents posted on forums is more difficult than mining regular, formal texts such as news reports. Forum posts usually are short and colloquial, and may contain typos, grammatical errors, forum-specific terms and symbols, and noise such as ads and irrelevant messages. Third, sentiment analysis must consider domain specific characteristics. In the health domain, for example, many sentimental words are used for descriptions of symptoms rather than for expressing personal feelings. A negative sentiment word may not necessarily indicate a negative sentiment. For example, the sentence "When (you're) not feeling well, sweating and shaking, a portable blood glucose meter will help" is actually a neutral, objective expression although negative words are used.

Sentiment analysis on Chinese health forums is even more challenging because the performance of existing natural language processing (NLP) tools is limited and standard Chinese sentiment lexicons do not yet exist. Few studies have been done in this area. The objective of this research is to propose an effective and efficient approach for sentiment analysis on Chinese health forums.

The main contribution of our study is three-fold. First, we explored the characteristics of Chinese health forum data and examined the impact of the distribution of sentiment categories on classification performance. By manually labelling a large number of forum posts, we found that the distribution of different sentiment categories was extremely unbalanced with a very small percentage of negative posts. Our experimental results showed that such a distribution could undermine the classification performance and a balanced training set could produce a better classifier. Second, we examined a number of hybrid approaches that combine different language model based approaches for sentiment analysis on Chinese health forums. Third, we evaluated the effects of different model settings on classification performance and found the optimal settings for improving the overall accuracy of the hybrid approaches. Some of the settings in our study of Chinese health forum posts were different from what was reported in previous studies of movie reviews.

The rest of the paper is organized as follows. Section 2 reviews the related work and identifies research gaps. Section 3 presents our framework for sentiment analysis of

Chinese health forums. Section 4 reports on experimental results. Section 5 discusses the results. Section 6 concludes the paper and suggests future directions.

2 Related Work

The sentiment analysis in our study is to determine the polarity orientation, positive or negative, of a given text (i.e., a forum post). There are two main approaches for this task, namely, the *lexicon-based approach* and the *text classification approach*.

The *lexicon-based approach* uses a dictionary of sentiment words with orientations and strength (e.g., −4 for "hate" and +2 for "inspire") [15]. By aggregating scores of all words, the overall score is derived as positive (+) or negative (−). This is simple, but it cannot be applied in our study as few Chinese sentiment lexicons are available.

The *text classification approach,* a supervised learning approach, is to build classifiers from labeled instances [13], which is the focus of our study. Based on the language models used for feature learning, it can be further categorized into three types: N-gram model and its variants, structured language models, and neural net models.

N-gram Model and Variants. The N-gram model is one of the most widely used models for feature representation. It assumes that the probability of a given word is only conditional on its preceding n-1 word, where n could be 1 (the unigram model), 2 (the bigram model), 3 (the trigram model), or any whole number. This approach converts a collection of text documents into feature vectors by recording the n-gram frequency counts, and uses these vectors as input to classifiers. Wang and Manning proposed an n-gram based method called *NBSVM*, which combines Naive Bayes log-count ratio and Support Vector Machine via linear interpolation [16], and achieves outstanding performance across datasets. However, it remains an open question to determine the optimal n for sentiment analysis. Pang et al. showed that unigrams alone perform better than combining unigrams and bigrams on a movie review dataset [13]. Wang and Manning found that the inclusion of bigrams gives consistent performance gains compared with unigrams alone [16]. Mesnil et al. improved the performance on the Internet Movie Database (IMDB) dataset by adding trigrams [9].

Despite the simplicity, efficiency and accuracy of the n-gram models, their feature spaces grow linearly with the vocabulary size, which often leads to data sparsity. They also simply count the word frequency without considering word semantics.

Structured Language Model. The Structured Language Model (SLM) identifies syntactic structure of sentences by combining automatic parsing and language modeling [2]. Socher et al. developed a *Sentiment Treebank* approach to determining sentiment of sentences represented as a parser tree [14]. With rules for combining sentiment polarity of two semantic units, one can derive the polarity of words, phrases, and finally the whole sentence using a "bottom-up" method. It performs well on treebank sentences and is good at finding negations. However, its applicability is limited in the Chinese context since the performance of existing NLP tools for Chinese dependency parsing is not satisfactory, especially for long sentences.

Neural Net Language Model. The Neural Net Language model (NNLM) overcomes the curse of dimensionality in n-gram models by learning fixed-dimensional distributed representation of words [4]. The widely adopted NNLMs are RNNLM, Word2Vec, and Paragraph Vector.

- *RNNLM.* There are two architectures for NNLM, feedforward and recurrent (See Fig. 1). The feedforward neural network model (FNNM) is limited in the same way as in N-gram model where only preceding $n-1$ words in the history are taken as context. Mikolov et al. proposed RNNLM, a recurrent neural network based language model, where the history is represented by neurons with recurrent connections and hence the context length is unlimited [11]. Plenty of empirical evidence suggests that RNNLM outperforms n-grams significantly.
- *Word2Vec.* Word2Vec is a well-known RNN based implementation of distributed word representation with two novel architectures: CBOW (Continuous Bag-of-Words Model) and Skip-gram (Continuous Skip-gram Model) (Fig. 2) [10]. CBOW sums up or averages the context on the projection layer and ignores word order as BoW model does. To improve the efficiency of the two models, binary Huffman tree based *hierarchical softmax* is used as an approximation of the full softmax. In [12], Mikolov et al. further speeded it up with the *negative sampling* approach, which subsamples the frequent words instead of building a binary tree. Word2Vec can grasp semantic relationship between words, e.g., vector("king") − vector ("man") + vector("woman") ≈ vector("queen").
- *Paragraph Vector.* Paragraph Vector (PV) is an improved version of Word2Vec and maps *sentences, paragraphs, and documents* rather than only words to continuous vector representations. Hence, this approach is more suitable for sentiment analysis than Word2Vec [6]. PV adopts similar architectures and efficiency tricks as Word2Vec, except that it adds a paragraph vector as the context during training. Le and Mikolov reported that for the PV approach, Skip-gram is better than CBOW using hierarchical softmax, and it is the new state of the art in sentiment analysis on the above mentioned two movie review datasets.

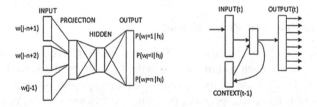

Fig. 1. Feedforward neural network (left) vs. Recurrent neural network (right) [11].

Based on our literature review we found that most prior language model based sentiment analysis studies have been done in the business and entertainment domains such as product reviews and movie reviews, little has been done in the medical and health domain. Among the state-of-the-art approaches, NBSVM, RNNLM, and PV can be applied for feature learning using limited Chinese resources. However, each

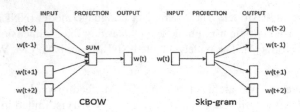

Fig. 2. Two model architectures for Word2vec [10].

approach needs to adjust several parameters for optimal performance including different history lengths in n-grams (e.g., unigrams, bigrams, trigrams, etc.), two architecture options (CBOW and Skip n-gram), as well as two efficiency tune-ups for PV. Different types of approaches can also be combined to produce better performance. For example, Mesnil and Mikolov reported that combining all three approaches yields the best performance on an English movie review dataset [9]. However, it is still not clear under which conditions and with what kind of combination these advanced techniques could achieve the best performance for sentiment analysis on Chinese health forums. Hence, we propose the following research questions:

- How can we apply the state-of-the-art language model based approaches for sentiment analysis on Chinese health forums?
- Which hybrid approach performs the best?
- How do different model settings affect sentiment classification performance?

3   Research Design

In this section, we present the process for sentiment analysis on Chinese health forums, including Data Collection and Preprocessing, Design of Data Sampling Strategy, Evaluation of Individual Approaches, and Combination of Different Models.

3.1   Data Collection and Preprocessing

Data for sentiment analysis can be collected from a health related forum platform using a web crawler. Usually each forum has a specific focus (e.g., diabetes, heart diseases, and arthritis). A text parser is then used to extract specific attributes from posts, including the forum ID, URL, post ID, post title, post time, and text content.

Data preprocessing consists of two tasks: data cleansing and word segmentation. Data cleansing includes removing duplicate posts and irrelevant information added by the platform (e.g., date of the last edit), and integrating each post into one paragraph. Word segmentation is an essential step for feature extraction in applications of mining Chinese text. Unlike English that uses space to naturally separate words, there are no delimiter characters in Chinese. In our study, we used NLPIR (http://www.nlpir.org/), a widely adopted NLP toolkit, for Chinese word segmentation.

3.2   Design of Data Sampling Strategy

Most prior sentiment analysis studies employing language model based approaches have used movie review data, where instances are evenly distributed between positive and negative sentiment classes [8, 9, 12]. However, many datasets have an unbalanced distribution among classes. A classifier trained with unbalanced data may have bias towards the majority class [1]. To address this issue, a balanced sample can be generated out of the data by designing a proper sampling strategy [7]. However, it remains unknown whether, when tested with a real, unbalanced set, the classifier trained with a balanced training set would produce better predictive accuracy than with the real, unbalanced training set, as the performance also depends on the domain, feature learning approaches, and the classification approach [1].

Hence, the sentiment distribution of the health forum data must be analyzed first by manually labelling a large sample of posts. An appropriate data sampling strategy can then be designed based on the analysis result. Specifically, if sentiment polarity in the data is evenly distributed, a simple random sampling approach will produce a balanced training set. Otherwise, an undersampling strategy [7], which randomly draws a matching number of instances out of the majority class with the minority class, can be used to create a balanced training set. Then we compare the performance of a balanced training set with the unbalanced one, and the one shows an higher accuracy on the real unbalanced test dataset is selected as the final approach.

3.3   Evaluation of Individual Feature Learning Approaches

Feature learning is the prerequisite for classification. In our study, features are learned using the state-of-the-art language model based approaches: NBSVM (n-gram), RNNLM (neural net), and PV (neural net). As mentioned above, the performance of NBSVM and PV can be affected by specific settings. Hence, we test the performance of NBSVM under three most widely adopted settings: unigrams, unigrams + bigrams, and unigrams + bigrams + trigrams. We evaluate the performance of PV under four (2X2) possible settings with two architectures (CBOW and Skip-gram), and two alternative efficiency tune-ups (hierarchical softmax and negative sampling).

3.4   Combination of Different Approaches

In statistics and machine learning studies, combining different learning methods often produces better performance than using a single approach. In this study, we examine hybrid approaches that combine the three language models (NBSVM, RNNLM, and PV), each of which is under their best settings derived from the previous individual approach evaluation step. The final output is generated by a weighted linear combination of each approach; and the weight of each model is set according to its accuracy on the validation set. The performance of all possible combinations is then evaluated.

The learned features are represented as vectors and used as input to a classifier, which assigns a label for each instance. In both the individual approach evaluation and the model combination steps, we adopt a logistic regression classifier as it shows similar performance with linear SVM but requires less training time. The accuracy rate is calculated based on manually labeled data to assess the performance.

4   Experiments

4.1   Datasets

To evaluate our proposed hybrid approach for sentiment analysis on Chinese health forums, we collected posts from an online diabetes forum (http://bbs.tnbz.com/), which is popular among diabetes patients in China. We collected 184,708 posts in total. The date range was between September 2005 and December 2013.

We manually labeled each instance (i.e., forum post) to prepare for the training and test datasets. Our aim is to identify the negative posts to help prioritize patients in need, which is especially beneficial to the health domain. Rather than simply classifying the instances into either negative or non-negative like in many prior studies [8, 9, 12–14], we labeled it as negative, positive, or neutral. To ensure coding reliability, we first sampled 1,000 posts and hired 3 coders to label the sample. Fleiss' kappa was calculated as a measure of inter-coder agreement. The kappa values were 0.76 for the coding of three categories (negative, positive, neutral) and 0.70 for two categories (negative, non-negative), both of which indicate high inter-coder reliability.

The coding result of a much larger sample of 50,000 posts shows that the data are distributed quite unbalanced, i.e., there are only a small percentage of negative posts (see Table 1). This is interesting because we expected that there were many negative posts in health related forums, where people share their feelings (e.g., worries, frustration, and anxiety) about their health conditions. Such an unbalanced distribution makes it extremely difficult to find enough negative posts for training the classifier and may significantly lower the performance.

Table 1. Sentiment polarity distribution in the health forum dataset

	Negative	Non-negative	
		Positive	Neutral
# posts	2,806 (5.6 %)	998 (2 %)	46,196 (92.4 %)

As our data was distributed unbalanced, the undersampling strategy was selected over the simple random sampling strategy. We evaluated the performance of each language model based approach using both balanced and unbalanced training sets.

- Balanced training set: 2,520 (90 % of 2,806) negative and non-negative instances;
- Balanced testing set: 280 (10 % of 2,806) negative and non-negative instances;
- Unbalanced training set: 2,520 negative and 42,340 non-negative instance.

For the unsupervised PV approach, we used all 50,000 instances without class labels. For approaches with several possible settings, we randomly assigned a specific one (i.e., *skip n-gram* architecture with *negative sampling* efficiency tune-up for PV

approach, and using *unigrams, bigrams, and trigrams* as history length for NBSVM).
Table 2 reports the accuracy of different models trained using balanced and unbalanced
sets and tested using a balanced set. Tests using unbalanced sets produced similar
results, which suggests that a balanced training set can deliver better performance and
generalizes well to the real unbalanced test set.

Table 2. Accuracy with different training sets

	RNNLM	PV	NBSVM
Balanced training set	75.02 %	82.46 %	82.71 %
Unbalanced training set	53.46 %	58.27 %	56.24 %

4.2   Evaluation

Performance of Individual Approaches. We evaluated the performance (accuracy)
of individual approaches under all possible settings as shown in Table 3. Statistical
analyses were performed using a one-tailed paired sample t test. Among the three
approaches, NBSVM shows the highest accuracy, followed by PV, and then RNNLM.

We also explore the effects of different settings on these approaches. For the two
architectures of PV, Skip n-gram significantly outperforms CBOW, which is consistent
with previous findings using movie review data [6]. As for the two speed tune-ups, the
accuracy of negative sampling (NS) is significantly higher than that of hierarchical
softmax (HS). Moreover, NS requires much less training time (30 min) than HS
(90 min) in our experiments using one CPU only. Thus NS + Skip n-gram is the best
setting for PV in terms of both effectiveness and efficiency.

Table 3 also reflects the impact of different lengths of n-grams on NBSVM, where
unigrams (U) and unigrams + bigrams (UB) outperform unigrams + bigrams + trigrams
(UBT) significantly, and there is no significant difference between U and UB while UB
produces a slightly higher accuracy rate. In terms of efficiency, U takes slightly less
training time than UB as it has smaller size of feature space. Hence, both U and UB
could be the best settings for NBSVM.

Table 3. Accuracy of individual approaches with ten-fold cross validation

Approach			Accuracy	p-value
RNNLM			75.02 %	–
PV	Hierarchical Softmax (HS)	CBOW	78.34 %	0.008
		Skip n-gram	**79.98 %****	
	Negative Sampling (NS)	CBOW	81.32 %	0.003
		Skip n-gram	**82.46 %****	
NBSVM	Unigrams (U)		83.64 %	–
	Unigrams + Bigrams (UB)		**83.73 %**	–
	Unigrams + Bigrams + Trigrams (UBT)		82.71 %	–

*p < 0.05; * * p < 0.01.

Performance of Hybrid Approaches. We evaluated the performance of the hybrid models to find whether combining different models produces higher accuracy and to assess the contribution of each individual approach (see Table 4).

We first evaluated the performance of the combination of two models. Among such combinations, PV + NBSVM produced the highest accuracy, followed by RNNLM + NBSVM, and RNNLM + PV, indicating that NBSVM contributes most to the overall performance. Moreover, the significant difference between the performance of PV + NBSVM and RNNLM + NBSVM suggests the importance of PV.

The performance of three-model combination was worse than PV + NBSVM, indicating that the RNNLM reduces the overall accuracy. Still, no significant difference was found between the accuracy under unigram and unigram + bigram settings of NBSVM, while the latter shows a slightly higher average accuracy.

Overall, the PV + NBSVM (UB) approach performed the best with a 2.47 % increase in accuracy from NBSVM (UB), the best state-of-the-art individual approach.

Table 4. Accuracy of hybrid approaches using ten-fold cross validation

Model combinations	Accuracy	p-value
RNNLM + PV	82.50 %	–
RNNLM + NBSVM (Unigrams)	83.68 %	0.1277
RNNLM + NBSVM (Unigrams + Bigrams)	84.09 %	
PV + NBSVM (Unigrams)	85.59 %	0.0738
PV + NBSVM (Unigrams + Bigrams)	**86.20 %**	
RNNLM + PV + NBSVM (Unigrams)	85.30 %	0.2216
RNNLM + PV + NBSVM (Unigrams + Bigrams)	82.50 %	

5   Discussion

Two findings distinguish our sentiment analysis on Chinese health forum data from prior studies of movie reviews in English:

First, the effect of the length of n-grams is found to be different from previously reported. Our experiments on the NBSVM approach show that both unigrams (U) and unigrams + bigrams (UB) are better than unigrams + bigrams + trigrams (UBT). However, a previous study using the IMDB dataset shows that UBT is the best among the three, followed by UB, and then U [9].

Second, we found that the effects of the two efficiency tune-ups used in the PV approach are also different. Our experiments show that when using the PV approach for sentiment analysis on Chinese health forum data, negative sampling (NS) produces higher accuracy than hierarchical softmax (HS) does. Yet in a previous study, HS is selected as a better choice for learning paragraph vector [6].

To find out the causes for the accuracy differences, we compared two types of errors under different settings, i.e., the ratio of positive posts misclassified as negative (i.e., false negative) and the ratio of negative posts misclassified as positive (i.e., false positive). Table 5 shows that the differences are mainly caused by a higher false positive error in UBT, and a higher false negative error in HS.

We further analyzed the impact of post length on accuracy. In our training set, the average lengths of positive and negative posts are 579 and 364, respectively. We first examined the posts misclassified by UBT/HS but correctly classified by UB/NS. As shown in Table 6, posts misclassified by UBT generally are shorter than those in the training set, indicating that UBT may not work well for short posts. This is because a Chinese medical term usually consists of multiple characters, each of which is a word by itself, and is longer than its English counterpart. For example, "糖尿病," the Chinese term corresponding to the single-word term "diabetes" in English, has three characters. As a result, a short post in Chinese may not be long enough to generate as many trigram features as in English.

We then analyzed posts misclassified by HS but correctly classified by NS, both of which use the Skip n-gram architecture. Because the skip n-gram architecture is essentially an n-gram model with a history length of at most 5 in our experiment, which is a stricter matching criterion than trigrams, these misclassified posts should be shorter than the average posts in the training set. However, as shown in Table 6, the false negative posts in HS, on average, are longer than those in the training set. Looking into these posts, we found that the longer average length is caused by a small percentage of rather long posts (i.e., 20 % posts longer than 1100), indicating that HS does not work well for long posts.

Table 5. Types of errors in different settings

Approach	Settings	False positive	False negative
NBSVM	Unigrams + Bigrams (UB)	18.93 %	12.14 %
	Unigrams + Bigrams + Trigrams (UBT)	**22.86 %**	10.71 %
PV	NS	15.35 %	19.64 %
	HS	16.43 %	**23.57 %**

Table 6. Average length of posts misclassified in UBT/HS only

	False positive	False negative
UBT	311	67
HS	319	567

Examples of posts misclassified by UBT/HS but correctly classified by UB/NS are shown in Table 7. Note that we use "/" to show word segmentation returned by the NLPIR tool in the original Chinese posts, and use "()" to indicate the originally omitted words in the translated version.

Table 7. Examples of posts misclassified by UBT/HS but correctly classified by UB/NS

App	Err	Original post	Translation
UBT	False Pos.	糖/妈妈/们/请/帮帮/我/最/好/是/生/过/的/。/。/我/是/个/糖/妈妈/现在/怀孕/8/个/月/了/宝宝/马上/要/降生/了/在/怀孕/期间/发生/过/6–7/次/低血糖/低血糖/发生/的/时候/大多/都/是/3点/多/请问/对/孩子/有/影响/吗/?/?/我/好/怕/我/低血糖/宝宝/生/下来/会/脑瘫/啊/有/过来/的/妈妈/告诉/下/会/发生/这样/的/情况/吗/?/?/?/?	Could any diabetic mothers help me? It would be better if you already have a baby…I was diagnosed with gestational diabetes in my 8th month of pregnancy and would give birth soon. Hypoglycemia has occurred 6-7 times during my pregnancy and it happens mostly at 3:00 PM. Would it have any impact on the baby?? I'm afraid that my baby will be born with cerebral palsy since I have a low blood glucose level (.) Could any experienced mom tell me whether it will happen????
	False Neg.	肾功能不全/:/上/星期六/和/老伴/同/测/了/个/尿/四/样/,/今天/见/报告单/上/写/着/"/肾功能不全/"/,/但/指标/都/正常/,/虚惊/一/场	Renal insufficiency: My wife and I did a urine test last Saturday. The report showed that it was renal insufficiency. However, all indicators were normal. It turned out to be a false alarm.
HS	False Pos.	俞老/,/请/教/:/我/是/11月/4日/看/了/DM/的/宣传/海报/上/说/的/症状/和/偶/一样/,/口渴/,/喝/大量/的/水/,/消瘦/,/马上/到/了/医院/检查/:/先是/查/了/尿/尿糖/:/3 +/胆红素/:/阴性/酮/体/:/微量/蛋白质/:/1 +/亚硝酸盐/:/阴性/血红蛋白/:/微量/白细胞/:/阴性/PH/:/5.5/尿/比重/:/1.030/红细胞计数/:/0/白细胞计数/:/0…………/后面/的/就/不/写/了/,/看/完/尿/,/医生/让/偶/做/了/生化/血/葡萄糖/:/14.91/总胆固醇/:/4.99/甘油三酯/:/1.84/高密度脂蛋白胆固醇/:/1.19/低密度脂蛋白胆固醇/:/3.40C/肽/:/1.724/胰岛素/:/67.20/医生/说/我/是/糖尿病/。/俞老/,/有/几/个/问题/请教/,/感谢/!/1/,/我/不/要/做/葡萄糖/耐量/测试/就/确定/是/DM/了/吗/?/2/,/我/尿/里/有/蛋白/,/为什么/医生/不/让/偶/做/微量/检查/?/是/不/是/我/	Dr. Yu, I have some questions to ask you. I saw the DM poster on November 4. I had the symptoms mentioned in the poster: thirsty, drinking plenty of water, and weight loss. I went to the hospital immediately, and did a urine test: glycosuria: 3+ (,) bilirubin: negative(,) ketones: trace(,) protein: 1 + (,) nitrite: negative(,) hemoglobin: trace(,) WBC: trace(,) urine specific gravity: 1.030(,) RBC count: 0(,) WBC count: 0········ The rest is omitted here. After the urine test, the doctor asked me to do a biochemical test: blood glucose: 14.91(,) total cholesterol: 4.99(,) triglycerides: 1.84(,) high-density lipoprotein cholesterol: 1.19(,) low-density lipoprotein cholesterol: 3.40C(,) peptide: 1.724(,) insulin: 67.20(.)

(Continued)

Table 7. (*Continued*)

App	Err	Original post	Translation
		肾/有/病/了/,/这个/是/我/最/担心/的/,/家族/里/有/人/得/过/./怕/怕/。	The doctor said that I have diabetes. Thus, Dr. Yu, I have some questions to ask you and thank you in advance: 1. Is it certain that I have DM without doing a glucose tolerance test? 2. Why did the doctor not ask me to do a micro inspection since I have protein in my urine? Is there something wrong with my kidney? This is my greatest worry since I have a family history of kidney diseases. It is scary.
	False Neg.	建议/版/主/详细/介绍/一下/活力/试纸/行货/、/水货/和/假货/的/识//学会/识别/行/、/水/、/假货/试纸/的/本领/,/对/想/省/银子/的/DMer/十分/重要/。。	(I) suggest that moderators explain in detail about the recognition of properly licensed, parallel and counterfeit active test strips. Learning to recognize properly licensed, parallel and counterfeit test strips is important to DMers who want to save money.

6 Conclusion and Future Directions

This paper presents our research of sentiment analysis on online Chinese forums that are related to health topics. Our research generates three major findings. First, based on the manual labeling process on a large number of posts we found that the distribution of sentiment categories (positive, negative) in the health-related forum posts is extremely unbalanced. Using different data sampling strategies, we found that the sentiment category distribution can dramatically affect the classification performance and a balanced training set could produce higher accuracy than the unbalanced one. Second, we found that hybrid approaches combining different language models outperform individual approaches for sentiment analysis on Chinese health forums. Finally we evaluated the effects of different model settings for each approach and applied the optimal settings to the hybrid approaches to improve the overall accuracy. Some of the settings in our study of Chinese health forum posts were different from what was reported in previous studies of movie reviews. In the future, we will extend our work by incorporating prior knowledge into these models to further improve the performance of sentiment analysis.

Acknowledgments. This work was supported by the National High-tech R&D Program of China (Grant No. SS2015AA020102), National Basic Research Program of China (Grant No. 2011CB302302), the 1000-Talent program, and the Tsinghua University Initiative Scientific Research Program. We appreciate the research assistance provided by Qingbo Cao, Yanshen Yin, and Xinhuan Chen at Tsinghua University.

References

1. Chawla, N.V.: Data mining for imbalanced datasets: an overview. In: Maimon, O., Rokach, L. (eds.) Data Mining and Knowledge Discovery Handbook, pp. 853–867. Springer, New York (2005)
2. Chelba, C., Jelinek, F.: Recognition performance of a structured language model. arXiv:cs/0001022 (2000)
3. Fox, S.: The social life of health information 2011. Pew Internet & American Life Project Washington, DC (2011)
4. Hinton, G.E.: Learning distributed representations of concepts. In: Proceedings of the Eighth Annual Conference of the Cognitive Science Society, vol. 1, p. 12, Amherst, MA (1986)
5. Huh, J., Yetisgen-Yildiz, M., Pratt, W.: Text classification for assisting moderators in online health communities. J. Biomed. Inform. **46**(6), 998–1005 (2013)
6. Le, Q.V., Mikolov, T.: Distributed representations of sentences and documents. In: Proceedings of the 31th International Conference on Machine Learning, ICML 2014, Beijing, China, 21–26 June 2014. JMLR Proceedings, vol. 32, JMLR.org (2014)
7. Lee, C.Y., Lee, Z.J.: A novel algorithm applied to classify unbalanced data. Appl. Soft Comput. **12**(8), 2481–2485 (2012)
8. Maas, A.L., Daly, R.E., Pham, P.T., Huang, D., Ng, A.Y., Potts, C.: Learning word vectors for sentiment analysis. In: Proceedings of the 49th Annual Meeting of the Association for Computational Linguistics: Human Language Technologies, vol. 1, pp. 142–150. Association for Computational Linguistics (2011)
9. Mesnil, G., Ranzato, M., Mikolov, T., Bengio, Y.: Ensemble of generative and discriminative techniques for sentiment analysis of movie reviews. CoRR bs/1412.5335 (2014)
10. Mikolov, T., Chen, K., Corrado, G., Dean, J.: Efficient estimation of word representations in vector space. CoRR abs/1301.3781 (2013)
11. Mikolov, T., Karafiát, M., Burget, L., Cernocký, J., Khudanpur, S.: Recurrent neural network based language model. In: INTERSPEECH 2010, 11th Annual Conference of the International Speech Communication Association, Makuhari, Chiba, Japan, pp. 1045–1048, 26–30 September 2010
12. Mikolov, T., Sutskever, I., Chen, K., Corrado, G.S., Dean, J.: Distributed representations of words and phrases and their compositionality. In: Advances in Neural Information Processing Systems, pp. 3111–3119 (2013)
13. Pang, B., Lee, L., Vaithyanathan, S.: Thumbs up?: sentiment classification using machine learning techniques. In: Proceedings of the ACL-02 Conference on Empirical Methods in Natural Language Processing, vol. 10, pp. 79–86. Association for Computational Linguistics (2002)
14. Socher, R., Perelygin, A., Wu, J.Y., Chuang, J., Manning, C.D., Ng, A.Y., Potts, C.: Recursive deep models for semantic compositionality over a sentiment treebank. In: Proceedings of the Conference on Empirical Methods in Natural Language Processing (EMNLP), vol. 1631, p. 1642. Citeseer (2013)

15. Taboada, M., Brooke, J., Tofiloski, M., Voll, K., Stede, M.: Lexicon-based methods for sentiment analysis. Comput. Linguist. **37**(2), 267–307 (2011)
16. Wang, S., Manning, C.D.: Baselines and bigrams: simple, good sentiment and topic classification. In: Proceedings of the 50th Annual Meeting of the Association for Computational Linguistics: Short Papers, vol. 2. pp. 90–94. Association for Computational Linguistics (2012)
17. Xu, Y., Wang, L., He, J., Bi, Y., Li, M., Wang, T., Wang, L., Jiang, Y., Dai, M., Lu, J., et al.: Prevalence and control of diabetes in Chinese adults. JAMA **310**(9), 948–959 (2013)

Clinical and Medical Data Mining

Clustering Analysis on Patient-Physician Communication and Shared Decision-Making During Cancer Prognosis Discussion

Yikang Li[1], Yuxuan Liu[2], Nan Kong[3(✉)], and Cleveland G. Shields[4]

[1] Department of Industrial Engineering, Tsinghua University,
Beijing, China
liykl2@mails.tsinghua.edu.cn
[2] School of Industrial Engineering, Purdue University,
West Lafayette, IN, USA
liu1118@purdue.edu
[3] Weldon School of Biomedical Engineering, Purdue University,
West Lafayette, IN, USA
nkong@purdue.edu
[4] Department of Human Development and Family Studies, Purdue University,
West Lafayette, IN, USA
cgshields@purdue.edu

Abstract. We conducted clustering analyses to verify whether common patterns can be identified from two distinct types of end-stage cancer prognosis discussion information, including patient-centered communication and shared decision making data. We applied hierarchical clustering on patient-centered communication measurement data and frequent itemset hierarchical clustering on coded shared decision-making interaction information. Our results suggested modest association between the two data sets in clustering assignments when measuring it with a normalized mutual information index. However, we could not find any noticeable overlap between the two assignments.

Keywords: Cancer · Patient-centered communication · Shared Decision-Making · Prognosis discussion · Clustering analysis

1 Background and Introduction

Ineffective discussion between patients and physicians in their medical encounters remain to be one singular significant contributor [1] to poor communication and shared decision-making. During these medical encounters, it is common for patients not to understand their diagnostic findings, prognosis, and treatment options. Often lack of understanding or misunderstanding may hinder patient and clinician actions (e.g., [2]). Meanwhile, although guidelines exist for physicians in the discussions [3, 4], there is no firm evidence supporting any one approach [5]. Moreover, shared decision-making is known to improve the quality of care and patient health outcomes [6], as the process by which healthcare providers include patients in decisions about healthcare. The foundation of shared decision-making is collective participation where physicians and

© Springer International Publishing Switzerland 2016
X. Zheng et al. (Eds.): ICSH 2015, LNCS 9545, pp. 85–98, 2016.
DOI: 10.1007/978-3-319-29175-8_8

patients use their knowledge, experience, and values of involvement to evaluate and choose best available treatment options [7]. Patient perceptions on their involvement in care are associated with increased patient satisfaction, pain management, and treatment adherence [8–10].

In the aspect of communication, both patient and physician factors affect the discussion effectiveness [11]. It is evident that such effectiveness is dependent on patient's cultural and social background, often different focus of the patient and her physician, as well as physician's patient-centered communication skills. Using cancer prognosis discussion as an example, Cassileth et al. [12] and Jenkins et al. [13] reported that cancer patients in western cultures prefer understanding their diagnostic findings, prognosis, and probability of successfully treating their disease. However, not all cultures endorse such a preference. Mitchell [14] reported that physicians from non-western cultures may be more reluctant to disclose prognostic information than western physicians. Meanwhile, the discussion may also be hampered by the different focus of the patient and the physician [15]. Patients are often focused on the impact of cancer on their lives and their discomfort and pain. Physicians, by contrast, are focused on the illness, particular on its progression and treatment.

Furthermore, physician's communication skills, especially the ability of achieving patient-centered communication, are critical to the discussion effectiveness. Eliciting and validating patient concerns, two major communication skills, are a multi-faceted construct that includes physicians' eliciting and understanding patients' perspective, understanding the patients' psychological context, developing a shared understanding of the problem, and sharing decision-making power if patients desire [16]. In the literature, eliciting and validating patient concerns has proved to be the most reliable and valid component of measuring patient-centered communication, and is known to be associated with greater satisfaction with visits [17]. Another set of measures reflect various aspects of the physician's voice tone, including attentiveness, anxiety, and hostility. Other measures include physician use of certainty language, prognosis communication assessment, as well as a few miscellaneous ones. The above measures can serve as important indicators that differentiate physicians in terms of their communication skills and styles in prognosis discussion. In addition, they have been shown to be indicative to communication effectiveness and patient satisfaction [18, 19]. Nevertheless, given that these measures are mainly derived for assessing the communication outcomes, effectiveness and satisfaction, it remains unclear whether they are still indicative when studying the aspect of shared decision-making.

On the other hand, several measures of shared decision-making focus on overall ratings of physician decision-making and provide rich data for shared decision-making in medical encounters. The OPTION (observing patient involvement) scale is widely used to rate the overall shared decision-making process and focus on the physician's ability to invite patients to participate in the visit [20]. Some other scales assess patients' perception of shared decision-making; e.g., [21, 22]. Because shared decision-making is a simultaneous process of transferring information between the physician and the patient, it is important to identify specific behaviors that achieve this two-way exchange and thus also focus on the behaviors of the patient [23]. Further, Shields et al. [24] explored the assessment of the interplay between patient and physician behaviors.

The authors developed the Medical Interaction Decision-Making (MIDM) coding scheme. MIDM is intended to code specific physician and patient behaviors (e.g., what topics being discussed, in what sequence, and for how long) during decision-making episodes. Subsequently, it allows researchers to define key behaviors associated with shared decision-making, the relationship between physician behaviors and patient behaviors, and the contexts in which these decisions occur. Although several measures of shared decision-making have been proposed, it remains unclear how detailed behavior information from the shared decision -making process may influence patient-centered communication.

To answer the above questions, we in this paper conducted clustering analysis to explore the association between the differences among physicians in their communication and the differences in their shared decision-making with patients. More specifically, we tested the hypothesis that the groupings of physicians in terms of attributes from the two aspects are identical. We analyzed the data collected from a previous study by co-author Shields and his colleagues [18] that examines the discussion of prognosis during oncology visits, and thus focusing on end-stage cancer consultation. We also analyzed the data collected for another previous study by co-author Shields and his colleagues [24] that develops the MIDM to code the behavior data during shared decision-making. We believe this exploratory study would offer insights into how easily to train physicians to behave and communicate well in a consultation session with cancer that informs prognosis and discuss care options. A main methodological challenge is to perform clustering analysis on resultant high-dimensional shared decision-making data (i.e., detailed behavior data).

The remainder of the paper is organized as follows. In Sect. 2, we provide detailed description on the data analyzed. In Sect. 3, we report and discuss our data analysis. In Sect. 4, we conclude the paper by outlining the limitations of the work and future research directions.

2 Methods

2.1 Human Subject Study Design

In a pilot human subject study, co-author Shields and his colleagues recruited 46 physicians, 23 primary care physicians and 23 oncologists, through the Family Practice Research Network in a Midwestern state and through senior specialists at a regional medical center. In the same pilot study, co-author Shields and his colleagues also recruited three male actors to portray stage IV lung cancer patients seeking a new consultation. These actors are called standardized patients (SP). The SP method has been extensively used in primary care research [16, 17, 25–27] but has not been used to examine oncology patient visits.

The SP cover story in this pilot study was that he had moved from another part of the country to live closer to his daughter. The SP medical record attested to the SP's previous treatment for lung cancer. SPs were coached to give information about themselves in response to questions, but not to give too much unsolicited information.

The SP's background was that he had been a manager of a small motel until he became ill. He had first gone to the physician for care because of back pain, which turned out to be lung cancer. He had radiation treatment for his cancer, but no chemotherapy or surgery. Because he felt better following the radiation treatment, he was not fully aware that the cancer had not been cured. He stated that he had not been told his diagnosis when he was first treated. He presented to the physician with new pain in the front of his chest that he was unaware was likely a new metastasis of his cancer. The purpose of this scenario was to invoke a sense of urgency for the physicians to treat or refer the SP. Because the SP was both unaware of his prognosis and the likelihood that his new pain was indicative his cancer had metastasized further, physicians would need to explain these facts to the SP in order to plan treatment, or refer him to an oncologist in the case of primary care physician visits.

In the study, the SPs were first trained to adhere to role with a model transcript full of biological data. Then they made unannounced visits to consenting physicians. For the visits, the SPs carried 2 digital recorders that fit into their pockets in order to record the visit surreptitiously. The SPs turned on the audio recorders in their cars before they approached the physicians' offices to avoid detection. To prepare the physician-patient interaction during each visit, the SP was given a complete script detailing with the clinical and personal history responses to potential physician questions or actions. Prior to each visit, the physician received a complete medical record with purpose of making the SPs' diagnosis and stage of cancer believable. The audio recordings were reviewed by the study organizers and the SPs were debriefed weekly to optimize their role fidelity. In a follow-up study, Shields et al. [28] reported that the SPs adhered to their roles with 94 % accuracy based on a 1–5 Liker-type rating scale, and were detected in only 14 % of the visits, a level found in similar studies (e.g., [29]).

2.2   Data Description

With the study, two types of data were obtained. The first type of data contains variables known as influential factors to the effectiveness of patient-centered communication effectiveness and visit satisfaction. The second type of data contains variables detailing patient and physician behaviors and interactions during shared decision-making. The final data set contained 35 records, which involves 18 primary care physicians and 17 oncologists, due to physician withdrawal and departure, as well as recording incompleteness. In other words, these 35 records used in analysis have complete information for the aforementioned two data types.

Description of Data Set 1. Data set 1 contains 13 predictive variables related to patient-centered communication. The majority of them fall into four categories of eliciting/validating patient concerns (1 variable), voice tone (3 variables), physician use of certainty language (1 variable), and assessment of prognosis communication (2 variables). Other variables include total interaction time, patient's word count, as well as physician's gender, age and occupation. Table 1 lists the descriptive statistics about these predictive variables. All variables were standardized to the range of 0 to 1.

Table 1. Descriptive statistics of data set 1 (n = 35)

Category	Variable name	Characteristic	Oncologist (n = 17)			Family physician (n = 18)		
			Mean	SD	Range	Mean	SD	Range
Eliciting/validating patient concerns	elicit_val	Average score of 19 items of 1–5 scale	1.074	0.672	0.167–2.333	1.486	0.626	0.75–2.667
Voice tone	attentive	Average scores among four raters using 1–7 scale	4	0.848	2.75-5.5	3.917	0.752	3–5
	anxious		2.941	1.088	2–5	2.722	0.669	1–4
	Hostile		2.235	0.903	1–5	2	0.767	1–4
Physician use of certainty in lang.	P_WC	Integer word count	1452	982	486–4249	1612	578	669–2764
	youdying	Binary indictor	0.588	0.507	{0,1}	0.222	0.428	{0,1}
Assessing prognosis communication	prog_sum	Aggregate score of items of 1–5 scale	12.41	6.89	3–27	8.56	6.32	2–23
	prog_freq	Integer	4.471	2.154	1–9	3.278	2.218	1–8
	D_WC	Integer word count	2044	1124	4595–5290	2030	1178	728–5394
Miscellaneous	totaltime	Integer (in mins)	29.28	12.88	14.5–56	31.15	13.57	15–72.5
	age	Integer	47.06	7.56	35–68	48.5	10.30	31–72
	male	Binary indicator	0.706	0.47	{0,1}	1	0	{0,1}

Eliciting/Validating Patient Concerns. Nineteen items were used to measure eliciting/validating patient concerns. These items implies whether physicians conducted preliminary information elicitation, further exploration, and validation to discussion topics such as mood/depression, family support, disease's impact on life, previous physicians, and scans done since diagnosis. Each item was quantified with a 1–5 scale and the average scores were reported.

Voice Tone. Three measures were used to characterize physician's voice tone. They are anxious/attentive/hostile tones. A number of independent raters listened to the audio recordings and coded for the voice tone using a 1–7 scale. For example, to measure attentiveness voice tone, each physician was rated on four separate items: warmth, concern, worry, and openness. The average was then taken.

Physician Use of Certainty in the Language. The amount and percentage of certainty words said by physicians in an encounter with SPs were tallied. These certainty words include absolute, certain, clear, complete, confident, definite, and sure. Individuals who used more certainty-conveying words seek causal understandings [30], an important task for physician making diagnoses. However, because those who have a need for certainty tend to be less tolerant of ambiguity, they may curtail data gathering and engage in premature closure [31]. In addition, an indicator was recorded on whether the physician used phrases to strongly indicate the mortality possibility to SPs.

In addition, we included 1 variable measuring the total physician-patient interaction time (in minutes), 1 variable measuring patient engagement by counting the words he/she spoke during the interaction (integer), 3 variables indicating the physician's age (integer), gender (1 being Male and 0 being Female), and occupation (1 being an oncologist and 0 being a family physician).

Description of Data Set 2. Shields et al. [24] analyzed 40 complete recordings to assess the reliability and validity of the MIDM, which was developed to code behaviors associated with decision-making and the relationship between physician behaviors and patient behaviors. The patient-physician interactions were first categorized into 12 discussion topics, including Appointment, Depression, Family, Counseling, Medical Issue, Medications, Pain Management, Referral, Scanning Tests, Other Tests, and Treatment. Within each topic, physician behavior information was further coded based on the manual of MIDM [32]. The 10 possible codes include Cut-Off (i.e., Cut-Off – MD interrupts or blocks PT's further expression or statement; could cause the MD to change the subject), Init (i.e., Initiate – MD makes a suggestion/recommendation to the patient first; to first bring up the topic), DG PT (i.e., Disagree with Patient – MD has different views, emotions, and/or opinions about a given plan/action), AG PT (i.e., Agree with Patient – MD has similar views, emotions, and/or opinions about a given plan/action), Rec (i.e., Recommendation – MD recommends, proposes, or suggests an action of any kind on the patient's behalf; MD gives advice to PT about treatment, medication, and plans for the next appointment), Opt (i.e., Gives Options – MD lists treatment or medication options for the patient; just stating the options is enough to be coded, even without a response from the patient), Val (i.e., Validation – MD makes an empathic response to PT's expression or statement; acknowledges the patient's expression in an empathic way), Risks (i.e., Risks – MD explains or tells PT about risks or possible side effects), Expl (i.e., Explanation – MD provides the PT information about a treatment plan or medication), and Ask FB (i.e., Feedback – MD gets the patient's thoughts on treatment and planning and encourages patient involvement).

Patient behavior information was also further coded. The possible codes include Go-Along (i.e., Go-Along – Patient does not provide a verbal agreement or disagreement when MD makes a recommendation; this does not necessarily mean patient agrees), Init (i.e., Initiate – Patient brings up a topic to MD first, examples in the transcript are PT usually initiates family member involvement), Intr MD (i.e., Interrupts MD – Patient tries to speak while the doctor is talking), DG Plan (i.e., Disagree with Plan MD suggests – Patient has different views, emotions, and/or opinions about a given plan/action), AG Plan (i.e., Agree with Plan MD suggests – Patient has different views, emotions, and/or opinions about a given plan/action), Give Info (i.e., Gives Information – this usually occurs when MD is talking about a recommendation or asking for feedback and PT is giving information to MD; PT may also tend to give information to PT when they bring up a new topic or ask for clarification), A/R (i.e., Ask/Request – this usually occurs in response to a suggestion/recommendation that MD makes), A/C (i.e., Ask/Clarification – Patient asks MD for more information because s/he does not fully understand what is being said when asking a question).

Such detailed behavioral information was quite unstructured if being handled directly. We thus further transformed the coded information to form a data matrix. First, we ignored the patient's behaviors due to the fact that they were SPs and thus should be relatively similar between physicians. Then, for each topic, we recorded 1 if one physician's behavior appeared when discussing the topic and 0 otherwise.

Moreover, for each topic, we recorded the total number of physician and patient exchanges about the topic throughout the session. Next we recorded the order by which each topic appeared during the session. The resultant data matrix is of 120 columns. Similar to preprocessing the data of the first type, we standardized variables that are not valued between 0 and 1.

2.3   Clustering Analysis

We applied hierarchical clustering to partition physician prognosis communication patterns based on data set 1 and applied frequent itemset hierarchical clustering to partition their shared decision-making interactions based on data set 2. We then compared the two clustering assignments to identify associations between patient-centered communication measures and shared decision-making behaviors.

Clustering Analysis on Data Set 1. We viewed the data in data set 1 as generic data because the variables are general performance measures/indices. We applied hierarchical clustering to find the natural clusters among all the 35 physicians. Hierarchical clustering [33] and k-means are two well-known methods to perform clustering on data of generic data type. In addition, distribution-based clustering methods such as the EM method [34] are applicable.

Hierarchical clustering is a widely used clustering analysis method which seeks to build a hierarchy of clusters. There are two types of hierarchical clustering approaches: agglomerative and divisive. Agglomerative hierarchical clustering takes a bottom-up approach, i.e., each observation is in its own cluster at the beginning, and pairs of clusters are merged recursively according to the dissimilarity between the two clusters. Divisive hierarchical clustering take a top-down approach, i.e., all observations start with a single cluster, and splits are performed repeatedly based on the similarity between the subsets of observations. We chose hierarchical clustering over other plausible methods for the following reasons. First, our sample size is relatively small, so we do not have to pay much attention to the algorithm efficiency. Second, the shape of the clusters may not be globular so it is appealing to use single links for hierarchical clustering. Third, hierarchical clustering can perform much better than k-means in handling clusters of differing sizes and densities. Fourth, hierarchical clustering does not make any assumption on distribution of the observations. Finally, hierarchical clustering is more interpretable and visualizable with the hierarchy, which may be beneficial to explaining the results.

In our study, we regarded each physician record as a point in the Euclidean space of 13 dimensions. When computing the distance between clusters, we used single link ($\min\{d(a,b): a \varepsilon A; b \varepsilon B\}$) as the distance of the pair of clusters avoid the problem of derived clusters being non globular.

Clustering Analysis of Data Set 2. We regarded the codes (a hierarchy containing topics and behaviors within each topic) in data set 2 as words shown in the documents/texts. The value of each feature indicates whether the corresponding topic/behavior combination appears in the sample patient-physician interaction. In addition, there are many zeros in the data matrix, and we are more interested in whether a pair of samples both have ones in a feature as opposed to both having zeros. Thus, data set 2 has a pattern that is commonly detected in data of text type.

With more than 100 features but only 35 samples, we dealt with a clustering problem with high dimensionality. By simple observation, we concluded some features were not indicative as the corresponding topics were either talked by nearly all physicians or none. We thus applied Term Frequency Inverse Document Frequency (TF-IDF) index [35] to quantify the importance of each feature and prune those unimportant features. We then applied Frequent Itemset Hierarchical Clustering (FIHC) [36] to perform the clustering for data set 2. FIHC defines globally frequent itemsets to do future feature selection, which implies that only features that frequently appear together are used in the clustering. The feature selection process improves the accuracy of clustering and thus enhances the efficiency of the algorithm. With the clustering results obtained, we identified what common features led to a set of physicians grouped together. The definition of cluster frequent items solved the problem satisfactorily and gave us meaningful cluster descriptions. FIHC is sensitive to the setting of global minimum support, so in our study we performed parameter tuning, i.e., finding a relatively wide range of global minimum support in which the number and collection of clusters is nearly invariant. We used normalized mutual information to calculate the similarity between clustering results of different global minimum supports and finally found a stable clustering result. We coded the FIHC algorithm using MATLAB in our actual implementation.

2.4   Preparation of a Fair Comparison Between the Two Clusterings

In order to make a fair comparison between the two clustering results based on the two data sets, we used a normalized mutual information index [37] to make further specifications on the two clustering analyses to ensure relative stability in the derived clustering assignments. The use of this index is both for determining the global support value for the FIHC used in the second clustering analysis and assessing the association between the two clustering results.

We introduce the normalized mutual information index between two clusterings, namely C and C'. First we define $P(i) = \frac{|C_i|}{n}$ and $P(i,j) = \frac{|C_i \cap C'_j|}{n}$, where clusters $C_i \in C$, $C'_j \in C'$, and n is the total number of records. We further denote K and L to be the number of clusters in respective clusterings C and C'. The entropy associated with one clustering is defined as $H(C) = -\sum_{i=1}^{K} P(i) \cdot \log_2 P(i)$, which is a measure for the uncertainty about the cluster of a randomly picked element. Similarly, we can define $H(C')$ with the specification of L. The mutual information measure between the two clusterings is thus defined as $I(C, C') = \sum_{i=1}^{K} \sum_{j=1}^{L} P(i,j) \cdot \log_2 \frac{P(i,j)}{P(i)P(j)}$, which describes how much we can reduce the uncertainty about the cluster of a random element when knowing its cluster in another clustering of the same set of elements. Using the above two definitions, we can quantify the normalized mutual information as $NMI(C, C') = \frac{I(C,C')}{\sqrt{H(C)H(C')}}$.

We believe that the normalized mutual information index has several advantages over those measures that are based on counting pairs (e.g., Chi Squared Coefficient, Rand Index, Fowlkes-Mallows Index, etc.) or on set overlaps (e.g., F-measure, Maximum-Match-Measure, Van Dongen-Measure, etc.). First, it does not rely on strong assumption such as independence of the clustering. Second, it can handle clustering results with different numbers of clusters. Third, alternative methods based on counting overlaps tend to ignore the unmatched parts of the clusters, which is unreasonable. Fourth, the result is not affected by swapping the positions of any pair of clusters. We coded the comparison algorithm using MATLAB in our actual implementation.

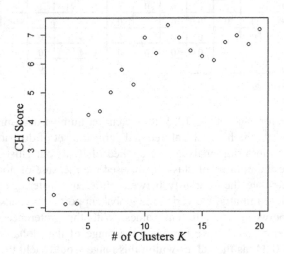

Fig. 1. CH Score vs. the number of clusters (K)

3 Results and Discussion

For data set 1, we applied hierarchical clustering to generate a hierarchical tree. We then used the CH index [38] to determine the most appropriate number of clusters, which yielded the largest CH score. We provide more specifications on the CH index in the following. Ideally, we'd like to generate clusterings that simultaneously have a small Between-cluster Variation (B) and a small Within-cluster Variation (W). This is the idea between the CH index. For clusterings coming from K clusters, we record its CH score to be $CH(K) = \frac{B(K)/(K-1)}{W(K)/(n-K)}$. To choose K, one would just pick some maximum number of clusters to be considered K_{max}, and choose the value of K with the largest score CH(K) between 0 and K_{max}. In our implementation, we used the HCLUSTER function in R with method = single and CLUES package with disMethod = Euclidean to calculate the CH score. See Fig. 1 for the CH(K) results. We concluded that the most appropriate

Table 2. Determine an appropriate global support value in FIHC

Global support value (× 100)	21	22	23	24	25	26	27	28	29	30	31	32	33	34
21	1	1	0	0	0	1	0	1	0	0	0	0	0	0
22	1	1	0	0	0	1	0	1	0	0	0	0	0	0
23	0	0	1	1	1	0	0	1	0	0	0	0	0	0
24	0	0	1	1	1	0	0	1	0	0	0	0	0	0
25	0	0	1	1	1	1	1	1	0	0	0	0	0	0
26	1	1	0	0	1	1	0	1	0	0	0	0	0	0
27	0	0	0	0	1	0	1	1	0	0	0	0	0	0
28	1	1	1	1	1	1	1	1	0	0	0	0	0	0
29	0	0	0	0	0	0	0	0	1	1	1	0	0	0
30	0	0	0	0	0	0	0	0	1	1	1	0	0	0
31	0	0	0	0	0	0	0	0	1	1	1	0	0	0
32	0	0	0	0	0	0	0	0	0	0	0	1	1	0
33	0	0	0	0	0	0	0	0	0	0	0	1	1	0
34	0	0	0	0	0	0	0	0	0	0	0	0	0	1

number of clusters for data set 1 is 12. With the cluster number determined, we chose a cut-off line to truncate the hierarchical tree and derived a set of decision rules.

For the second clustering analysis, we applied FIHC as our clustering method. In order to determine the number of clusters, we used the measure of normalized mutual information to calculate the similarity between different clusterings with the global support value varied. Initially, we varied the global support value between 0.1 and 0.4 with 0.03 apart between two adjacent values. With the preference that the cluster number is between 5 and 15, we narrowed the range of the global support value to between 0.21 and 0.34, as the values within this range would yield the cluster number to be between 5 and 15. Subsequently, we checked the 14 possible global support values with 0.01 apart within the range. For each pair of the 14 values, we performed the calculation of the normalized mutual information index to assess the association between them. See Table 2 for the comparison results. In each cell of the table, a labeling of 1 implies that the pair of the global support values would yield strong association between the two clusterings (with the normalized mutual information index greater than 0.8); and 0 otherwise. From the table, we found that when the global support value is between 0.21 and 0.28, the clusterings were similar to each other (or say stable). Note that most of the ones appear in the corresponding 8 by 8 submatrix (i.e., shared area consisting of the first 8 rows and 8 columns). We thus set the global support value to be 0.25 as the center of the stable area, and obtained 12 clusters for data set 2 with the use of the FIHC algorithm. Note that we obtained 12 clusters with both data sets.

Table 3 reports the clusterings for the two data sets. Coincidentally, the cardinality values for both clusterings are 12. When first looking at the two clusterings, we could only find a few cases where a pair of physicians being grouped together in both clusterings but could not find any agreement on a trio of physicians being grouped together in both assignments. For example, there are 3 one-element clusters in the clustering based on data set 1 whereas there are 6 such clusters based on data set 2. However, only 2 of such clusters are identical between the two clusterings. For clusters with more than 1 element, there is no identical cluster that appears in both clusterings. Additionally, some elements appear in clusters with few elements based on data set 1 whereas they appear in clusters with many elements based on data set 2; e.g., element no. 7 is in a cluster by itself with the clustering based on data set 1; it is contained in a large cluster with the clustering based on data set 2.

Given the ambiguous nature in directly comparing the two clusterings, we thus next calculated normalized mutual information index to quantify the association between the two clusterings. The index is valued 0.478, which shows modest association between the two clusterings. Our association assessment suggests some association between the measures/indices in the two categories: patient-centered communication and shared decision-making. However, we are unable to judge the stability of the association given the current size of the data sets and coding schemes. Furthermore, because we can barely find similar clusters in both assignments, we thereby conjectured that a physician's detailed behaviors in shared decision-making may not be well aligned with his/her communication effectiveness.

Table 3. Clustering comparison for data sets 1 and 2

Data set 1		Data set 2	
Cluster no.	Physician no.	Cluster no.	Physician no.
1	**11**	1	**11**
2	**28**	2	**28**
3	**7**	3	**7**, 2,6,13,21,22,24,32,34,35
4	**10**,32	4	**10**,3,15,19,29
5	**5**,2,23	5	**5**
6	**14**,21,29	7	**14**,9,12,18,25,31
7	**16**,8,3	6	**16**,17,20,23
8	17,24,35	8	4,8
9	1,13,15,25	9	**1**
10	**27**,12,9,33	10	**27**,26
11	**30**,20,22,34	11	**30**
12	4,6,18,19,26,31	12	33

4 Conclusions and Future Research

Using a rigorous study design that controlled for patient-to-patient differences in prognosis discussion, we examined the association between physician behaviors in a shared medical decision-making process and physician measures on patient-centered communication. Faced with the challenges that the coded behavior data is sequence data of high-dimensionality with unequal dimensions among subjects, we applied frequent itemset hierarchical clustering. Our analysis suggested that the physician behavior data set (i.e., data set 2) likely contains different features that influence the prognosis discussion effectiveness and patient visit satisfaction from the physician prognosis communication data set (i.e., data set 1). Even though it becomes increasingly convenient to analyze the natural language appearing in shared decision-making, it may still be challenging to achieve better discussion effectiveness and satisfaction by standardizing physician's behavior in shared decision-making. Reversely, our analysis also suggested that the differences in physician's communication style may not be easily taken into consideration when optimizing his/her shared decision-making process. Note that the shared decision-making process could significantly be diversified in real settings as we only used standard patients in our study.

While it is our ultimate goal to operationalize the shared decision making process by real-time controlling the discussion process, it may be more difficult than our initial thought because it remains largely unclear how the different patterns in physician's behaviors in shared decision-making interact with the different patterns in physician's communication styles (i.e., voice tones, certainty in language use, etc.). In our future study, we hope to conduct a similar association assessment study based on a larger-scale human subject study and perhaps on a different kind of medical encounter. For example, we will consider the data set of more than 100 recordings collected by co-author Shields in the past few years on pain management discussions. In addition, we plan to conduct a more thorough investigation on different coding schemes of the shared decision-making interaction sequences. Finally, we plan to conduct a supervised learning study as we have recently obtained outcome data on patient visit satisfaction, with the hypothesis that carefully coded behavior data can improve the prediction of the visit satisfaction outcomes as opposed to using patient-centered communication measures alone.

References

1. Rhoades, D.R., McFarland, K.F., Finch, W.H., Johnson, A.O.: Speaking and interruptions during primary care office visits. Fam. Med. **33**(7), 528–532 (2001)
2. Zapka, J.G., Carter, R., Carter, C.L., Hennessy, W., Kurent, J.E., Desharnais, S.: Care at the end of life: focus on communication and race. J. Aging Health **18**, 791–813 (2006)
3. Baile, W.R., Buckman, R., Lenzi, R., Glober, G., Beale, E.A., Kudelka, A.P.: SPIKES – a six-step protocol for delivering bad news: application to the patients with cancer. Oncologist **5**(4), 302–311 (2000)
4. Clayton, J.M., Hancock, K.M., Butow, P.N., Tattersall, M.H.N., Currow, D.C.: Clinical practice guidelines for communicating prognosis and end-of-life issues with adults in the advanced stages of a life-limiting illness, and their caregivers. Med. J. Aust. **186**(12 Suppl), S77–S108 (2007)
5. Hagerty, R.G., Butow, P.N., Ellis, P.M., Lobb, E.A., Pendlebury, S.C., Leighl, N., MacLeod, C., Tattersal, M.H.N.: Communicating with realism and hope: incurable cancer patients' views on the disclosure of prognosis. J. Clin. Oncol. **23**(6), 1278–1288 (2005)
6. Guadagnoli, E., Ward, P.: Patient participation in decision-making. Soc. Sci. Med. **47**(3), 329–339 (1998)

7. Brock, D.W.: The ideal of shared decision making between physicians and patients. Kennedy Inst. Ethics J. **1**(1), 28–47 (1991)

8. Gattellari, M., Butow, P.N., Tattersall, M.H.: Sharing decisions in cancer care. Soc. Sci. Med. **52**(12), 1865–1878 (2001)

9. Upshur, C.C., Bacigalupe, G., Luckmann, R.: "They don't want anything to do with you": patient views of primary care management of chronic pain. Pain Med. **11**, 1791–1798 (2010)

10. Wilson, S.R., Strub, P., Buist, A.S., Knowles, S.B., Lavori, P.W., Lapidus, J., Vollmer, W.M.: Better outcomes of asthma treatment (BOAT) study group: shared treatment decision making improves adherence and outcomes in poorly controlled asthma. Am. J. Respir. Crit. Care Med. **181**(6), 566–577 (2010)

11. Steinmetz, D., Walsh, M., Gabel, L.L., Williams, P.T.: Family physicians' involvement with dying patients and their families. attitudes, difficulties, and strategies. Arch. Fam. Med. **2**, 753–760 (1993)

12. Cassileth, B.R., Zupkis, R.V., Sutton-Smith, K., March, V.: Information and participation preferences among cancer patients. Ann. Intern. Med. **92**(6), 832–836 (1980)

13. Jenkins, V., Fallowfield, L., Saul, J.: Information needs of patients with cancer: results from a large study in UK cancer centers. Br. J. Cancer **84**(1), 48–51 (2001)

14. Mitchell, J.L.: Cross-cultural issues in the disclosure of cancer. Cancer Pract. **6**(3), 153–160 (1998)

15. Donabedian, A.: Aspects of Medical Care Administration: Specifying Requirements for Health Care. Harvard University Press, Cambridge (1973)

16. Epstein, R.M., Frank, P., Fiscella, K.M., Shields, C.G., Meldrum, S.C., Kravitz, R.L., Duberstein, P.R.: Measuring patient-centered communication in patient-physician consultations: theoretical and practical issues. Soc. Sci. Med. **61**, 1516–1528 (2005)

17. Fiscella, K.M., Meldrum, S.M., Franks, P.M., Shields, C.G., Duberstein, P.P., McDaniel, S.H., Epstein, R.M.: Patient trust: is it related to patient-centered behavior of primary care physicians? Med. Care **42**, 1049–1055 (2004)

18. Shields, C.G., Coker, C.J., Poulsen, S.S., Doyle, J.M., Fiscella, K., Epstein, R.M., Griggs, J. J.: Patient-centered communication and prognosis discussions with cancer patients. Patient Educ. Couns. **77**, 437–442 (2009)

19. Fang, S., Shi, W., Shields, C.G., Kong, N.: A preliminary variable selection based regression analysis for predicting patient satisfaction on physician-patient cancer prognosis communication. In: Zheng, X., Zeng, D., Chen, H., Zhang, Y., Xing, C., Neill, D.B. (eds.) ICSH 2014. LNCS, vol. 8549, pp. 171–180. Springer, Heidelberg (2014)

20. Elwyn, G., Hutchings, H., Edwards, A., Rapport, F., Wensing, M., Cheung, W.Y., Grol, R.: The OPTION scale: measuring the extent that clinicians involve patients in decision-making tasks. Health Expect. **8**(1), 34–42 (2005)

21. Sainfort, F., Booske, B.C.: Measuring post-decision satisfaction. Med. Decis. Making **20**(1), 51–61 (2000)

22. Scholl, I., Koelewijn-van Loon, M., Sepucha, K., Elwyn, G., Légaré, F., Härter, M., Dirmaier, J.: Measurement of shared decision-making – a review of instruments. Z Evid Fortbild Qual Gesundhwes **105**(4), 313–324 (2011)

23. Kasper, J., Légaré, F., Scheibler, F., Geiger, F.: Turning signals into meaning – 'shared decision making' meets communication theory. Health Expect. **15**(1), 3–11 (2012)

24. Shields, C.G., Newman, L., Elias, C.: Interactions between Physicians and Patients during Decision-Making: Assessed with the Medical Interaction Decision-Making Coding System. Working Paper (2015)

25. Tamblyn, R., Berkson, L., Dauphinee, W.D., Gayton, D., Grad, R., Huang, A., Isaac, L., McLeod, P., Snell, L.: Unnecessary prescribing of NSAIDs and the management of NSAID-related gastropathy in medical practice. Ann. Intern. Med. **127**(6), 429–438 (1997)

26. Kravitz, R.L., Epstein, R.M., Feldman, M.D., Franz, C.E., Azari, R., Wilkes, M.S., Hinton, L., Franks, P.: Influence of patients' requests for direct-to-consumer advertised antidepressants: a randomized controlled trial. J. Am. Med. Assoc. **293**(16), 1995–2002 (2005)

27. Peabody, J.W., Luck, J., Glassman, P., Dresselhaus, T.R., Lee, M.: Comparison of vignettes, standardized patients, and chart abstraction a prospective validation study of 3 methods for measuring quality. J. Am. Med. Assoc. **283**(13), 1715–1722 (2000)

28. Shields, C.G., Finley, M.A., Elias, C.M., Coker, C.J., Griggs, J.J., Fiscella, K., Epstein, R. M.: Pain assessment: the roles of physician certainty and curiosity. Health Commun. **28**(7), 740–746 (2013)

29. Franz, C.E., Epstein, R., Miller, K.N., Brown, A., Song, J., Feldman, M., Kelly-Reif, S., Kravitz, R.L.: Caught in the act? Prevalence, predictors, and consequences of physician detection of unannounced standardized patients. Health Serv. Res. **41**(6), 2290–2302 (2006)

30. Pennebaker, J.W., Chung, C.K., Ireland, M., Gonzales, A., Booth, R.J.: Operator's manual: Linguistic Inquiry and Word Count: LIWC 2007 (2007). homepage.psy.utexas.edu/homepage/faculty/pennebaker/reprints/

31. Pennebaker, J.W., King, L.A.: Linguistic styles: language use as an individual difference. J. Pers. Soc. Psychol. **77**(6), 1296–1312 (2007)

32. Newman, L., Elias, C., Shields, C.G.: MIDM – Medical Interactive Decision Making. Internal Reference (2015)

33. Rokach, L., Maimon, O.: Clustering Methods. Data Mining and Knowledge Discovery Handbook, pp. 321–352. Springer, New York (2005)

34. Dempster, A.P., Laird, N.M., Rubin, D.B.: Maximum likelihood from incomplete data via the EM algorithm. J. Roy. Stat. Soc. B **39**(1), 1–38 (1977)

35. Salton, G., Buckley, C.: Term-weighting approaches in automatic text retrieval. Inf. Process. Manage. **24**(5), 513–523 (1998)

36. Fung, B.C.M., Wang, K., Ester, M.: Hierarchical document clustering using frequent itemsets. SIAM **3**, 59–70 (2003)

37. Estévez, P., Tesmer, M., Perez, C., et al.: Normalized mutual information feature selection. IEEE Trans. Neural Networks **20**(2), 189–201 (2009)

38. Calinski, T., Harabasz, J.: A dentrite method for cluster analysis. Commun. Stat. **3**(1), 1–27 (1974)

Need for a Specialized Metamodel for Biomedical and Health Informatics Domain

Rishi Kanth Saripalle[(✉)]

School of Information Technology, Illinois State University, Normal, IL 61790, USA
rishi.saripalle@ilstu.edu

Abstract. The history of computing has taught the software community significant lessons and few of them in a hard way. After spending numerous resources, the community has realized the need for establishing standards or specification for efficiently handling interoperability issues across diverse applications and tools. For example, UML for model driven development, and XML for information exchange. The domain of biomedical informatics is traversing through a similar path where numerous resources are employed for achieving interoperability among heterogeneous biomedical applications. To mitigate this issue and learning from previous experiences, the biomedical domain has to establish a modeling standard for design and development of its software applications and tools. Towards this goal, this research article proposes a minimal metamodel for the domain of biomedical and health informatics based on MOF and UMLS Semantic Network.

Keywords: UML UMLS · MOF UMLS · Biomedical modeling · UMLS metamodel · Biomedical metamodel · MOF biomedical metamodel

1 Introduction

The domain of computing has very rich history with great achievements, major setbacks which further fueled its success and, importantly, lessons to learn from its history. However, few of these lessons are learned in a very hard way – interoperability issues. To overcome this issue, the software community has defined standards, allowing the domain experts to design diverse applications based on these agreed standards and in turn easing interoperability issues. For example, Unified Modeling Language (UML) [1], a defacto standard for object-oriented (OO) modeling was defined to unify diverse OO methodologies, standards, and languages. Further, experts defined Meta Object Facility (MOF) [2], a standard meta-meta model that allows experts to instantiate MOF to build OO based metamodels such as UML. The role of a metamodel is to define the semantics for how elements in a metamodel get instantiated. In the modeling hierarchy, MOF is at the top and is exploited to define OO metamodels such as UML, i.e. UML is an instance of MOF. The UML is instantiated to define domain model, which in turn are used to capture domain data. We will utilize MOF for your research objective. Another lesson learnt similar to UML can be found in design and development of XML. In terms of utilization of UML and XML, most prominent standards such as HL7 Clinical Document Architecture [3], and

© Springer International Publishing Switzerland 2016
X. Zheng et al. (Eds.): ICSH 2015, LNCS 9545, pp. 99–104, 2016.
DOI: 10.1007/978-3-319-29175-8_9

Continuity Care Document [4] are represented using XML and HL7 Reference Information Model [3] is represented using UML. This shows the influence and dominance of these standards in the biomedical domain and importance of establishing a modeling standard itself.

The biomedical and health informatics domain, will be referred as biomedical domain for the rest of the paper, is going through a similar problem – interoperability issues with diverse data across diverse applications. In order to integrate diverse data across systems, the biomedical experts have implemented standard semantic terminologies. The goal is to tag the data with standard semantics and then integrate the data. Currently, the domain has numerous semantic standards (~60) and are facing interoperability issues of their own, as a biomedical concept can be represented differently (structure, semantic, and grammar) across various standards. To overcome this issue, the National Library of Medicine has initiated Unified Medical Language System (UMLS) [5, 6], whose goal is to integrate the biomedical concepts across the disparate semantic standards. UMLS is composed of two major components: Metathesaurus (META) and Semantic Network (SN). UMLS META – holds nearly two million concepts that are linked using twelve millions relationships. It has been successfully employed in various biomedical applications such as text processing [7] and EHR applications [8] to name a few. UMLS SN – a semantic graph formed by defining semantic types (ex. Finding) and semantic relationships (ex. disrupts). The UMLS-SN captures very rich biomedical knowledge and its sole goal is to provide consistent categorization of *all* the concepts in UMLS-META. UMLS-SN also provides additional semantics *acting* as a meta-structure to the UMLS-META [6]. The biomedical experts provided a standard semantic knowledge in the form of UMLS-SN for interoperability issues across semantic standards, *but* failed to provide a standard similar to UML or XML dedicated to biomedical domain for designing interoperable software applications.

The lessons learned from history of computing, combined with evidence to ease interoperability issues by establishing a modeling standard and absence of such as standard in the biomedical domain presents a perfect opportunity to design and establish a standard biomedical metamodel. To achieve this goal, we will be exploring the idea of combining the rich knowledge captured in UMLS-SN and MOF, a meta-meta modeling standard. The yield of this combination, an OO based Biomedical and Health Informatics metamodel (BHIM) similar to UML will serve two purposes. First, expressing UMLS-SN knowledge as a metamodel using a well-established standard will expose it to other industrial/research areas dominated by metamodels and model driven development. This is evident in the knowledge representation domain, where they have identified the influence of modeling and have proposed Ontology Definition Metamodel [9] – a metamodel – an instance of MOF - but based on Resource Description Format, RDF Schema and Web Ontology Language standards. Second, the availability of a metamodel will allow expert to define diverse software applications that are interoperable as they are based on an agreed standard. The rest of the article supports the proposed research and is organized in three sections. Section 2 will briefly discuss previous research efforts. Section 3 will provide the design approach for BHIM and finally, Sect. 4 discusses the future work and concludes the article. Due to the page limitation and also as it is an ongoing research, the complete results could not be expressed in this article.

2   Previous Work

In the previous research effort [10], the author has designed and implemented a UML Profile for UMLS-SN, named UMLS-SN:UP, to capture UMLS-SN knowledge for biomedical application modeling. This work exploited UML Profile feature to convert UMLS-SN semantic concepts to metamodeling elements. The semantic types are translated into stereotypes that extend the UML Class, semantic relationships are translated into stereotypes that extend the UML Association and "isa" is translated into stereotype that extend the UML Generalization. As UML Profile is dependent on UML, the developed UMLS-SN:UP is dependent on UML. Other research works that were proposed over the years on UMLS are: focused on expanding the current UMLS-SN to include new types [11–13]; realize the UMLS-SN using OWL [14, 15]; divide UMLS-SN into manageable views [16]; converting it into OO database model [17]; validating and verifying the UMLS-SN [18], etc. But the goal of the proposed research is to establish a standalone metamodel for efficient and interoperable biomedical software modeling by using UMLS-SN knowledge and MOF.

3   Biomedical and Health Informatics Metamodel (BHIM): MOF + UMLS-SN

In this section we will discuss our approach in combining the UMLS-SN knowledge and MOF to design and develop a standard minimal metamodel for modeling biomedical applications and tools. The research will be utilizing Cohesive Partitioning technique [16], a methodology that divides the UMLS-SN into 28 semantic-type collections, where each collection has 4–5 semantic types. This methodology allows UMLS-to be more manageable and user friendly. The following procedure is followed to design the proposed metamodel.

- First, the Core metamodel is defined that will form the foundation of the BHIM. This Core metamodel contains basic metaelements that are used by other metamodels.
- Second, the Relationship metamodel is defined that captures BiomedicalAssociation entity. This metaelement captures links/associations between modeling elements and has two named ends that link them to instances of the metaelement Classifier.
- Finally, the UMLSSN metamodel translates the UMLS-SN knowledge into metaelements using the Core and Relationship metamodels as shown in Fig. 1.

The Core metamodel captures the main metaelements of our BHI metamodel as shown in Fig. 2 (top). These metaelements were identified based on the current standards and previous metamodels based on MOF from various domains. The primary metaelement is Element, an abstract structure that is generalized from three metaelements: ModelElement, Classifier and Feature. Classifier is further specialized to define abstract metaelement BiomedicalEntity – captures the essence of class (instances with similar feature or attributes or characteristics) - similar to UML Class; and DataTypes – captures data types such as string, integer, etc. The abstract metaelement Feature is specialized to define Attribute - a named entity to capture Classifier attributes. A Feature is owned (owner) by a

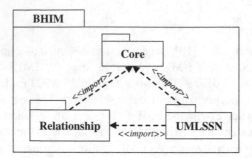

Fig. 1. A high-level architectural view of BHIM and interactions between its metamodels.

Classifier, which can have zero or more Feature, but a Feature belong to at most one Classifier. That means an attribute belongs to a Classifier or BiomedicalEntity.

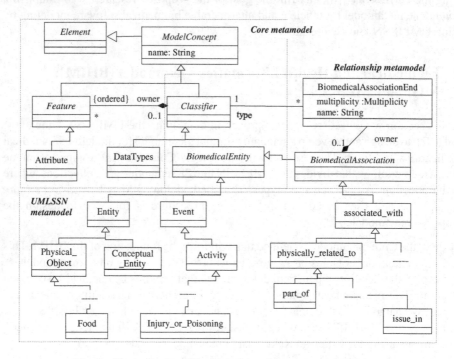

Fig. 2. Biomedical and Health Informatics metamodel (BHIM).

The Relationship metamodel as shown in Fig. 2 (right) captures metaelements that allows use to define relationships between Classifiers. The abstract metaclass BiomedicalAssociation, which needs to be specialized, defines a semantic relationship between Classifiers and must have two or more ends. The BiomedicalAssociationEnd is an endpoint of an association that connects the BiomedicalAssociation to a Classifier. They are part/owned by the BiomedicalAssociation and are responsible for associating the BiomedicalAssociation with the owned Classifier.

The UMLSSN metamodel imports Core and Relationship metamodels and extends their metaelements as shown in Fig. 2 (bottom). The UMLSSN semantic types such as Entity, Event, Physical Object, Activity, etc. extend the abstract BiomedicalEntity to form concrete metaelements i.e. can be instantiated to form domain model classes. For example, Activity metaclass – from semantic type Activity (due to space constraints, the semantic type and relationship definition and explanation cannot be included) - will capture all the domain classes that deal with operations a machine or an organism carries out. Similarly, the sematic relationships such as associated_with, part_of, issue_in, etc. extend BiomedicalAssociation to form concrete meta-associations. For example, associated_with - the semantic relationship associated_with - will capture all relationships between classes (of type BiomedicalEntity) that have significant interactions. The constraints on various metaelements in BHIM such as a BiomedicalAssociation must have at least two BiomedicalAssociationEnds or BiomedicalAssociationEnd must have a unique name within the BiomedicalAssociation, etc. are specified using Object Constraint Language (OCL). Due to space constraints, the complete Fig. 2 and the OCL constraints could not be explained in detail.

Now, the proposed BHIM is an instance of MOF (M3 – meta-meta model) and is in par with UML in the modeling hierarchy (M2 – metamodel) and is as shown in Fig. 3. The experts can use BHIM to design diverse biomedical applications (M1 – domain models) that are interoperable and these domain models can then be implemented to capture real data (M0 – domain data), similar to UML or XML.

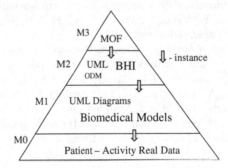

Fig. 3. Biomedical and Health Informatics metamodel (BHIM) in the modeling hierarchy.

4   Conclusion and Future Work

This paper proposes a conceptual minimal metamodel for promoting a model drive development approach for biomedical applications in order to curb interoperability issues. The proposed metamodel is developed based on the MOF and UMLS-SN, which can be used of a wide variety application and tool development. The BHIM serves three purpose: a formally defined metamodel will have a potential increase in the reuse of solutions; promotes interoperability between diverse applications; and bridges the gap between UMLS-SN and model driven development - a sound and popular approach in industry and research.

In the future work, we will investigate to add additional aspects of the biomedical domain from other knowledge sources and also, expand the current metamodel with other metaelements such as package, constraint, namespace, etc. that could not be scoped into the current research minimal metamodel. Additionally, we intend to implement tools that experts can use to design biomedical application using the proposed metamodel.

References

1. Object Management Group. OMG Unified Modeling Language (2015)
2. Object Management Group. OMG Meta Object Facility (MOF) Core Specification (2015)
3. Boone, K.W.: The CDA ™ book. Springer (2011)
4. Ferranti, J.M., Musser, R.C., Kawamoto, K., Hammond, W.E.: The clinical document architecture and the continuity of care record: a critical analysis. J. Am. Med. Inform. Assoc. **13**(3), 245–252 (2006)
5. Humphreys, B.L., Lindberg, D.A.B., Schoolman, H.M., Barnett, G.O.: The unified medical language system: an informatics research collaboration. J. Am. Med. Assoc. **5**(1), 1–11 (1996)
6. Bodenreider, O.: The unified medical language system (UMLS): integrating biomedical terminology. Nucleic Acids Res. **32**, 267–270 (2003)
7. Savova, G.K., Masanz, J.J., Ogren, P.V., Zheng, J., Sohn, S., Kipper-Schuler, K.C., et al.: Mayo clinical text analysis and knowledge extraction system (ctakes): architecture, component evaluation and applications. J. Am. Med. Inform. Assoc. **17**(5), 507–513 (2003)
8. Plaza, L., Diaz, A.: Retrieval of similar electronic health records using UMLS concept graphs. In: Hopfe, C.J., Rezgui, Y., Métais, E., Preece, A., Li, H. (eds.) NLDB 2010. LNCS, vol. 6177, pp. 296–303. Springer, Heidelberg (2010)
9. Object Management Group. Ontology Definition Metamodel (2009)
10. Saripalle, R.: UMLS semantic network as a UML metamodel for improving biomedical ontology and application modeling. J. Health Inform. Syst. Inform. **10**(2), 34–56 (2015)
11. Chen, Y., Gu, H., Perl, Y., Halper, M., Xu, J.: Expanding the extent of a UMLS semantic type via group neighborhood auditing. J. Am. Med. Inform. Assoc. **16**(5), 746–757 (2009)
12. Morrey, C.P., Perl, Y., Halper, M., Chen, L., Gu, H.H.: A chemical specialty semantic net work for the unified medical language system. J. Cheminform. **4**(1), 9 (2012)
13. Chen, Y., Gu, H., Perl, Y., Geller, J.: Overcoming an obstacle in expanding a UMLS semantic type extent. J. Biomed. Inform. **45**(1), 61–70 (2012)
14. Ozdemir, B.G., Baykal, N.: Alternative representations of unified medical language system semantic network elements in web ontology language. In: Innovations in Intelligent Sys-tems and Applications, pp. 545 – 549, IEEE (2011)
15. Kashyap, V., Borgida, A.: Representing the UMLS semantic network using OWL: (Or What's in a semantic web link?). In: Fensel, D., Sycara, K., Mylopoulos, J. (eds.) ISWC 2003. LNCS, vol. 2870, pp. 1–16. Springer-Verlag, Heidelberg (2003)
16. Zong, C., Perl, Y., Halper, M., Geller, J., Huanying, G.: Partitioning the UMLS semantic network. IEEE Trans. Inf. Technol. Biomed. **6**(2), 102–108 (2002)
17. Gu, H., Perl, Y., Geller, J., Halper, M., Liu, L., Cimino, J.J.: Representing the UMLS as an object-oriented database: modeling issues and advantages. J. Am. Med. Inform. Assoc. **7**(1), 66–80 (1999)
18. Geller, J., He, Z., Perl, Y., Morrey, C.P., Xu, J.: Rule-based support system for multiple UMLS semantic type assignments. J. Biomed. Inform. **46**(1), 97–110 (2003)

Predicting Pre-triage Waiting Time in a Maternity Emergency Room Through Data Mining

Sónia Pereira[1], Filipe Portela[1,2(✉)], Manuel F. Santos[1],
José Machado[1], and António Abelha[1]

[1] Algoritmi Centre, University of Minho, Braga, Portugal
b7004@dps.uminho.pt, {cfp,mfs}@dsi.uminho.pt,
{jmac,abelha}@di.uminho.pt
[2] ESEIG, Porto Polytechnique, Porto, Portugal

Abstract. An unsuitable patient flow as well as prolonged waiting lists in the emergency room of a maternity unit, regarding gynecology and obstetrics care, can affect the mother and child's health, leading to adverse events and consequences regarding their safety and satisfaction. Predicting the patients' waiting time in the emergency room is a means to avoid this problem. This study aims to predict the pre-triage waiting time in the emergency care of gynecology and obstetrics of Centro Materno Infantil do Norte (CMIN), the maternal and perinatal care unit of Centro Hospitalar of Oporto, situated in the north of Portugal. Data mining techniques were induced using information collected from the information systems and technologies available in CMIN. The models developed presented good results reaching accuracy and specificity values of approximately 74 % and 94 %, respectively. Additionally, the number of patients and triage professionals working in the emergency room, as well as some temporal variables were identified as direct enhancers to the pre-triage waiting time. The implementation of the attained knowledge in the decision support system and business intelligence platform, deployed in CMIN, leads to the optimization of the patient flow through the emergency room and improving the quality of services.

Keywords: Data mining · Classification algorithms · Gynecology and obstetrics care · Maternity care · Emergency room · Triage system · Interoperability · IDSS

1 Introduction

Crowding and prolonged waiting times in the emergency department (ED) of a hospital unit has been considered a major problem. This problem can possibly lead to adverse events and consequences towards the patient safety as well as the quality of services [1, 2]. Addressing these concerns and therefore, optimizing patient flow through the ED can be enhanced by providing improved services such as adequate staffing, destination management and hospital bed access [2, 3]. A new approach to increase patient satisfaction in the emergency room is to estimate the waiting time [4]. The prediction of waiting times helps staff to prioritize patients and operations, as well as avoiding patients leaving the ED

© Springer International Publishing Switzerland 2016
X. Zheng et al. (Eds.): ICSH 2015, LNCS 9545, pp. 105–117, 2016.
DOI: 10.1007/978-3-319-29175-8_10

unanswered [5, 6]. Furthermore, it may improve morale and reduce the patient tendency to seek further opinions, as well as minimize the complaints and litigation [7]. Regarding maternity services, delivering the best emergency care is fundamental since it has the potential to affect the mother and child's health at a crucial time. These good practices can be achieved by taking advantage of the information technologies currently available in the healthcare sector, capable of providing complete and reliable information aiding clinical and administrative decisions [8].

The emergency care of gynecology and obstetrics (GO) of Centro Materno Infantil do Norte (CMIN), the maternal and perinatal care unit of Centro Hospitalar of Oporto (CHP), owns a pre-triage system for sorting patients in emergency (URG) and consultation (ARGO) classes. The system was developed in CHP and it is a part of the Intelligent Decision Support System (IDSS) implemented in CMIN [9]. In order to improve the ED quality services by reducing crowding and upgrading the resource management, the current study induces data mining (DM) techniques using real data available in CMIN to predict the patients' waiting time at pre-triage - the time elapsed since the patient arrives to ED until she is called to go to the triage room. The required information is provided by the systems used in CMIN to collect medical data. Nursing System (SAPE) is a decision support system that allows producing and storing clinical information. In addition, the Electronic Health Record (EHR) records the patient data and their admission form. By combining the information collect by these systems in several scenarios and inducing data mining (DM) algorithms, the case study managed to achieve useful knowledge to support the CMIN's emergency care services. The best DM achieved results demonstrate the reliability of the variables provided by the information systems, reaching accuracy and specificity values of approximately 74 % and 94 %, respectively.

This article includes five sections in addition to the introduction. The second section presents the context and related work. The study materials and methods are described in section three. Section four states the data mining process following the Cross Industry Standard Process for Data Mining (CRISP-DM) phases. Formerly, section five contains a discussion about the obtained results, while the last section includes a set of considerations as well as possible directions for future work.

2   Background and Related Work

2.1   Context

The quality of care and patient's safety are the primary focus in clinical environments. Moreover, the patient's satisfaction is also an important outcome [10]. GO triage are trouble with reports of low satisfaction and long length of waiting times, making healthcare providers struggle with time management and budgetary constraints [11].

CMIN, as one of the four constituent hospitals of CHP, is prepared to provide neonatology, obstetrics and gynecology services and accompany the women and child conditions since the early pregnancy until the first stages of child growth. Its triage room provides outpatient care for women who require evaluation of labor, assessment of fetal wellbeing and acute obstetric issues. Studying the clinical and environmental information available at the patient's arrival and identifying its relation with the waiting times can be crucial to improve the unit services and therefore the patient's quality care and satisfaction.

2.2 Pre-triage System for Gynecology and Obstetrics Care in CMIN

In a hospital environment a vast number of triage systems are used. The most common are those with five levels of severity such as the Emergency Severity Index (ESI), the Manchester Triage System (MTS) and the Canadian Triage Acuity Scale (CTAS) [9]. These systems are limited as tools to use in Maternity Care due to their lack of flexibility. Since they were meant to be used in general emergency units, their guidelines do not have an appropriative degree of generalization to GO services [12].

Accordingly, CMIN healthcare professionals and Information System researchers developed a pre-triage system specific for GO, where the queries are focused on the particular type of patients that attend these services, i.e. pregnant women. This system is implemented in CMIN since 2010, and classifies patients according to the severity of their clinical condition, establishing clinical priorities and not diagnosis [13]. The system is inserted in the Intelligent Decision Support System (IDSS) and provides the triage result based on a set of predefined questions in the form of rules of a decision tree. The IDSS is an interactive and adaptable system, which uses artificial intelligence techniques and decision models to analyze a vast amount of variables to answer a question. The presence of the IDSS offers a better understanding of the patient's real state. In opposition to the MTS, triage is done by physicians and nurses [14].

Regarding the procedure, when a patient is admitted in the GO emergency room needing urgent care (i.e. women who arrive by ambulance or present serious conditions) she is immediately assisted, without any triage. In the remaining cases, the patients have to wait to be called to the triage room. Women in need of urgent care are classified as URG, while non-urgent cases are sent to consultation (ARGO). After the triage moment, the patients return to the waiting room where they remain until being called to the respective care [13, 15]. This study focus on the prediction of the patient's waiting time before the triage, i.e., when the patient is waiting to be called to the triage room.

2.3 Integration, Archive and Diffusion of Medical Information

As mentioned in the previous section, the current study depends of the combination of the information provided by the information systems implemented in the healthcare institution. The SAPE resulted from the Information Systems in Nursing. It records clinical episodes associated with each patient as an alternative to the traditional way of information on paper [16]. EHR stores and retrieves detailed patient information, as the admission form, helping monitoring, improving and reporting data on health care quality and safety [17]. These heterogeneous systems are only able to provide the information needed since they are connected by the Agency for Integration, Archive and Diffusion of Medical Information (AIDA), which allows the interoperability of the hospital existing systems [15]. AIDA is a platform based on the use of pro-active agents, being responsible for tasks such as communication with systems, sending and receiving information and responding to requests of information. This multi-agent system enables the standardization of clinical systems and overcomes the medical and administrative complexity of the different sources of information from the hospital, thereby allowing a suitable information management [18, 19].

2.4 Knowledge Discovery and Data Mining in Healthcare

The Knowledge Discovery in Databases (KDD) process can be described as an automatic, exploratory analysis and modeling of large data repositories, which identifies meaningful and potentially useful information [20, 21]. The KDD process is a set of five steps, beginning with the selection of the data set. The next step includes cleaning and processing the data, to make it consistent. Then, the data is transformed according to the study goal. Data mining (DM) is the core step, which results in the discovery of hidden knowledge. Finally, follows the interpretation and evaluation of the patterns attained [22]. This study follows this process to discover new knowledge, using DM classification algorithms in order to attain data models.

Data mining techniques have been used in many domains to solve classification, segmentation, association, diagnosis and prediction problems [23]. In healthcare, data mining has recently been used to reduce the number of adverse events, anticipate patient's future behavior and find solutions regarding the institution's management, providing organizations with quality services and clinical decisions at affordable costs [24, 25].

In CHP several data mining models are induced in Intensive Care Units [35] to predict patient outcome, readmissions, length of stay, organ failure, among others in real-time [16, 26–28]. Regarding the maternity care, many studies have been conducted that resorted to DM techniques to solve health services limitations. For instance, the induction of DM models to predict preterm and full term births, as it remains a complex clinical problem for families and the healthcare system [29]. In the CMIN, data mining models were already used to predict events in the Voluntary Interruption of Pregnancy [30] and to categorize GO patients through a clustering based approach [31].

3 Study Description

In order to achieve knowledge from the available data, the study follows the KDD process described in Sect. 2.4. The DM step applies the Cross Industry Standard Process for Data Mining (CRIP-DM), a sequence of six phases well-structured and defined, which works as guidelines for data miners [32].

CRISP-DM organizes the DM process into six phases: business understanding, data understanding, data preparation, modeling, evaluation and deployment. These phases provide a path to follow while planning and implementing a DM project [33].

The DM models were induced using different classification algorithms: Decision Trees (DT), Generalized Linear Models (GLM), Support Vector Machine (SVM), Naïve Bayes (NB) and Neural Networks (NN). The selection of these techniques was based on the playability of the models and engine efficiency, given the data.

The dataset studied consists of 78186 admissions on the gynecology and obstetrics care emergency room in CMIN, comprising a period between 2010-01-06 and 2015-06-25, a total of 1850 days and 32207 women patients.

4 Data Mining Process

In the following section the data mining step of the KDD process is described, according to the CRISP-DM phases.

4.1 Business Understanding

The business goal of the present study is the prediction of pre-triage waiting times in the emergency room of the gynecology and obstetrics care unit in CMIN. Moreover, the study pretends to identify the relation between the environmental and personal information available at the patient's admission and the actual waiting time, in order to improve the triage process in any maternity care.

Therefore, the DM goal is to develop accurate models able to predict the pre-triage waiting time from the collected data. Acceptable models with decent statistical metrics lead to an improvement in the quality of services.

4.2 Data Understanding

In this phase, the relevant variables from the two data sources were collected, forming the dataset. A total of 13 variables were considered. Some of them were temporal features: the day of the week, the part of the day, the month, the day of the month, the part of the month, the trimester, the hour and the season of the year, concerning each particular entry. In addition, the dataset is composed by the identification number (ID) of the triage professional, the number of triage professionals working (NTP) and the number of patients waiting in the room (NPW). All these variables were selected to understand how the environment influences the waiting time. Finally, it also covers two patient's characteristics: the age and the gestation weeks (in case of pregnancy).

Table 1 shows the different classes of some used variables and the percentage of their occurrence, which provides a better interpretation of the dataset. In turn, Table 2 present statistical measures concerning the numerical variables studied.

Table 1. Classes and occurrences of some variables used in the dataset

Variable	Class	Percentage
Day of the Week	Sunday	10.14 %
	Monday	18.51 %
	Tuesday	14.51 %
	Wednesday	15.27 %
	Thursday	15.36 %
	Friday	14.95 %
	Saturday	11.26 %

(Continued)

Table 1. (*Continued*)

Variable	Class	Percentage
Part of the Day	Morning	44.49 %
	Evening	55.26 %
	Night	0.25 %
Part of the Month	First Third	29.91 %
	Second Third	36.32 %
	Last Third	33.77 %
Trimester	First Quarter	25.40 %
	Second Quarter	28.22 %
	Third Quarter	24.11 %
	Last Quarter	22.27 %
Station	Winter	28.02 %
	Spring	28.92 %
	Summer	24.50 %
	Autumn	22.56 %

Table 2. Statistical measures of the numerical variables of the dataset

Variable	Min	Max	Avg	Std Dev
NTP	1	21	5.24	2.85
NPW	1	24	2.18	1.48
Age	8	92	32.01	10.44
Gestation Weeks	0	42	11.39	15.48

The target variable *Waiting Time* was convened in classes, time intervals, in order to run the classification algorithms. Initially, it was simply divided in two classes: 0 being the waiting time between the minimum value and the average, and 1, the waiting time superior to the average. This approach allowed examining the viability of the study itself and confirming that the selected variables are indeed suitable to predict the pre-triage waiting time. In a second stage, the target variable was distributed in four different classes, obeying the normal distribution of the target variable. Table 3 present both distributions of the target classes. These two approaches are properly addressed through the DM process.

Table 3. Both distribution of the target variable in classes

Approach	Class	Distribution	Percentage
2 classes	0	0–17 min	64.94 %
	1	18–340 min	35.06 %
4 classes	0	0–13 min	51.28 %
	1	14–17 min	13.66 %
	2	17–20 min	7.46 %
	3	21–340 min	27.60 %

4.3 Data Preparation

The information provided by the information systems required some transformations to reach the dataset exposed in Sect. 4.2.

In a pre-processing phase, some variables were attained from raw content. This phase was extremely important to create the scenarios and it required the development of several procedures. For instance, the temporal variables, such as the day of the week or the part of the month, were obtained by arranging the patients' admission date of the entrance records. Similarly, the number of patients and triage professions required creating some procedures to count the pre-triage entries meeting the required conditions, and organize the information differently. The patient age was acquired through the transformation of the birth and episode dates. Later, some null/noise values were deleted from the dataset to ensure the information consistency, remaining 78186 pre-triage records. The entire dataset was prepared and processed through Oracle SQL Developer. The dataset was then replicated and studied with different displays of the target variable mentioned in the previous subsection.

4.4 Modeling and Evaluation

In the modeling phase, the DM models were induced using the DM techniques: GLM, SVM, DT, NB and NN. The sampling method applied was the Holdout sampling, where 30 % of the data was used for testing, and the remaining entries compose the training set. Finally, different variables' scenarios were combined to identify which variables influence the pre-triage waiting time on the GO emergency room. The ten considered scenarios were:

S0: {All variables}
S1: {Day of the week, Part of the day, Trimester, Hour, Season}
S2: {NTP, NPW}
S3: {Age, Gestation Weeks, Day of the week, Part of the day, Trimester, Hour, Season, NTP, NPW}
S4: {Month, Day of the month, Hour, ID professional, NPW}
S5: {Age, Day of the week, Part of the day, Day of the month, Part of the month, Season, NTP}
S6: {Month, Day of the month, Part of the month, Trimester, Season}
S7: {Day of the week, Part of the day, Hour}
S8: {Age, Gestation Weeks, Day of the month, Season, NTP, NPW}
S9: {Age, Gestation Weeks, Trimester, NTP, NPW}

The DM models were induced in both target approaches. Thus, each Data Mining Model (DMM) can be identified by Eq. 1.

$$DMM_m = DMT_y \times A \times T_s \times S_i \tag{1}$$

DMT_Y refers to the DM technique, A_t is the target approach, T_s represents the sampling method and S_i identifies the scenario. A total of 100 models were induced (10 scenarios * 5 techniques * 1 sampling method * 2 target approaches).

All models were induced using the R Studio with the configurations presented in Table 4, concerning the DM classification algorithms.

Table 4. Algorithms settings

Technique	R algorithm	Setting	Value
DT	Ctree	Subset	Null
		Weights	Null
		Xtrafo	Ptrafo
		Ytrafo	Ptrafo
NB	naiveBayes	Subset	Null
		Laplace	0
GLM	Glm	Subset	Null
		Weights	Null
		Family	Binomial
SVM	Ksvm	Scaled	True
		Type	C-bsvc
		Kernel	Vanilladot
NN	Nnet	Size	4
		Rang	0.1
		Decay	5e-04
		Max It	200

The statistic metrics described in Eqs. 2, 3 and 4 were considered to evaluate the induced models. These metrics were estimated through the results provided by the confusion matrix (CMX) of each model.

$$Sensitivity = TP/(TP + FN) \tag{2}$$

$$Specificity = TN/(TN + FP) \tag{3}$$

$$Accuracy = TP/(TP + FT + TN + FN) \tag{4}$$

CMX contains four types of results: the number of True Positives (TP), False Positives (FP), True Negatives (TN) and False Negatives (FN). The CMX along with these metrics were obtained automatically using the package 'caret' in R Studio.

The best results concerning the first target approach are exposed in Table 5. It contains the top 4 scenarios and the best DM techniques to each of them.

Table 5. Best statistic results in view of the first target approach (2 classes)

DMT	Accuracy	Specificity	Sensitivity	DMT	Accuracy	Specificity	Sensitivity
Scenario 0				*Scenario 2*			
DT	0.7135	0.9078	**0.3534**	DT	0.7105	**0.9394**	0.2859
NB	0.7038	0.9163	0.3102	GLM	**0.7131**	0.9237	**0.3225**
GLM	**0.7282**	**0.9304**	0.3323	NN	0.7106	0.9337	0.2965
Scenario 3				*Scenario 4*			
DT	0.7170	0.9288	0.3236	DT	**0.7118**	0.9270	0.3159
GLM	0.7261	**0.9274**	0.3383	GLM	0.7028	0.9198	**0.3179**
NN	**0.7381**	0.9366	**0.3473**	NN	0.7117	**0.9303**	0.3093

The results are satisfactory enough to prove that there is a relation between the variables studied and the pre-triage waiting time. The second target approach, which divides the target in 4 classes, was pursued. In this case, since the target is not binary, the only metric used to evaluate the models was the accuracy. Accordingly, the results are presented in Table 6.

Table 6. Best accuracy results in view of the second target approach (4 classes)

Scenario	DMT	Accuracy
0	NB	0.6134
3	DT	**0.6243**
9	DT	0.6088

The best results were achieved in the first approach, reaching a specificity value of 93.94 %. These high values of specificity mean that the models are highly capable predicting class 0, pre-triage waiting times shorter than the average waiting time.

In a clinical environment, the first approach will provide to the healthcare professions a larger confidence (almost 94 %) predicting smaller times, the second approach represents a valuable resource to the service, since nearly 62 % of the triage events fit this profile (four classes).

Overall, the DM model that attained the best outcomes was scenario 3, inducing the neural network algorithm, obtaining an accuracy of 73.81 %, representing a high assertiveness. The best accuracy results provided by the second approach have statistical value, since the dataset has a four class target, but are not enough to be considered worthy clinical achievements.

4.5   Deployment

After a careful review to the results, the best DM models as well as the processed data are reported to the maternity care unit of CMIN, being implemented in the IDSS and the Business Intelligence (BI) platform already deployed in the hospital, correspondently [34]. The BI platform assists the healthcare professionals and the administrators in their decision making, regarding the services and the patients. The study will contribute to the improvement of the pre-triage system and the conditions regarding the Gynecology and Obstetrics emergency room.

5 Discussion

In the evaluation phase the study achieved satisfactory results regarding the dataset which divides the target variable *Waiting Time* in two classes (lesser than 17 min or greater than 18 min). The best 3 models are highlighted in Table 7.

Table 7. Top 3 models that present the higher values of accuracy, sensitivity and specificity in view of the first target approach (2 classes)

S	DMT	Accuracy	Specificity	Sensitivity
0	GLM	0.7289	0.9304	0.3323
3	DT	0.7170	0.9288	0.3236
3	NN	**0.7381**	**0.9366**	**0.3473**

Overall, the specificity values are far higher than the sensitivity ones, allowing the gynecology and obstetrics care unit to identify upfront the patients which waiting time for pre-triage will be shorter, and subsequently, to organize the resources accordingly.

Regarding the studied variables, the scenarios 0, 2, 3, 4 and 9 achieved the best outcomes. Thus, the variables directly proportional to the pre-triage waiting time are the number of patients present in the waiting room (NPW), the number of triage professionals working at the moment (NTP) and some temporal variables – the hour of the day, the day of the month and the season of the year. This information benefits the maternity emergency room workflow, since it can identify outstanding situations, and therefore, improve the healthcare services.

The dataset that divides the target variable into 4 groups (obeying its normal distribution) obtained good results in a statistical point of view, since it is not a binary prediction. Nevertheless, the best accuracy value achieved is 62.43 %, not being good enough to be used in the maternity care decision support systems.

The analysis of the patient records from January 2010 to June 2015 also allows detecting some weaknesses in the pre-triage system implemented in CMIN. Since the system only distinguishes patients in two levels of priorities (URG and ARGO), adverse events may occur in this categorization. Besides, some triage professionals force a different output than would be expected by the pre-triage system.

6 Conclusions and Future Work

This study aimed the prediction of pre-triage waiting times in the emergency room of gynecology and obstetrics care unit. A dataset was built from real data recorded in the SAPE and EHR systems of Centro Materno Infantil do Norte (CMIN), the maternal and perinatal care unit of Centro Hospitalar of Oporto (CHP), collecting personal and environmental variables available at the patient's admission. After inducing several data mining techniques on different combinations of the dataset variables (scenarios), satisfactory results were achieved. The best DM model was acquired by inducing Neural Networks algorithm through the variables composing scenario 3, achieving an accuracy of approximately 74 % and a specificity of 94 %, when dividing the target variable in two classes. These results lead to quality improvements in the emergency room of the maternity care.

This study also was important to identify which variables most contributes to change the waiting time. This information is valuable to the ED. They have now a new tool able to give to them an idea of the patient waiting time basing their analysis in the data associated to the critic variables.

The Data Mining models induced and the variables identified as critical are the most important contribution of this work.

Alongside, another study is being conducted to predict the post-triage waiting time (the time between the moment of pre-triage and the doctor's admission) in CMIN. As for future work, both studies will be implemented in the IDSS and BI platform used in the maternity unit, optimizing patient flow through the ED and therefore, improving their safety and satisfaction.

Acknowledgments. This work has been supported by FCT - Fundação para a Ciência e Tecnologia within the Project Scope UID/CEC/00319/2013.

References

1. Bergs, J., Verelst, S., Gillet, J.-B., Deboutte, P., Vandoren, C., Vandijck, D.: The number of patients simultaneously present at the emergency department as an indicator of unsafe waiting times: a receiver operated curve-based evaluation. Int. Emerg. Nurs. **22**, 185–189 (2014)
2. Hoot, N., Aronsky, D.: Systematic review of emergency department crowding: causes, effects and solutions. Ann. Emerg. Med. **52**, 126–136 (2008)
3. Stover-Baker, B., Stahlman, B., Pollack, M.: Triage nurse prediction of hospital admission. J. Emerg. Nurs. **38**(3), 306–310 (2012)
4. Sun, Y., Teow, K., Heng, B., Ooi, C., Tay, S.: Real-time prediction of waiting time in the emergency department, using quantile regression. Ann. Emerg. Med. **60**(3), 299–308 (2012)
5. Boudreaux, E., O'Hea, E.: Patient satisfaction in the emergency department: a review of the literature and implications for practice. J. Emerg. Med. **26**(1), 13–26 (2004)
6. Shaikh, S., Witting, M., Winters, M., Brodeur, M., Jerrad, D.: Support for a waiting room time tracker: a survey of patients waiting in an urban ED. J. Emerg. Med. **44**(1), 225–229 (2013)
7. Taylor, C., Benger, J.: Patient satisfaction in emergency medicine. J. Emerg. Med. **21**, 528–532 (2004)
8. Khodambashi, S.: Business process re-engineering application in healthcare in a relation to health information systems. Procedia Technol. **9**, 949–957 (2013)

9. Pereira, E., Brandão, A., Salazar, M., Portela, F., Santos, M., Machado, J., Abelha, A., Braga, J.: Pre-triage decision support improvement in maternity care by means of data mining. In: Integration of Data Mining in Business Intelligence Systems, pp. 175–192 (2014)

10. Paul, J., Jordan, R., Duty, S., Engstrom, J.: Improving satisfaction with care and reducing length of stay in an obstetric triage unit using a nurse-midwife-managed model of care. J. Midwifery Women's Health 58(2), 1–7 (2013)

11. Zocco, J., Williams, M., Longobucco, D., Bernstein, B.: A systems analysis of obstetric triage. J. Perinat. Neonatal Nurs. 21(4), 315–322 (2007)

12. Murray, M., Bullard, M., Grafstein, E.: Revisions to the Canadian emergency department triage and acuity scale implementation guidelines. Cjem 6(6), 421–427 (2004)

13. Abelha, A., Pereira, E., Brandão, A., Portela, F., Santos, M., Machado, J., Braga, J.: Improving quality of services in maternity care triage system. Int. J. E-Health Med. Commun. 6(2), 10–26 (2015)

14. Abelha, A., Quintas, C., Cabral, A., Salazar, M., Machado, H., Machado, J., Neves, J., Santos, M.F., Portela, C.F., Pina, C.: Data acquisition process for an intelligent decision support in gynecology and obstetrics emergency triage. In: Cruz-Cunha, M.M., Varajão, J., Powell, P., Martinho, R. (eds.) CENTERIS 2011, Part III. CCIS, vol. 221, pp. 223–232. Springer, Heidelberg (2011)

15. Abelha, A., Pereira, E., Brandão, A., Portela, F., Santos, M., Machado, J.: Simulating a multi-level priority triage system for Maternity Emergency. In: European Simulation and Modelling Conference (2014)

16. Portela, F., Cabral, A., Abelha, A., Salazar, M., Quintas, C., Machado, J., Santos, M.: Knowledge acquisition process for intelligent decision support in critical health care. In: Healthcare Administration: Concepts, Methodologies, Tools, and Applications, p. 270 (2014)

17. Abelha, A., Analide, C., Machado, J., Neves, J., Santos, M., Novais, P.: Ambient intelligence and simulation in health care virtual scenarios. In: Camarinha-Matos, L.M., Afsarmanesh, H., Novais, P., Analide, C. (eds.) EFCN 2007, Part I. IFIP, vol. 243, pp. 461–468. Springer, New York (2007)

18. Abelha, A., Machado, J., Santos, M., Allegro, S., Rua, F., Paiva, M., Neves, J.: Agency for integration, diffusion and archive of medical information. In: IASTED International Conference - Artificial Intelligence and Applications (2002)

19. Peixoto, H., Santos, M., Abelha, A., Machado, J.: Intelligence in Interoperability with AIDA. In: 20th International Symposium on Methodologies for Intelligent Systems (2012)

20. Fayyad, U., Piatetsky-Shapiro, G., Smyth, P.: From data mining to knowledge discovery in databases. AI Mag. 17(3), 37 (1996)

21. Lin, J., Gan, W., Hong, T.-P., Tseng, V.: Efficient algorithms for mining up-to-date high-utility patterns. Adv. Eng. Inform. 29(3), 648–661 (2015)

22. Maimon, O., Rokach, L.: Introduction to Knowledge Discovery and Data Mining. In: Maimon, O., Rokach, L. (eds.) Data Mining and Knowledge Discovery Handbook, pp. 1–17. Springer, New York (2005)

23. Xia, J., Xie, F., Zhang, Y., Caulfield, C.: Artificial intelligence and data mining: algorithms and applications. In: Abstract and Applied Analysis (2013)

24. Srinivas, K., Rani, B.K., Govrdhan, A.: Applications of data mining techniques in healthcare and prediction of heart attacks. Int. J. Comput. Sci. Eng. 2(2), 250–255 (2010)

25. Yoo, I., Alafaireet, P., Marinov, M., Pena-Hernandez, K., Gopidi, R., Chang, J.-F., Hua, L.: Data mining in healthcare and biomedicine: a survey of the literature. J. Med. Syst. 36, 2431–2448 (2012)

26. Braga, P., Portela, F., Santos, M., Rua, F.: Data mining models to predict patient's readmission in intensive care units. In: ICAART - International Conference on Agents and Artificial Intelligence, Angers, France (2014)
27. Portela, F., Santos, M.F., Machado, J., Abelha, A., Silva, Á.: Pervasive and intelligent decision support in critical health care using ensembles. In: Bursa, M., Khuri, S., Renda, M.E. (eds.) ITBAM 2013. LNCS, vol. 8060, pp. 1–16. Springer, Heidelberg (2013)
28. Veloso, R., Portela, F., Santos, M., Sila, Á., Rua, F., Abelha, A., Machado, J.: A clustering approach for predicting readmissions in intensive medicine. Procedia Technol. **16**, 1307–1316 (2014)
29. Beta, J., Akolekar, R., Ventura, W., Syngelaki, A., Nicolaides, K.: Prediction of spontaneous preterm delivery from maternal factors, obstetric history and placental perfusion and function at 11–13 weeks. Prenat. Diagn. **31**(1), 75–83 (2011)
30. Brandão, A., Pereira, E., Portela, F., Santos, M., Abelha, A., Machado, J.: Managing voluntary interruption of pregnancy using data mining. Procedia Technol. **16**, 1297–1306 (2014)
31. Pereira, S., Portela, F., Santos, M., Abelha, A., Machado, J.: Clustering-based approach for categorizing pregnant in obstetrics and maternity care. In: C3S2E, Yokohoma, Japan, pp. 1–5 (2015)
32. Shafique, U., Qaiser, H.: A comparative study of data mining process models (KDD, CRISP-DM and SEMMA). Int. J. Innov. Sci. Res. **12**(1), 217–222 (2014)
33. Shearer, C.: The CRISP-DM model: the new blueprint for data mining. J. Data Warehouse. **5**(4), 13–22 (2000)
34. Pereira, E., Brandão, A., Portela, F., Santos, M., Machado, J., Abelha, A.: Business intelligence in maternity care. In: IDEAS - International Database Engineering and Applications Symposium, Portugal (2014)
35. Portela, F., Santos, M.F., Machado, J., Abelha, A., Silva, Á., Rua, F.: Pervasive and Intelligent Decision Support in Intensive Medicine – The Complete Picture. In: Bursa, M., Khuri, S., Renda, M. (eds.) ITBAM 2014. LNCS, vol. 8649, pp. 87–102. Springer, Heidelberg (2014)

A Game Theoretic Predictive Modeling Approach to Reduction of False Alarm

Fatemeh Afghah[1]($\boxtimes$), Abolfazl Razi[1], S.M. Reza Soroushmehr[2,3],
Somayeh Molaei[2,3], Hamid Ghanbari[4], and Kayvan Najarian[2,3,5]

[1] Electrical Engineering and Computer Science Department,
Northern Arizona University, Flagstaff, Arizona 86011, USA
{fatemeh.afghah,abolfazl.razi}@nau.edu
[2] Department of Emergency Medicine, University of Michigan,
Ann Arbor, Michigan 48109, USA
{ssoroush,smolaei,kayvan}@med.umich.edu
[3] Michigan Center for Integrative Research in Critical Care: MCIRCC,
University of Michigan, Ann Arbor, Michigan 48109, USA
[4] Internal Medicine, University of Michigan, Ann Arbor, Michigan 48109, USA
ghhamid@med.umich.edu
[5] Computational Medicine and Bioinformatics Department,
University of Michigan, Ann Arbor, Michigan 48109, USA

Abstract. False alarm is one of the main concerns in intensive care units which could result in care disruption, sleep deprivation, insensitivity of care–givers to alarms and so on. Many approaches such as improving the quality of physiological signals by filtering and developing more accurate sensors have been proposed in the last two decades to suppress the rate of false alarm. Moreover, some multi–parameter/feature methods have been developed to classify the alarms more accurately. One of the main problems facing these methods is that they neglect those features that individually have low impact on the accuracy. In this paper, we propose a model based on coalition game that considers the inter–features mutual information which results in gaining the accuracy of the classification. Simulation results on a database produced by four hospitals shows the superior performance of the proposed method compared to other existing methods.

Keywords: False alarm · Feature selection · Coalition game theory · Classification

1 Introduction

In order to monitor a patient and also for the sake of diagnostic, prognostic and treatment, many monitoring and therapeutic devices are utilized in intensive care units (ICUs). These devices are also used to measure vital signs, support or replace impaired or failing organs and administer medications to patients [12]. Each of these devices might generate optic/acoustic alarms due to patient's physiologic condition, patient movement, motion artifact, malfunction of individual sensors and imperfections in the patient–equipment contact [18]. Many of the alarms (80 % to 99 % [9]) could be false and/or clinically insignificant

© Springer International Publishing Switzerland 2016
X. Zheng et al. (Eds.): ICSH 2015, LNCS 9545, pp. 118–130, 2016.
DOI: 10.1007/978-3-319-29175-8_11

which are not related to patients' condition. These alarms could compromise quality and safety of care, which could result in many problems such as "alarm fatigue" among care–givers as well as the possibility of missing a real event due to care–givers insensitivity to these unreliable alarms known as "cry–wolf" effect.

Dealing with false alarms is widely considered the number one hazard imposed by the medical technology and an important concern in ICUs [9]. Many approaches have been utilized to decrease the number of false alarms such as adding short delay [9], improving the quality of signals, improvements in sensor technology and utilizing advanced multi–parameter models [3,21]. An overview on clinical situation and different aspects of false alarm problem can be found in [9,13].

Using a machine learning approach, Li and Clifford have designed a framework for false alarm reduction on arrhythmia patients. They extracted 114 features from electrocardiogram (ECG), arterial blood pressure (ABP), and Photoplethysmogram (PPG or PLETH), that measures oxygen saturation level (SpO2), and used a genetic algorithm to select a subset of these features. Using a relevance vector machine (RVM) as a classifier, false alarm suppression was reported to be 86.4%, 100% and 27.8% respectively for asystole, extreme extreme bradycardia and extreme tachycardia. An automated method for false arrhythmia suppression was proposed in [5] that is based on quality assessment of normal and abnormal rhythms of ECG signals. In this method an ECG signal is downsampled to 125 Hz and then QRS detection algorithms are applied. After that baseline wander is filtered and different signal quality indexes (SQI) are calculated and used in a support vector machine (SVM) classifier where the obtained accuracy, sensitivity and specificity are respectively 0.990, 0.985, and 0.994. Different approaches including k–nearest neighbors (KNN), Naive Bayes, Decision Tree, SVM and multi–layer Perceptron have been tested on a database from MIMIC II for alarms classification, where the features have been extracted from age, sex, Central venous pressure (CVP), SpO2, ABP, ECG and pulmonary arterial pressure (PAP) [4]. The suppression rate for true alarm detection is between 2.33% and 17.73% for 5 alarms and false alarm suppression rate is between 71.73% to 99.23%. Charbonnier and Gentil have proposed a trend extraction that tracks the changes in signals using a fuzzy decision approach [6] and could filter 81% of the false alarm without filtering any true alarms where they tested their method on a small number of examples.

The above models considers a number of features/parameters extracted from multiple continuously–measured physiological signals, such as ECG and ABP to create more reliable alarms. The major problem faced by these multi–parameter approaches is the presence of many parameters/features that individually have low impact on the model performance, and as such they might not be included in the model, while when coupled with other such parameters could significantly improve the performance of the accuracy and specificity of the alarm detection algorithms. Besides statistical evidence to this observation, the fact that physicians, by visual interpretation of the patterns in all patients' signals, can very often correctly decide on the validity of the alarms caused by individual machines/monitors, suggests when a suitable combination of all data/features are included in a model, false alarms can be reduced significantly [7].

Several data mining and feature reduction algorithms have been utilized in analysis of big data sets to improve the prediction accuracy and reliability through reducing the feature space to a more concise and relevant set of attributes [11,16,17,22,26]. However in the majority of these conventional methods, each of the features is evaluated separately, and as such, the possible correlation among them is neglected. Specifically, the existing methods either only account for the effect of individual features on the target or consider the inter–feature mutual information to obtain higher performance; however, it is often the case that a set of features together have a considerable effect on the classifier, while each individual attribute in the set does not. Therefore, these features will most likely be filtered out resulting in significant degradation in the performance [10].

Cooperative game theoretic approach has been recently utilized in feature selection algorithms [8,19,20]. In this paper, we propose a coalition based game–theoretic predictive modeling approach to suppress the false alarm for five types of life threatening arrhythmias including asystole, extreme bradycardia, extreme tachycardia, ventricular tachycardia, and ventricular flutter/fibrillation. Three main signals of ECG, ABP, and PLETH are used as the inputs of our proposed model. In the first stage (i.e. signal analysis) wavelet coefficients of each signal at different levels of decomposition are calculated. Then, a number of statistical features such as mean, variance, median, kurtosis and entropy of the resulting wavelet coefficients are calculated for each level. The calculated coefficients along with the other parameters are used as features for our proposed coalition game theoretic approach in which different combinations of features are considered for creating a predictive model that assesses the validity of the alarms. The proposed method accounts for intricate and intrinsic interrelation among all potentially effective combinations of the features by measuring the contribution of features both individually and in group with others in order to identify the most informative grouping. A main capability of the proposed method is finding discriminating combined/sub–sets of apparently low–impact features, which despite their weak individual contribution to the classifier could have a quantifiable impact on the specificity and accuracy of the alarm detection approaches when grouped with other features.

The rest of this paper is organized as follows. Section 2 introduces the proposed signal analysis and feature extraction techniques. An introduction to coalition game theory followed by the description of the proposed game theoretic based feature selection method are presented in Sect. 3. The numerical analysis results are presented in Sect. 4, followed by conclusion in Sect. 5.

2   Signal Analysis and Feature Extraction

A set of wavelets defines a special filter bank which can be used for signal component analysis and the resulting wavelet transform coefficients can be further applied as signal features for classification. Here, we applied a discrete wavelet transform (DWT) on the 1–D input signals, ECG, PLETH and ABP. The DWT is selected because of its advantages over other transforms due to its ability to separate details in signals. Very fine details can be isolated using small wavelet and rough details can be captured using large wavelets [24]. DWT decomposes each input signals into two approximations and detailed coefficient components. Approximation set is obtained by applying a high–pass filter at low scales and details coefficients are computed by applying a low–pass filter at high scales. We used Daubechies 8 (db8) for ECG signal as there is a good match between the shape of ECG signal and this wavelet. Also we used Daubechies 4 for PLETH and ABP signals for the same reason. DWT is a shifted and scaled by power of two of mother wavelet as:

$$\psi_{i,j}(t) = 1/\sqrt{2^i}\psi(\frac{t - j \times 2^i}{2^i}) \tag{1}$$

where i, j are scale and shift parameters respectively and ψ for a Daubechies wavelet of class D-2N is defined as:

$$\psi(t) = \sqrt{2}\sum_{k}(-1)^k h_{2N-1-k} \times \phi(2t - 1), \tag{2}$$

$$\phi(t) = \sqrt{2}\sum_{k} h_k \times \phi(2t - k)$$

where h shows a high pass filter.

Wavelet coefficients are calculated by convolving the high pass filter, h, and the corresponding low pass filter, $g_k = h_{2N-1-k}$, with a signal and then the results are down–sampled. Each of the three mentioned signals is decomposed into 6 levels by convolving the high–pass and low–pass filters. The calculated coefficient are shown as $X = [E_1, ..., E_l, A_1, ..., A_l, P_1, ..., P_l]$ where l shows the number of decomposition levels, (here $l = 6$). E_i, A_i and P_i respectively show the wavelet coefficients of ECG, ABP and PLETH signals. For $i = l$ each of these parameters shows the details coefficients and for $i \neq l$ each of them shows the approximate coefficient. Approximate and details coefficients can be respectively calculated from (3) and (4)

$$a_i(t) = \sum_{k} a_{i-1}(t)h_{2t-k} \tag{3}$$

$$d_i(t) = \sum_{k} a_{i-1}(t)g_{2t-k} \tag{4}$$

where a_{-1} shows the input signal (i.e. ECG, ABP or PLETH). Including all wavelet coefficients as features to the classification setup is not efficient and may significantly decrease the generalization property of the trained model due to over-fitting. Therefore, we further reduce the number of features by extracting representative statistical and information–theoretic properties of the wavelet vectors as summarized in Table 1. In calculating information–theoretic properties (e.g. Entropy), we assume that the wavelet vector elements are derived from an unknown probability distribution.

In Table 1, features 1 to 10 are typical statical properties of the signal, where μ_n is the nth standardized sample moment defined in

$$\mu_n = \frac{\Sigma_{i=1}^{N}(X_i - \bar{X})^n}{N}, \bar{X} = \frac{\Sigma_{i=1}^{N}X_i}{N} \tag{5}$$

In (5), $X_1, \ldots, X_N$ are the Nth wavelet coefficients associated with each signal probe. *Kurtosis* and *skewness* define the shape of probability distributions such that *kurtosis*, defined in (6) measures the peakedness of distribution and is defined as the ratio of the forth standardized moment to the square of variance.

$$\kappa(X) = \frac{E[(X - \mu)^4]}{\left(E[(X - \mu)^2]\right)^2} = \frac{\mu_4(X)}{\sigma_4(X)} \tag{6}$$

Likewise, *skewness* is a measure of the symmetry of distribution around zero and is defined as

$$\lambda(X) = E\left[\left(\frac{X - \mu(X)}{\sigma(X)}\right)^3\right] = \frac{\mu^3(X)}{\sigma^3(X)} \tag{7}$$

Harmonic mean is defined as $\frac{N}{\sum_{i=1}^{N} 1/X_i}$. *Interquartile range* is calculated based on the difference between the 75th and 25th percentiles. Shannon entropy is an information theoretic property of the square of coefficients approximated by their sample counterparts and calculated as

$$H(X^2) = -\sum_{i=1}^{N} X_i^2 \log_2 X_i^2 \tag{8}$$

Table 1. Statistical and Information-theoretic features of wavelet vectors.

No	Feature	No	Feature	No	Feature
1	mean	13	skewness	25	$n_{S(10)}$
2	mode	14	harmonic mean	26	$n_{S(100)}$
3	median	15	interquartile range	27	$n_{S(1000)}$
4	max	16	Shannon Entropy	28	$n_{S(10000)}$
5	min	17	Log Entropy	29	$n_{S(25000)}$
6	range	18	$n_{T(1)}$	30	$n_{S(50000)}$
7	variance	19	$n_{T(10)}$	31	$n_{S(65000)}$
8	std (σ)	20	$n_{T(100)}$	32	an_1
9	μ_3	21	$n_{T(500)}$	33	an_2
10	μ_4	22	$n_{T(1000)}$	34	an_3
11	coefficient of var	23	$n_{T(5000)}$	35	an_5
12	kurtosis	24	$n_{S(1)}$	36	an_{10}

Log energy is defined as $\sum \log X_i^2$. $n_T(\alpha)$, defined in (9), counts the number of times that the value of wavelet coefficients exceed the threshold α.

$$n_T(\alpha) = \sum_{i=1}^{N} \mathbb{1}(|X_i| > \alpha) \qquad (9)$$

In (9), $\mathbb{1}(.)$ shows the indicator function. Also, $n_S(\alpha)$ is defined as

$$n_S(\alpha) = N - 2\sum_{i=1}^{N} \mathbb{1}(X_i^2 \leq \alpha^2) + 2\alpha^2 \sum_{i=1}^{N} \mathbb{1}(X_i^2 > \alpha^2) + \sum_{i=1}^{N} [X_i^2 \times \mathbb{1}(X_i^2 \leq \alpha^2)]$$
$$(10)$$

Finally, $an_p(X) = \sqrt[p]{\sum_{i=1}^{N} |X_i|^p}$ is the p-norm of the vector of the absolute values of the coefficients. Hereafter, features 1 to 15 are called as *Feature set 1:Statistical*, which includes statistical information and features 16 to 36 as *Feature set 2:Entropy*, which mainly includes information-theoretic and geometrical properties of the coefficients.

3   Feature Selection

Here, we map the coalition game–theoretical methodology to the feature selection problem by considering the competing features as the game players, where the features can be classified in different coalitions by noting their impact on the classifier and also by their interdependency.

3.1   Coalition-Based Game-Theoretic Feature Selection

Cooperative game theory has been recently utilized in feature selection algorithms [8,19,20,25]. Unlike non-cooperative games in which the players act individually [2], *coalition game* refers to a class of game theoretic approaches that studies the set of joint actions taken by a group of players. These games are defined based on exhaustive scenarios that players may form a group and how the total shared payoff is divided among the members. For a transferable utility coalition (TU–coalition) game with n players, let N denote the set of players, $N = \{1, 2, ..., n\}$. A coalition of players, S defines a sub-set of N, $S \subseteq N$. In general, for a n–player game there exists 2^n possible coalitions of any size. The empty coalition is denoted by ϕ, while grand coalition refers to the coalition of all players, N.

The n–player coalition game can be defined with the pair of (N, v), where $N = \{1, 2, ..., n\}$ is the set of players and the *characteristic function*, v is a real–valued function defined on the set of all coalitions, $v : 2^N \rightarrow \mathbb{R}$. For a coalition S, $S \subseteq N$, the characteristic function, $v(S)$ represents the total payoff that can be gained by the members of this coalition. This function satisfies the following conditions,

- characteristic function of an empty coalition is zero, $v(\phi) = 0$, and
- if S_i and S_j, $(S_i, S_j \subseteq N)$ are two disjoint coalitions, the characteristic function of their union has super–additivity property, meaning that $v(S_i \cup S_j) \geq v(S_i) + v(S_j)$.

Here, we model the features as the players of the game, and the characteristic function of a coalition, v is measured by contribution of its members (features) to the performance of the classifier (e.g. success rate in supervised learning). Different possible grouping of the features are examined to recognize the optimal coalition. The contribution of feature i in classification accuracy when it joins a coalition S is defined by *marginal importance* as follows

$$\Delta_i(S) = v(S \cup \{i\}) - v(S) \tag{11}$$

A solution of a coalition game is determined by how the coalition of players can be formed and how the total payoff of a coalition is divided among the members. Let's define the value function, γ that assigns an n–tuple of real numbers, $\gamma(v) = (\gamma_1(v), \gamma_2(v), ..., \gamma_n(v))$ to each possible characteristic function, in which $\gamma_i(v)$ measures the value of player i in the game with characteristic function v. If the following axioms are satisfied, Shapley value can be utilized as a fair unique solution of the coalition game [23]. The Shapley axioms for $\gamma(v)$ are

- Efficiency (group rationality): $\sum_{i \in N} \gamma_i(v) = v(N)$, meaning that the summation of values for all players is equal to the value of grand coalition.
- Symmetry: If for players i and j, $i, j \in N$ and for every coalition S not containing i and j we have $v(S \cup \{i\}) = v(S \cup \{j\})$, then $\gamma_i(v) = \gamma_j(v)$.
- Dummy player: If for player i and for every coalition S not containing i, we have $v(S) = v(S \cup \{i\})$, then $\gamma_i(v) = 0$
- Additivity: For characteristic functions u and v, we have $\gamma(u+v) = \gamma(u) + \gamma(v)$, meaning that the value of two games played at the same time is equal to summation of their values if played at different times.

The Shapley value of player i is defined as the weighted mean of its marginal importance over all possible subsets of the players.

$$\gamma_i(v) = \frac{1}{n!} \sum_{\pi \in \Pi} \Delta_i(S_i(\pi)), \tag{12}$$

where Π is the set of all $n!$ permutations over N and $S_i(\pi)$ is the set of features (players) preceding player i in permutation π.

Since in feature selection, the order of features in a coalition does not change the value of coalition, the calculations in (12), can be further simplified by excluding the permutation of coalitions in the average:

$$\gamma_i(N, v) = \frac{1}{n!} \sum_{S \subseteq N/i} \Delta_i(S) |S|_i (n - |S| - 1))!, \tag{13}$$

where $S \subseteq N/i$ represents the coalitions that player i does not belong to. It is equivalent to the weighted average of coalitions, where the weight of each coalition is the number of its all possible permutations.

As shown in (12) and (13), the Shapely value solution accounts for all possible coalitions that can be formed by the players [23]. Since in false alarm detection problem, the data set includes a large number of features, thereby calculating the Shapley value would be computationally intractable. Furthermore, considering the coalitions of a large number of features or all of them is practically unnecessary, since the maximum number of feature may interact with one another is much less than the total number of features. Therefore, we utilize the Multi–perturbation Shapley value measurement with coalition sizes up to L rather than the original Shapely value, which is determined using an unbiased estimator based on Shapley value [14,15].

In our proposed algorithm, at each round, the features are randomly divided into groups of size L. Then, we calculate the corresponding Multi-perturbation Shapely value of feature i inside its group, $\gamma_i'(v)$ considering all possible coalitions of size $1 \leq l \leq L$. This is equivalent to randomly sampling from uniformly distributed feature i, $\gamma_i'(v)$ is calculated as follows.

$$\gamma_i'(v) = \frac{1}{|\Pi_L|} \sum_{\pi \in \Pi_L} \Delta_i(S_i(\pi)), \tag{14}$$

where Π_L denotes the sampled permutation on sub–groups of features of size L. There is an essential trade–off to set L in the proposed method. Large L values consider higher order relations, while increasing the complexity of finding Multi–perturbation Shapely value at each subgroup. We conjecture that the optimum value of L for our datasets taking into account various factors such as the nature of data, number of features, and the inter-feature dependence is in the range of 3 to 6. This is confirmed by simulation results in Sect. 4. It is worth noting that in most feature selection algorithms, each feature is being considered separately or equivalently $L = 1$.

Since the size of subgroups and the role of each group at the classification for the normalized data is almost equal, at the end of each iteration, the n_e less effective features are removed from the list, regardless of the enclosing subgroup. In order to minimize the impact of individual grouping, at the end of each iteration, we do not remove all features with Multi perturbation shapely value below threshold as in [15]. Rather, we remove only n_e features with the lowest Multi–perturbation Shapely value (if below Multi–perturbation Shapely threshold γ_m). We choose n_e a small number, because (i) the complexity reduces linearly with

Table 2. Alarms definition

Alarm Type	Definition
Asystole	There is no QRS for at least 4 s
Extreme Bradycardia	Heart rate < 40 bpm for 5 consecutive beats
Extreme Tachycardia	Heart rate higher > 140 bpm for 17 consecutive beats
Ventricular Tachycardia	At least 5 ventricular beats with heart rate > 100 bpm
Ventricular Flutter/Fibrillation	Fibrillatory, flutter, or oscillatory waveform for at least 4 s

n_e and (ii) the features with lower Multi–perturbation Shapely value may have a higher impact, when belong to another group in the next iterations. After removing the less contributing features, we randomly permute the remained features and repeat regrouping. Therefore, over the long run, the features are most likely to visit any other features, since $L \ll N$. We terminate the algorithm if one of the following two conditions are violated; (i) the minimum number of features n_m is reached or (ii) the classification accuracy of all remaining features fall below a threshold T.

4   Numerical Analysis Results

The database used for this study, which is publicly available through Physionet [1], was produced by four hospitals in the USA and Europe , using monitors with different manufacturers, unit–specific protocols, software versions and unit types. The definition of the alarm is presented in Table 2 [1]. The total number of records is 219 and for each alarm a label including 'true', 'false', or 'impossible to tell' has been assigned by expert annotators. Interference from pacemakers and other noise artifacts may be present in the ECG signals.

Experimental results are provided in this section for the proposed alarm validation method as well as other state–of–the–art explicit feature selection methods including Chi–square, Gain Ratio, Relief and Info Gain methods. The Chi–square method evaluates a subset of features by finding their corresponding chi–squared statistics with respect to the class. The Gain ratio (GR) is an information based method that minimizes the conditional entropy of class given the selected features. The Relief method is an iterative algorithm that

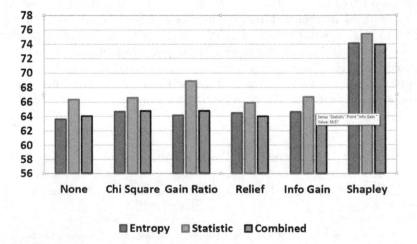

Fig. 1. True alarm recognition rate for the first 30 features using different feature selection methods with Bayes Net classification.

starts with an initial weights for features and then iteratively adjusts the weights by randomly choosing an instance from data and weighting each feature based on its corresponding distance between the selected data instance and the closest instances in different classes to highlight features with higher discriminative properties. The Information Gain Ratio maximizes the mutual information between the selected features and the class labels. The numerical results are obtained utilizing the proposed coalition–game theoretic method where the multi–perturbation Shapley value is calculated for coalitions' size up to 4, $L = 4$.

The alarm typing rate for all feature selection methods are evaluated in combination with Bayes Net classification as a representative classifier. In all simulations, the 30 most informative features are selected to compare the performance of different feature selection techniques. The comparison results in Fig. 1 suggest a considerable improvement for the proposed method in discarding the false alarms compared to the competitor methods. The alarm typing success rate for the proposed method is about 75 % meaning that only 25 % of alarms are deemed false, whereas the false alarm report rate for the best competitor method (Gain Ratio) is at least $100 - 68.88\% \approx 31\%$. The improvement is due to potential synergy impact of coalitions among features which is overlooked or not directly addressed in other methods. The proposed method outperforms the case of incorporating all wavelet coefficients (represented by None in Fig. 1) due to eliminating the irrelevant features. Another important observation in Fig. 1 is the obtained success rate using feature set 1 (Statistical features) is slightly better than that of feature set 2 (Entropy–based features), meaning that feature set 1 provides more useful information in recognizing the true alarms. Interestingly, this is consistent among all feature selection methods. Although feature set 2 is relatively successful in identifying the true alarms, however adding it to the statistical features does not enhance alarm typing success rate suggesting that it does not bear additional information. It is notable that the promising rate of 75 % is obtained using only 30 statistical features for any subject, which significantly reduces the risk of over fitting compared to using all 18000 wavelet coefficients for each signal.

Figure 2 presents the average appearance of the 15 extracted statistical features in the six DWT levels for three ECG, PLETH and APB signals in identifying alarm validity for different feature selection methods. The average over all methods is also depicted in Fig. 2. This figure reveals that all statistical properties contribute almost equally to the false alarm recognition. However, there is a significant difference in the contribution of various signal source levels. The average appearance of statistical features and signals are re–depicted in Fig. 3. It is clear from the results in Fig. 3 that the first level of discrete wavelet transform for *ECG* and *PLETH* signals play a more significant role in the alarm validation. Indeed, the collective contribution of levels 2 to 6 are less than the contribution of level 1 solely. However, all levels of signal *APB signal* contribute almost equally for alarm recognition.

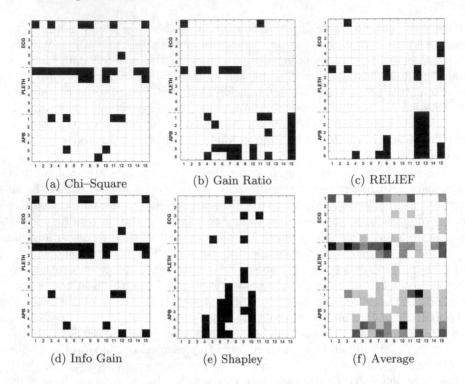

Fig. 2. Average appearance of the 15 extracted statistical features in the six DWT levels for three ECG, PLETH and APB signals

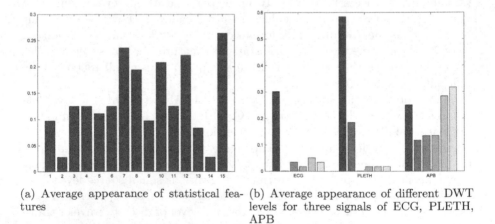

(a) Average appearance of statistical features

(b) Average appearance of different DWT levels for three signals of ECG, PLETH, APB

Fig. 3. Average results for different feature selection techniques

5 Conclusion

In this paper, we proposed a novel coalition–based game theoretic model to improve the accuracy of false alarm detection as one of the critical yet unresolved concerns in intensive care units. In this study, the three signals of ECG, PLETH and ABP from Physion Net's MIMIC II database were considered. First, each of these signals were decomposed into 6 levels using discrete wavelet transform, resulting in total of 18 vectors for each patient. Then, several statistical and information–theoretic features were extraced from these wavelet decomposed vectors in order to reduce the computational complexity and lower the possibility of overfitting in false alarm detection. Finally, these features were fed to the proposed game–theoretic feature selection method as the players of a coalition game. The impact of each feature in the game was defined as its contribution to improve the false alarm detection accuracy in interaction with other features when they form a coalition and it was measured by Multi–perturbation Shapely for coalitions of size 4. The proposed model can be applied to any commonly used classification methods. The numerical results in this paper were presented for Bayes Net classification technique. The results show the significant performance of the proposed model in false alarm detection comparing to other feature selection techniques including Chi–square, Gain Ratio, Relief and Info Gain methods.

References

1. Reducing false arrhythmia alarms in the ICU. http://www.physionet.org/challenge/2015/. Accessed 7 September 2015
2. Afghah, F., Razi, A., Abedi, A.: Stochastic game theoretical model for packet forwarding in relay networks. Springer Telecommunication Systems Journal, Special Issue on Mobile Computing and Networking Technologies (2011)
3. Ansermino, J.M.: Intelligent patient monitoring and clinical decision making. In: Ehrenfeld, J.M., Cannesson, M. (eds.) Monitoring Technologies in Acute Care Environments, pp. 401–407. Springer, New York (2014)
4. Baumgartner, B., Rodel, K., Knoll, A.: A data mining approach to reduce the false alarm rate of patient monitors. In: Engineering in Medicine and Biology Society (EMBC), 2012 Annual International Conference of the IEEE, pp. 5935–5938. IEEE (2012)
5. Behar, J., Oster, J., Li, Q., Clifford, G.D.: ECG signal quality during arrhythmia and its application to false alarm reduction. IEEE Trans. Biomed. Eng. **60**(6), 1660–1666 (2013)
6. Charbonnier, S., Gentil, S.: On-line adaptive trend extraction of multiple physiological signals for alarm filtering in intensive care units. Int. J. Adapt. Control Signal Process. **24**(5), 382–408 (2010)
7. Clifford, G., Aboukhalil, A., Sun, J., Zong, W., Janz, B., Moody, G., Mark, R.: Using the blood pressure waveform to reduce critical false ECG alarms. In: Computers in Cardiology, 2006, pp. 829–832. IEEE (2006)
8. Cohen, S., Dror, G., Ruppin, G.: Feature selection via coalitional game theory. Neural Comput. **19**(7), 1939–1961 (2007)
9. Cvach, M.: Monitor alarm fatigue: an integrative review. Biomed. Instrum. Technol. **46**(4), 268–277 (2012)

10. Fan, J., Samworth, R., Wu, Y.: Ultrahigh dimensional feature selection: beyond the linear model. J. Mach. Learn. Res. **10**, 2013–2038 (2009)
11. Guyon, I., Elisseeff, A.: An introduction to variable and feature selection. J. Mach. Learn. Res. **3**, 1157–1182 (2003). http://dl.acm.org/citation.cfm?id=944919.944968
12. Imhoff, M., Kuhls, S.: Alarm algorithms in critical care monitoring. Anesth. Analg. **102**(5), 1525–1537 (2006)
13. Imhoff, M., Kuhls, S., Gather, U., Fried, R.: Smart alarms from medical devices in the OR and ICU. Best Pract. Res. Clin. Anaesthesiol. **23**(1), 39–50 (2009)
14. Kaufman, A., Kupiec, M., Ruppin, E.: Multi-knockout genetic network analysis: the Rad6 example. In: IEEE Computational Systems Bioinformatics Conference, (CSB 2004), pp. 332–340 (2004)
15. Keinan, A., Sandbank, B., Hilgetag, C., Meilijson, I., Ruppin, E.: Axiomatic scalable neurocontroller analysis via the shapley value. Artif. Life **12**, 333–352 (2006)
16. Lazar, C., Taminau, J., Meganck, S., Steenhoff, D., Coletta, A., Molter, C., de Schaetzen, V., Duque, R., Bersini, H., Nowe, A.: A survey on filter techniques for feature selection in gene expression microarray analysis. IEEE/ACM Trans. Comput. Biol. Bioinform. **9**(4), 1106–1119 (2012)
17. Molina, L., Belanche, L., Nebot, A.: Feature selection algorithms: a survey and experimental evaluation. In: Proceedings 2002 IEEE International Conference on Data Mining, ICDM 2003, pp. 306–313 (2002)
18. Philip, E.: Evaluation of medical alarm sounds. Ph.D. thesis, New Jersey Institute of Technology, Department of Biomedical Engineering (2009)
19. Razi, A., Afghah, F., Belle, A., Ward, K., Najarian, K.: Blood loss severity prediction using game theoretic based feature selection. In: IEEE-EMBS International Conferences on Biomedical and Health Informatics (BHI 2014), pp. 776–780 (2014)
20. Razi, A., Afghah, F., Varadan, V.: Identifying gene subnetworks associated with clinical outcome in ovarian cancer using network based coalition game. In: 37th Annual International Conference of the IEEE Engineering in Medicine and Biology Conference (EMBC 2015) (2015)
21. Saeed, M., Villarroel, M., Reisner, A.T., Clifford, G., Lehman, L.W., Moody, G., Heldt, T., Kyaw, T.H., Moody, B., Mark, R.G.: Multiparameter intelligent monitoring in Intensive Care II (MIMIC-II): a public-access Intensive Care Unit database. Criti. Care Med. **39**(5), 952 (2011)
22. Saeys, Y., Inza, I., Larrañaga, P.: A review of feature selection techniques in bioinformatics. Bioinformatics **23**(19), 2507–2517 (2007)
23. Shapley, L.S.: A value for n-person games. In: Kuhn, H.W., Tucker, A.W. (eds.) Contributions to the Theory of Games, vol. 2, pp. 307–317. Princeton University Press, Princeton (1953)
24. Sifuzzaman, M., Islam, M., Ali, M.: Application of wavelet transform and its advantages compared to fourier transform (2009)
25. Sun, X., Liu, Y., Li, J., Zhu, J., Chen, H., Liu, X.: Feature evaluation and selection with cooperative game theory. Pattern Recogn. **45**(8), 2992–3002 (2012). http://dx.org/10.1016/j.patcog.2012.02.001
26. Tibshirani, R.: Regression shrinkage and selection via the lasso: a retrospective. J. Roy. Stat. Soc. **73**(3), 273–282 (2011)

Information Credibility: A Probabilistic Graphical Model for Identifying Credible Influenza Posts on Social Media

Qiaozhen Guo[1(✉)], Wei (Wayne) Huang[1], Kai Huang[2], and Xiao Liu[3]

[1] School of Management, Xi'an Jiaotong University, Xi'an, China
guoquaozhen@163.com, whuang@mail.xjtu.edu.cn
[2] School of Computer Science, Fudan University, Shanghai, China
khuangl4@fudan.edu.cn
[3] Department of Management Information Systems,
University of Arizona, Tucson, USA
xiaoliu@email.arizona.edu

Abstract. Social media is an important data source to compliment traditional epidemic surveillance. However, misinformation in social media hinders the exploitation of valuable information. Analysis of information credibility has drawn much attention of academia in recent years. In this paper, we focus on analyzing the credibility of influenza posts published on Sina Weibo. We propose a semi-supervised probabilistic graphical model to jointly learn the interactions between user trustworthiness, content reliability, and post credibility. To test the performance of the approach, we apply it to identify credible influenza posts published from May 2013 to June 2014 on Sina Weibo. Random Forests and the Bayesian Network are used as baselines for evaluation. The results show that our approach performs effectively with the highest average accuracy of 71.7 %, f-measure 51 %. Our proposed framework significantly outperformed the baselines in detecting credible influenza posts on Sina Weibo.

Keywords: Credibility · Trustworthiness · Reliability · Objectivity · Probabilistic graphical models · Sina weibo · Influenza

1 Introduction

With the advent of the web 2.0, social media has emerged as a primary source for sharing opinions and experiences. The openness of social media results in a large amount of user-generated content (UGC) that contain inaccurate information, rumors and spams. The incredible information may have negative effects on people's decision-making. It is critical to evaluate the credibility of social media content and avoid false information.

Social media information credibility is particularly important in healthcare domain. Social media data are playing a critical role in patient education and scientific research. It has been used to detect influenza epidemics [1], and extract drug-disease relations [2], and adverse drug reaction [3]. Inaccurate or incredible social media information may significantly impact patients' disease management and result in huge economic cost for public health system.

© Springer International Publishing Switzerland 2016
X. Zheng et al. (Eds.): ICSH 2015, LNCS 9545, pp. 131–142, 2016.
DOI: 10.1007/978-3-319-29175-8_12

Social media information credibility research has attracted attention from many researchers. The major research focuses are to measure the credibility of social media text, to select features for classifying credible and incredible content, and to improve classification methods [4]. The credibility of a post is commonly reflected by the trustworthiness of post authors (e.g., age, gender and location, number of followers) [17], the content reliability of posts (e.g., statement, language objectivity), and etc. [12, 17]. Features for credible content are often times associated. For instance, a statement is more likely to be credible if posted by a trustworthy user or expressed with objective language [17]. However, few considered the interactions between features.

Additionally, analyses of information credibility vary in different languages. They require different natural language processing techniques and features corresponding to specific linguistic contexts [5]. Some studies establish a general conceptual model for recalibrating credibility in different contexts and languages [6]. Most prior information credibility models were applied to English [7], German [8], and Arabic [1]. There were very few studies on Chinese social media credibility. Due to the expansion of Chinese content in recent years, there is a need for automating the task of measuring its credibility.

Our research focuses on measuring the credibility of Chinese text published on Sina Weibo. Sina Weibo[1] is a Chinese microblog service similar to Twitter, where each microblog contains a maximum of 140 Chinese characters. It has shown great promise in detecting epidemics such as influenza [1]. Weibo users post microblogs about influenza a lot during outbreaks, generating reports of epidemics that complement traditional surveillance resources. In addition, Sina Weibo enables real-time surveillance, making them extremely suitable for early stage influenza epidemic detection.

Although Sina Weibo based influenza surveillance potentially offers the advantages noted above, it might contain inaccurate information that biases the influenza epidemics detection results. To address this issue, we propose to develop a semi-supervised probabilistic graphical model to identify credible user-generated posts about influenza. As the significant and commonly used features in prior studies are post content features and user features [11–13, 17], our model jointly learns the interactions between user trustworthiness, content reliability, and post credibility.

The rest of this paper is organized as follows. Section 2 provides a review of relevant literature. We describe our research framework in Sect. 3. Section 4 reports our experiments and discusses the results. Finally, we conclude this paper in Sect. 5.

2   Related Work

There has been an increased interest in credibility research from different domains. The test beds utilized in prior studies generally come from three different types of sources: webpages [9], online discussion forums [10], Twitter [11]. Most of webpages are created by experts or authorities. Information on online discussion forums and Twitter is usually UGC, but the post length on forums is generally greater than that on Twitter.

---

[1] http://www.sina.com.cn.

Table 1. Prior information credibility research on social media

No.	Previous studies	Test bed	Focus	Features	Methods	Results	Language
[10]	Wanas et al. (2008)	Slashdot.org	Rating online discussion posts	Content features[a], User features[b]	Non-linear SVM	Accuracy: 50 % F1-measure: 49 %	English
[11]	Benevenuto et al. (2010)	Twitter	Detect spammers	Content features, User Features	Non-linear SVM	Micro-F1: 88 %	English
[1]	Al-Eidan et al. (2010)	Twitter	Measure the credibility of Arabic text content	Content features, User features	Set the weighted average of features credibility value as the credibility score	Precision: 52 % Recall: 56 %	Arabic
[12]	Castillo et al. (2011)	Twitter	Predict the credibility of the trend of topics	Content features, User features, Transmission features[c]	SVM, Decision trees, Decision rules, Bayes Network	Accuracy: 86 % Precision: 86 % Recall: 86 % F1-measure: 86 %	English
[13]	V. Quzvinianet al. (2011)	Twitter	Identify rumors	Content features, Transmission features	Bayesian classifiers and integration classifiers,	Precision: over 95 %; F1-measure: 90 %	English
[16]	Sondhi et al. (2012)	Medical webpages from Google	Predict reliability of webpages in the medical domain	Content features	SVM	Accuracy: 80 %	English
[15]	Pasternack, J. & Roth, D. (2013)	Internet web data	Analyze multi-source information credibility	Content features	Latent Credibility Analysis (LCA)	Average Accuracy: over 76 %	English
[17]	Mukherjee et al. (2014)	Healthboards.com	Extract rare or unknown side-effects of medical drugs	Content features, User features	Probabilistic Graphical model	Accuracy: 83 % Recall: 82 % F1-measure: 70 %	English

[a]Content features: keywords of domain lexicon, vocabulary, word stem, post length, whether there is emotional word (i.e., sentiment analysis), number of URLs on each post, number of hashtags in each post etc.
[b]User features: age, gender and location, number of posts, questions, replies, authority (or degree in social media), number of followers, and number of people the user follows etc.
[c]Transmission features: information extracted from the propagation tree that is built from the re-tweets.

Additionally, hierarchy on forums endows users different rights to posting, but users on Twitter can freely publish or share real-time messages as well as interact with others (Table 1).

A major objective of prior research is to analyze the credibility of posts about the trend of topics or popular events [1, 10–14]. Pasternack and Roth [15] evaluated the credibility of multi-source claims (i.e., claims generated from different data sources) about book authors, and populations. Some others assessed the reliability of medical webpages [16], and identified credible user statements about rare or unknown side effects of medications [17].

The most commonly used technique is text classification. Classification methods such as Support Vector Machines (SVM), decision trees, and Bayes Network have been adopted in recent studies. SVM and Bayesian classifiers are used to rate online discussion posts [10], and detect spams and rumors [11, 13], and predict reliability of webpages in medical domain [16]. Castillo et al. [12] used SVM, and decision trees, and Bayes Network to predict the credibility of the trending topics. Probabilistic graphical models were also proposed recently, such as the Latent Credibility Analysis (LCA) [15], where the credibility of each claim is a latent variable and the credibility of a source is captured by a set of model parameters. Mukherjee et al. [17] proposed a probabilistic graphical model to jointly learn the interactions between user trustworthiness, post language objectivity, and statement credibility in English context, inferring the credibility labels of user statements on drugs. Differently, we aim to jointly learn the interactions between user and content features in Chinese context, to identify the credibility label of each whole Sina Weibo post.

The significant features in prior studies can be categorized as post content features and user features. Post content features comprise of domain keywords [17], vocabulary [13], word stem [13], post length [12, 17], whether there is emotional word [12], number of URLs on each post [11], number of hashtags in each post [11]. User features are age [12, 17], gender and location [17], number of posts [11, 12, 17], questions [11, 17], replies [11, 12, 17], authority (or degree in social media), number of followers [12, 17], and number of followees [1, 11, 12, 17]. Wanas et al. [10] derived a set of features from post content including keywords relevance and originality, number of URLs, number of hashtags as well, and generated the threaded discussion structure for each post. Quzvinian et al. [13] analyzed the content features like vocabulary, stem words, hashtags, URL etc., and user features like number of posts, replies, and etc. Features of data sources and posts transmission were also utilized in some research [13, 14].

Most studies evaluated their performance using accuracy, precision, recall and F-measure. For classification methods, Castillo et al. [12] achieved an average accuracy of 86 %, precision of 86 %, recall of 86 %, and F-measure of 86 % in predicting the credibility of the trend of topics. Quzvinian et al. [13] obtained excellent performance in identifying rumors on Twitter with a precision of over 95 %, and F-measure of 86 %. Sondhi et al. [16] achieved an overall accuracy of 80 % in predicting reliable medical webpages. With graphical model, Gupta et al. [14] achieved an accuracy of 86 %. Mukherjee et al. [17] achieved an overall accuracy of 82 %, sensitivity of 83 %, recall of 82 %, and F-measure of 70 % in detecting credible user statements on rare or unknown side-effects of medications.

Most prior studies focus on credibility of text in English languages [10–17]. Few studies are performed on Chinese or considered on the interactions between features extracted. As features are interactive and associated, it will significantly increase the statistical power for credibility prediction if we can jointly model the features and their interactions. With this motivation, we try to devise a semi-supervised probabilistic graphical model to identify credible influenza posts on Sina Weibo. Our proposed model captures the important interactions among features between user trustworthiness, content reliability and post credibility, thus may identify credible post with better performance.

3   Research Framework

Our proposed research framework for identifying credible influenza posts is illustrated in Fig. 1. Major components are explained in detail below.

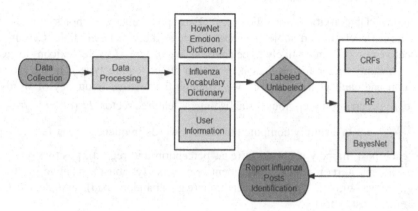

Fig. 1. Research framework for identifying influenza posts

3.1   Data Collection and Preprocessing

An automated crawler was developed to download posts from Sina Weibo. We used text parsers to extract specific fields including ID, URL, post time, post body content, and tags from each post, which were stored in our repository. We collected 128,260 posts about influenza from May 2013 to June 2014. Table 2 shows sample post content. For data preprocessing, we removed stop words, and performed part of speech (POS) tagging. We represented each post as a Bag-of-Words (BOW), and performed POS tagging with the Chinese POS tagger from the NLPIR/ICTCLA 2014 system[2].

Table 2. Sample posts extracted from Sina Weibo

No.	Post body content	Credible influenza post
1	鸭鸭,流感很厉害,多吃板蓝根! (Yaya, the flu is very severe, eat more radix isatidis!)	Yes (or 1)
2	禽流感,该吃点板蓝根神马的呀 (Bird flu, you should eat some radix isatidis)	Yes (or 1)
3	烦躁,喝袋板蓝根,降降火 (Agitated, drink bag of radix isatidis, calm inflammation)	No (or -1)

---

[2] http://ictclas.nlpir.org/.

3.2   Lexicon Based Feature Extraction

We propose a lexicon base approach to extract features for the user trustworthiness and content reliability. The content reliability is measured by language objectivity and statement credibility. User trustworthiness is captured by a set of user features. We create a feature vector for each post.

- Language Objectivity (Affect Features). Each post reflects author's attitude and emotion. Uncertain and subjective posts are less likely to be credible. Certain and objective posts are more likely to be credible. We use the HowNet lexicon[3] to create affect feature vector for each post. For each affect feature type f_i in the Hownet lexicon and each post content c_j, we compute the relative frequency of words of type f_i occurring in c_j, thus establishing a feature vector $F^L(c_j) = <freq_{i,j} = \frac{\#words\ in\ f_i}{length(c_j)}>$. We simply compute the relative words frequency of six feature types for each post, namely proposition (e.g., perception and regard), positive sentiment (e.g., accept, agree), negative sentiment (e.g., anxiety, abuse), positive evaluation (e.g., active, brave), negative evaluation (e.g., abandon, bad), and degree (e.g., extreme, most, very).
- Statement Credibility. Statements here refer to the lexicon-based keywords about influenza. To measure statement credibility, we established an influenza lexicon with information from Chinese Center for Disease Control and Prediction[4], and National Health and Family Planning Commission of the People's Republic of China[5]. The lexicon consists of keywords about influenza such as influenza, fever, headache, cough, and radix isatidis. For each post content c_j, we construct a statement credibility feature vector $<F^S(c_j)>$ using the words of the flu-related lexicon. If the words of the influenza lexicon appear in a post more frequently, the post will be more likely to be a credible influenza post. Sample words related to influenza are demonstrated in Table 3.
- User Features. User trustworthiness is mainly denoted by user' rank or authority in Sina Weibo. It can be measured by number of questions and answers posted), interaction features (e.g., replies, giving thanks), and demographic information (e.g., age, gender). We attempt to capture these aspects in per-user features $<F^U(u_k)>$.

Table 3. Sample influenza keywords

Type	Sample words
Verb	感染(infect) 治疗(treat)
Disease name	流感(influenza) 传染病(contagion) 病毒(virus) 甲型流感(influenza A)
Symptoms	高烧(high fever) 流涕(running nose) 咳嗽(cough)
Treatment name	利巴韦林(ribavirin) 甲基金刚烷胺(methyl amantadine) 板蓝根(radix isatidis) 抗体(antibody) 流感疫苗(influenza vaccine)

---

[3] http://www.cnki.net.
[4] http://www.chinacdc.cn.
[5] http://www.nhfpc.gov.cn.

3.3   A Probabilistic Graphical Model

Our model aims to capture interactions among user trustworthy, content reliability, and post credibility. We model these factors jointly through a probabilistic graphical model called Markov Random Field (MRF). MRF is a Markov network where a set of random variables having Markov property are described by an undirected graph. A Markov network can model dependencies among nodes in the network. Therefore, we adopt MRF to capture interactions between features, where each post is associated with a binary random variable. As to a given post, the corresponding variable should have value 1 if the post is credible, and -1 otherwise. Similarly, the values of content and user variables represent the reliability and trustworthiness of content and users. We formalize the problem of reliability prediction as a semi-supervised binary classification problem. Figure 2 demonstrates our model.

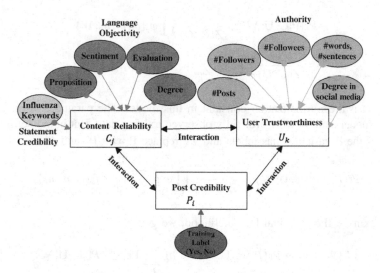

Fig. 2. Overview of the proposed model

The goal of the proposed system is to infer the credibility label of unlabeled posts given expert labeled posts and the observed features. Therefore, the MRF's nodes are connected by the following edges:

- Each user is connected to his or her post(s).
- Each post's content is connected to the post.
- Each user is connected to the content that appears in his or her post.

3.4   Probabilistic Inference

We model our learning task as a Markov Random Field (MRF), where the random variables are the users U, the distinct contents C, and the posts P. This is a semi-supervised model because a subset of posts is manually labeled based on expert databases. Let P^L be the set of posts labeled as yes (or 1, i.e., credible) or no (or -1, i.e., incredible), and let P^U be the set of unlabeled posts. The purpose of this model is to infer credible labels for the posts in P^U.

The cliques in this MRF model are triangles, each consisting of content c_j, a post p_i that contains that content, and a user u_k who wrote this post. $\varphi_i(c_j, p_i, u_k)$ denotes a potential function for clique i. Each clique has a set of associated features and their weight vector W. The individual features and their weight are defined as f_{il} and w_l. The features are composed of the language objectivity, statement credibility (similarity) and user features, which can be represented as: $F_i = F^L(c_j) \cup F^S(c_j) \cup F^U(u_k)$.

As some posts are labeled, we adopt the Conditional Random Fields (CRFs) [18] to compute the joint probability distribution $\Pr(P, C, U)$ and settle for the simple task of estimating the conditional distribution instead of using the standard MRF:

$$\Pr(P|C, U; W) = \frac{1}{Z(C, U)} \prod_i \varphi_i(c_j, p_i, u_k; W)$$

$$= \frac{1}{Z(C, U)} \prod_i \exp(\sum_l w_l \times f_{il}(c_j, p_i, u_k))$$

$Z(C, U)$ is the normalization constant in this model. The parameter estimation in the CRFs model usually works for fully observed training data. But in our setting, only a subset of the P variables has labels and we replace P with P^L and P^U:

$$\Pr(P^U, P^L|C, U; W) = \frac{1}{Z(C, U)} \prod_i \exp(\sum_l w_l \times f_{il}(c_j, p_i, u_k))$$

To maximize the marginal log-likelihood, we get:

$$LL(W) = \log \Pr(P^L|C, U; W) = log \sum_{P^U} \Pr(P^U, P^L|C, U; W)$$

Considering the observed values of P^L in the training data, the distribution over P^U is computed in the following equation:

$$\Pr(P^U, P^L|C, U; W) = \frac{1}{Z(P^L, C, U)} \prod_i \exp\left(\sum_l w_l \times f_{il}(c_j, p_i, u_k)\right)$$

To solve this maximization problem, we adopt the Expectation-Maximization (EM) method. The labels of the variables P^U are estimated from the posterior distribution using Gibbs sampling. The feature weights are estimated by maximizing the log-likelihood:

$$E - Step : q(P^U) = \Pr\left(P^U|P^L, C, U; W^{(v)}\right)$$

$$M - \text{Step} : W^{(v+1)} = argmax_{W'} \sum_{P^U} q(P^U) log Pr(P^L, P^U | C, U; W')$$

The update step to sample the labels of P^U variables by Gibbs sampling is given by:

$$Pr\left(P_i^U | C, U, P^L; W\right) \propto t_k \times \varphi_i\left(c_j, P_i, u_k; W\right)$$

Where t_k equals to 1 if p_i is assigned to be a credible influenza post in the previous EM iteration, otherwise t_k equals to 0. The Limited-memory Broyden-Fletcher-Goldfarb-Shanno (L − BFGS) method is used in the M-step. Therefore, the label of a post is determined by content credibility and the trustworthiness of the user.

3.5   Evaluation

We compare our model to two classic baselines commonly utilized in the literature, Random Forests (RF) and Bayesian Network (BayesNet), with the same features. It's worth mentioning that we don't report the performance of the Support Vector Machine (SVM) here, as it usually works similarly to the Bayesian Network dealing with binary classification. We leave it as the future work. To evaluate the performance of our model and the baselines, we use the standard measure accuracy, precision, recall, and f-measure, which are defined as follows:

$$accuracy = \frac{tp^9 + tn^{10}}{tp + tn + fp^{11} + fn^{12}}$$

$$precison = \frac{tp}{tp + fp}$$

$$recall = \frac{tp}{tp + fn}$$

$$f - measure = \frac{2 * precision * recall}{precision + recall}$$

We consider the posts labeled "yes" or 1 as positive ground truth, whereas all other posts labeled "no" or −1 are considered to be negative instances. We randomly selected 3000 out of 128260 posts and trained three medical research cooperators to label them. These 3000 labeled posts became the golden standard for credible influenza posts detection, among which 1217 posts are labeled as "yes" (i.e., positive), 1783 posts are labeled as "no" (i.e., negative). We then randomly selected another 3000 out of the remaining unlabeled 125260 posts as a subset of test set. We finally conducted 5-fold cross validation to obtain the evaluation results for credible influenza posts identification. Each time 80 % of the labeled posts and all the 3000 unlabeled were used as training set and 20 % of the labeled posts were used as test set. Our model and all the baselines used the same features and test sets.

4   Results and Discussions

Table 4 shows the evaluation results of our model and the baselines.

Table 4. Accuracy and precision of models

Method	Accuracy	Precision	Recall	F-measure
CRFs	0.711677	0.468085	0.563473	0.511336
RF	0.68343	0.416085	0.441317	0.428315
BayesNet	0.671677	0.409639	0.407186	0.408408

We find that our CRFs model achieves the highest accuracy, precision and f-measure compared to the baselines. Our model brings an accuracy improvement of 2.8 % and an overall 5.2 % increase in precision over the Random Forests baseline. It also achieves an accuracy improvement of 4 % and 5.8 % increase in precision over the Bayesian Network. Our model performs the best in identifying credible influenza posts on Sina Weibo.

To test performance significance, we adopted Fisher's Exact Test to test the following 3×2 contingency table for influenza posts identification based on the 3000 labeled posts. Table 5 demonstrates that the p value is below 0.01. The associations between methods and outcomes are significant.

Table 5. Performance significance test

Influenza posts detection	tp + tn	fp + fn
CRFs	2364	636
RF	2041	959
BayesNet	1954	1046
Sig. 0.000 (P Value) < 0.01		

5   Conclusion and Future Work

In this paper, we develop a semi-supervised probabilistic graphical model to identify credible influenza posts on Sina Weibo. Our model jointly learns the interactions among user trustworthy, content reliability, and post credibility. Compared to the baselines, our approach performs the best in identifying credible posts with an accuracy of 71.2 %. Our framework significantly outperforms the baselines.

To improve the performance, we would like to evaluate features such as the microblogging elements (hash tag, mention, and URL), and the transmission characteristics (the depth of the micro blog spread tree). There could be possible associations between them and credibility. In addition, a better natural language processing method for Chinese text as well as a more sophisticated information extraction approach can further improve our approach. Additionally, it's worth testing that what the results will be if only content features or user features are used in this proposed model. Also, as noted in Sect. 3.5, we will further study whether our model outperforms the Support Vector Machine (SVM) or not.

Finally, this model can be used in some other applications oriented use-cases, such as extracting adverse drug events, predicting influenza tendency. It can also be applied to analyze the credibility of online drugs and goods comments, which will contribute to the healthcare field and the general market surveillance.

Acknowledgements. We thank Jingwei Li, Qihui Xia, and Lidan Chen for the help with pre-processing and labeling data. We also show our great appreciation to professor Hsinchun Chen for the help with revising this paper. We finally would like to thank all the reviewers for their modification suggestions.

References

1. Al-Eidan, R., Al-Khalifa H., Al-Salman A.: Measuring the credibility of arabic text content in Twitter. In: 2010 Fifth International Conference on Digital Information Management (ICDIM), pp. 285–291. IEEE (2010)
2. Yang, C.C., Yang, H., Jiang, L., Zhang, M.: Social media mining for drug safety signal detection. In: Proceedings of the 2012 International Workshop on Smart Health and Wellbeing, pp. 33–40. ACM (2012)
3. Yang, H., Yang, C.C.: Harnessing social media for drug-drug interactions detection. In: 2013 IEEE International Conference on Healthcare Informatics (ICHI), pp. 22–29. IEEE (2013)
4. Gupta, A., Kumaraguru, P.: Credibility ranking of tweets during high impact events. In: Proceedings of the 1st Workshop on Privacy and Security in Online Social Media, p. 2. ACM (2012)
5. Yang, J., Counts, S., Morris, M.R., Hoff, A.: Microblog credibility perceptions: comparing the USA and China. In: Proceedings of the 2013 Conference on Computer Supported Cooperative Work, pp. 575–586. ACM (2013)
6. AlMansour, A.A., Brankovic, L., Iliopoulos, C.S.: A model for recalibrating credibility in different contexts and languages-a Twitter case study. Int. J. Digital Inf. Wirel. Commun. (IJDIWC) **4**(1), 53–62 (2014)
7. Walter, Z.: Web credibility and stickiness of content web sites. In: International Conference on Wireless Communications, Networking and Mobile Computing, pp. 3820–3823. IEEE (2007)
8. Juffinger, A., Granitzer, M., Lex, E.: Blog credibility ranking by exploiting verified content. In: Proceedings of the 3rd Workshop on Information Credibility on the Web, pp. 51–58. ACM (2009)
9. Vydiswaran, V., Zhai, C., Roth, D.: Content-driven trust propagation framework. In: Proceedings of the 17th ACM SIGKDD International Conference on Knowledge Discovery and Data Mining, pp. 974–982. ACM (2011)
10. Wanas, N., El-Saban, M., Ashour, H., Ammar, W.: Automatic scoring of online discussion posts. In: Proceedings of the 2nd ACM Workshop on information Credibility on the Web, pp. 19–26. ACM (2008)
11. Benevenuto, F., Magno, G., Rodrigues, T., Almeida, V.: Detecting spammers on Twitter. In: Collaboration, Electronic Messaging, Anti-abuse and Spam Conference (CEAS), vol. 6, p. 12 (2010)

12. Castillo, C., Mendoza, M., Poblete, B.: Information credibility on Twitter. In: Proceedings of the 20th International Conference on World Wide Web, pp. 675–684. ACM (2011)
13. Qazvinian, V., Rosengren, E., Radev, D.R., Mei, Q.: Rumor has it: identifying misinformation in microblogs. In: Proceedings of the Conference on Empirical Methods in Natural Language Processing, pp. 1589–1599. Association for Computational Linguistics (2011)
14. Gupta, M., Zhao, P., Han, J.: Evaluating event credibility on Twitter. In: SDM, pp. 153–164. SIAM (2012)
15. Pasternack, J., Roth, D.: Latent credibility analysis. In: Proceedings of the 22nd International Conference on World Wide Web, pp. 1009–1020. International World Wide Web Conferences Steering Committee (2013)
16. Sondhi, P., Vydiswaran, V., Zhai, C.: Reliability prediction of webpages in the medical domain. In: Baeza-Yates, R., de Vries, A.P., Zaragoza, H., Cambazoglu, B., Murdock, V., Lempel, R., Silvestri, F. (eds.) ECIR 2012. LNCS, vol. 7224, pp. 219–231. Springer, Heidelberg (2012)
17. Mukherjee, S., Weikum, G., Danescu-Niculescu-Mizil, C.: People on drugs: credibility of user statements in health communities. In: Proceedings of the 20th ACM SIGKDD International Conference on Knowledge Discovery and Data Mining, pp. 65–74. ACM (2014)
18. Lafferty, J., McCallum, A., Pereira, F.C.: Conditional Random Fields: Probabilistic Models for Segmenting and Labeling Sequence Data (2001)

Arrhythmia Classification Using Biosignal Analysis and Machine Learning Techniques

Jesus E. Nivia[1], Yesika M. Ramírez[1], and Jorge E. Camargo[2](✉)

[1] Systems and Industrial Engineering Department,
National University of Colombia, Bogotá, Colombia
{jenivial,yemramirezca}@unal.edu.co
[2] Laboratory for Advanced Computational Science and Engineering Research,
Antonio Nariño University, Bogotá, Colombia
jorgecamargo@uan.edu.co

Abstract. The Electrocardiogram (ECG) can provide valuable information for medical diagnosis and diseases prevention. This paper presents an algorithm for arrhythmia classification based on frequency domain analysis of ECG biosignals. Our approach includes the use of Support Vector Machines (SVM) to identify seven different types of beats and four types of arrhythmia. Different feature sets were tested using the MIT-BIH arrhythmia database and a classification accuracy of 95.79 % was achieved.

Keywords: Arrithmia detection · Biosignal analysis · Spectral frequency · SVM

1 Introduction

The hearts electrical activity produces signals that radiate through the surrounding tissue to the skin. In order to capture this signal, electrodes are attached to the skin and electrical signals are transmitted to an ECG monitor [12]. The analysis of the information provided by an electrocardiogram is a valuable tool in the diagnosis of heart diseases. An example of the utility of ECG signal analysis is arrhythmia detection. Abnormal changes in heart normal rhythm could result in a serious damage or even the death. Many approaches have been proposed for the detection of abnormal cardiac rhythms and automatic classification. Most of them are based on different strategies for extracting features from the ECG signal. Mohamed et al. [14] describe a feature extraction algorithm based on Daubechies wavelets in order to detect the QRS complex (Q, R and S waves).

Another automatic feature extraction method is presented in [13] by Chazal et al. Once fiducial points have been identified, the RR intervals are measured and the length of each QRS complex is calculated. Morphological features are extracted using two sampling windows that take 10 samples. The first window describes the behavior of the QRS, the second window describes the ST segment.

Most of the extracted features for automatic arrhythmia classification are based on standard features. Authors in [15] developed a detection system based

© Springer International Publishing Switzerland 2016
X. Zheng et al. (Eds.): ICSH 2015, LNCS 9545, pp. 143–153, 2016.
DOI: 10.1007/978-3-319-29175-8_13

on the Short-time Fourier transform (STFT) and the time frequency distribution (TDF) features, showing that the ECG signal could provide useful ECG information as the same as standard clinical features used by doctors.

In this paper, we describe a classification method that uses seven different beat types and four arrhythmia classes. A SVM is trained to perform the beat type classification task and a finite state machine is used for arrhythmia classification. The features are extracted using spectral methods and the interval between two successive beats.

The paper is organized as follows: Sect. 2 describes the background and related work focusing especially in the contributions that have been done in the analysis of biosignals and learning models for arrhythmia classification; Sect. 3 presents materials and methods used for the development of the proposed method; Sect. 4 shows experiments and results; and finally, in Sect. 5 conclusions and future work are presented.

2 Background and Related Work

In this section two approaches to analyze an ECG signal are presented, first the analysis from a doctor point of view is described, second the suitable use of spectral analysis for Arrhythmia detection is explained. Additionally, previous studies that proposed arrhythmia classification algorithms using machine learning techniques are summarized.

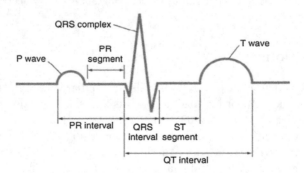

Fig. 1. Example of a normal complex QRS [6].

2.1 Standard Clinical ECG Features

In order to diagnosis a cardiac disease a doctor can extract useful information from an ECG record. Generally, the features extracted are measures of timing intervals and amplitudes. A normal cardiac complex consists of 5 waves called P, Q, R, S and T. A medical diagnosis is based on the presence or absence or certain waves and on measures of the length of fiducial points intervals [6]. Figure 1 shows an example of a normal QRS complex.

2.2 Spectral Analysis of the ECG

The frequency spectrum of a signal is a representation of its signal's power and phase distribution in the frequency domain. Particularly, ventricular arrhythmias manifest significant disturbances in the ECG [4]. These changes in the rhythm can even deform the signal to the point where the main fiducial points P, Q, R, S and T can not be recognized. For an arrhythmia detection, the spectral analysis of the ECG signal can provide useful information about the abnormalities presented in the morphology of the signal in the cases where the classic clinical approach becomes unpractical.

2.3 Learning Models for Arrhythmia Classification

The use of machine learning techniques has become an important tool to recognize diseases. For cardiac diseases, the application of learning models in the analysis of ECG signals is a key factor.

Authors in [7] compare the performance of three models based on neural networks for the classification of the arrhythmia types defined in the UCI dataset. The proposed models include a multilayer perceptron neural network (MLP), a generalized feed forward neural network, and a modular neural network. Using the records of an ECG of 12 leads and the MLP with 2 hidden layers, the obtained results show an accuracy of 86,67 %.

A learning model based on tree decision was presented by Mondal et al. in [9]. This model classifies correctly five types of arrhythmia using the length of fiducial points intervals, presence of P wave, and others features that are commonly used to make diagnosis.

A third example of learning models is the classification algorithm known as K-Nearest Neighbors (K-NN). This algorithm classifies unknown patterns measuring the distance between instances with respect to a trained pattern already known [8]. The distances are sorted and the first k samples are selected. Kirtania and Mali present in [10] the use of an optimal feature set and the implementation of the K-NN algorithm for the classification of five beat types achieving a precision of 98.87 %

Finally, authors in [11] describe the use of support vector machines for arrhythmia classification. Authors study different approaches to classify instances using strategies such as one against one, decision directed acyclic graph, fuzzy decision function and one against all. Authors claim that the performance evaluation was improved after applying Principal Component Analysis (PCA).

3 Materials and Methods

The classification method proposed in this paper is composed of three stages: (1) A pre-processing step is conducted to segment the ECG signal using methods applied to the frequency domain to extract a set of features; (2) The extracted features are used for training a set of support vector machines to perform beat classification; and (3) The detection of arrhythmic segments is carried out using a finite-state machine, which receives as input the outputs of the support vector machines. An overview of the method is depicted in Fig. 2.

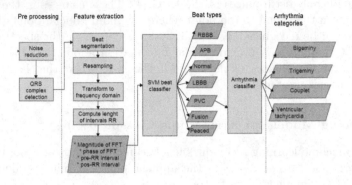

Fig. 2. Block diagram of the proposed arrhythmia classifier.

3.1   Dataset

The ECG records were selected from the MIT-BIH arrhythmia database [1], which contains 48 half-hour excerpts of two-channel ambulatory ECG recordings. Figure 3 illustrates an example of such signals. In this study, only records from the first channel were selected, each one with a signal frequency of 360 Hz. After the segmentation step, we obtained 102,250 beats instances. These instances contain seven ECG beat types, including the normal beat (N), the left bundle branch block beat (LBBB), the right bundle branch block beat (RBBB), the atrial premature beat (APB), the premature ventricular contraction (PVC), the peaced beat (P), and the fusion beat between a PVC and a Normal beat (F).

From the obtained set of records, 90 % of each beat type were used for training and 10 % for test, using the classical 10-fold cross-validation setup. The number of instances per beat type is presented in Table 1.

3.2   Signal Pre-processing and Feature Extraction

We pre-processed the ECG signal applying noise reduction, QRS complex detection, and beat segmentation for feature extraction. The first and second steps were carried out with the QRS detection algorithm developed by Pan and Tompkins [2]. The location of the R-peaks are used to divide the ECG signal into segments delimited by two successive RR intervals.

For feature extraction, each beat segment was re-sampled to reach a normalized length of 100 samples and transformed to the frequency domain using the Fast Fourier transform (FFT). Four features were extracted to train the beat classifier: The magnitude of FFT, phase of FFT, length of the pre-interval RR, and length of pos-interval RR.

Table 1. Beat types in the dataset

Beat type	Instances
Normal	7290
LBBB	806
RBBB	725
APB	253
PVC	707
Peaced	361
Fusion	79

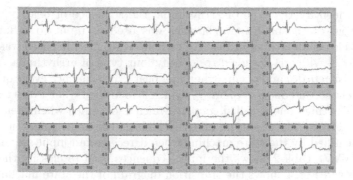

Fig. 3. MIT-BIH signals.

3.3 Beats Classification Using SVM

According to [4], the SVM is already regarded as the most efficient tool for classification problems. A SVM works in a high-dimensional feature space formed by a nonlinear mapping of the original N-dimensional input vector x, into a k-dimensional feature space through the use of a function $\varphi(x)$. The goal of a SVM is to find the hyperplane that best separates the feature vectors into different classes. The equation of that hyperplane is as follows:

$$y(x) = W^T \varphi(x) + w_0,$$

where $\varphi(x) = [\varphi_1(x), \varphi_2(x), ..., \varphi_k(x)]^T$, W is the weight vector of the network, $W = [w_1, w_2, ..., w_k]$, and w_0 is the bias. All mathematical operations are done using a kernel function $K(x, x')$, which is the inner product of the vector $\varphi(x)$. In the approach proposed the radial basis function kernel was used with parameters $C = 32$ and $\gamma = 0.5$. The C parameter controls the trade-off between the width of the separation margin and the γ parameter defines how big is the influence of a single training example.

$$K(x, x') = exp(\gamma|x - x'|),$$

Given that SVM separates data into two classes and there are seven types of beats to be classified, the implementation of a multi-class classifier was done by applying the *one against one* strategy. With n equals to the number of classes, n * (n − 1) / 2 classifiers were constructed and each classifier was trained with data from two classes.

A simple integration approach to define the winner class for each input feature vector consisted of considering a majority vote across all trained classifiers. The algorithm was implemented using the library *sklearn.svm*, which is a python wrapper for the *LibSVM* library [5].

3.4   Arrhythmia Classification Using a Finite-State Machine

In order to identify the type of arrhythmia, the sequence of beat types given by the output of the beat type classifier was used as input to a finite state machine, which is illustrated in Fig. 4. The finite state machine used was the one proposed in [3] which is designed to identify four type of arrhythmia. The first one is called *bigeminy* and occurs when in a beat type sequence every other beat is a PVC. The second one is *trigeminy*, which is identified when every third beat is a PVC. The third one is called *couplet*, which is obtained when there are two consecutive PVCs. The last type of arrhythmia is the ventricular tachycardia, which is identified by the state machine when it receives an input sequence beat type like *VVV. Table 2 shows the input sequences used to classify the type of arrhythmia and Fig. 4 shows the transition diagram of the state machine.

Table 2. Input sequences accepted by the finite state machine

Type arryhthmia	Regular expression
Bigeminy	*NV
Trigeminy	*NNV
Couplet	*VV
Ventricular Tachycardia	*VVV

Given the deterministic nature of a finite state machine, errors in arrhythmia classification occur depending on the input beat type sequence received from the SVM. In next section, experiments carried out to evaluate the accuracy of the SVM classifier are described.

4   Experiments and Results

4.1   Feature Combination

In order to test the performance of the SVM with different feature vectors, four feature sets were created.

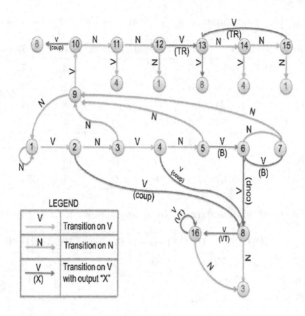

Fig. 4. Finite state machine [3].

- **Feature set 1**: consists of the FFT magnitude of the beat segment already re-sampled to 100 samples. This feature set give us a total of 101 attributes.
- **Feature set 2**: a vector with the FFT phase information is concatenated to the FFT magnitud for a total of 201 attributes.
- **Feature set 3**: formed by concatenating the length of the pre-RR and pos-RR interval to the previous set giving as result a vector of 203 attributes.
- **Feature set 4**: includes the FFT magnitud, the length of the pre-RR and pos-RR interval for a total of 103 attributes.

A set of experiments were conducted to evaluate accuracy for each of the 4 feature sets. We followed a 10-fold cross validation setup. Results are presented in

Table 3. Confusion matrix of the beat classifier for feature set 1

Type	APB	N	PVC	Peaced	Fusion	LBBB	RBBB
APB	168	69	3	0	0	2	11
Normal	16	7147	83	0	10	22	12
PVC	4	134	553	3	2	7	4
Peaced	0	8	7	346	0	0	0
Fusion	0	28	7	0	43	1	0
LBBB	0	42	11	0	0	752	1
RBBB	13	60	3	0	0	1	648

Table 4. Confusion matrix of the beat classifier for feature set 2

Type	APB	N	PVC	Peaced	Fusion	LBBB	RBBB
APB	167	71	5	0	0	3	7
Normal	28	7170	43	0	10	15	24
PVC	3	84	606	1	4	8	1
Peaced	0	20	5	335	0	1	0
Fusion	0	23	4	0	50	2	0
LBBB	1	55	5	1	0	743	1
RBBB	4	67	0	0	0	1	653

Table 5. Confusion matrix of the beat classifier for feature set 3

Type	APB	N	PVC	Peaced	Fusion	LBBB	RBBB
APB	185	59	3	0	1	1	4
Normal	17	7200	28	0	5	23	17
PVC	5	78	615	0	5	3	1
Peaced	0	22	3	336	0	0	0
Fusion	0	28	5	0	44	1	1
LBBB	0	50	4	2	0	748	2
RBBB	3	58	1	0	0	0	663

Tables 3, 4, 5 and 6, respectively. These tables show the corresponding confusion matrices, which allow to evaluate the performance of the classification algorithm.

4.2   Performance Evaluation

The results obtained for each SVM were evaluated using four measures: Precision, root mean squared error (RMSE), kappa statistic and area under ROC curve (Fig. 5).

Precision makes reference to the percentage of correctly classified instances.

The RMSE represents the sample standard deviation of the differences between predicted values and observed values, and is calculated as the square root of the mean/average of the square of all of the error.

$$RMSE = \sqrt{\frac{1}{N}\sum_{i=1}^{N}(y_i - \bar{y}_i)^2}$$

Finally, the kappa statistic is taken into account to compare the Observed Accuracy with the Expected Accuracy. Table 7 shows the results obtained for each SVM classifier trained with the features sets described in the previous subsection.

Table 6. Confusion matrix of the beat classifier for feature set 4

Type	APB	N	PVC	Peaced	Fusion	LBBB	RBBB
APB	177	63	0	0	0	0	13
Normal	17	7170	60	0	7	16	20
PVC	5	96	589	2	8	6	1
Peaced	0	17	6	338	0	0	0
Fusion	0	27	9	0	43	0	0
LBBB	0	40	9	1	2	754	0
RBBB	11	40	3	0	0	0	671

Table 7. Performance of the proposed feature sets

Feature set	Precision	RMSE	Kappa statistic
1	94.48 %	0.1256	0.88
2	95.13 %	0.1179	0.89
3	95.79 %	0.1096	0.90
4	95.31 %	0.1157	0.89

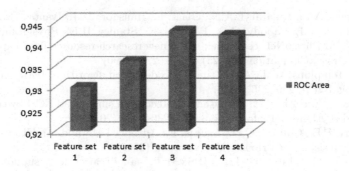

Fig. 5. Area under curves (AUC) for each feature set.

5   Conclusions and Future Work

This paper presented an arrhythmia classification method based on the biosignal analysis in frequency domain. Our study describes and proves the accuracy of an alternative solution to the standard clinical ECG assessment, which only relies on measures of the length of fiducial points intervals and amplitudes.

Four different feature sets were tested to train a Support Vector Machine that classifies seven different types of beat, including the normal beat (N), the left bundle branch block beat (LBBB), the right bundle branch block beat (RBBB), the atrial premature beat (APB), the premature ventricular contraction (PVC), the peaced beat (P) and the Fusion beat between a PVC and a Normal beat (F).

For identifying an arrhythmia category, the output of the SVM classifier was given as input to a finite state machine to classify four types of arrhythmia. Due to the deterministic nature of the state machines, results are dependent on the beat type input sequence to obtain a high accuracy. After performing different experiments for beat classification, a feature set consisted of a concatenated vector with FFT Magnitud, FFT Phase, length of pre-RR interval and length of pos-RR interval showed the best performance. Using a vector with this feature set, a precision of 95.7 % was achieved, a root mean squared error (RMSE) of 0.1096 and a Kappa statistic of 0.9086.

Given that atrial arrhythmias are difficult to detect through spectral methods but manifest significantly changes in the beat-to-beat timing, the inclusion of analysis in time domain is proposed for achieving a broader number of arrhythmia classes in the classifier.

Acknowledgements. We thank Dr. Guillermo Mora of the Internal Medicine Department, Faculty of Medicine at National University of Colombia for his contributions in the understanding of the medical concepts behind an arrhythmia.

References

1. Goldberger, A.L., Amaral, L.A.N., Glass, L., Hausdor, J.M., Ivanov, PCh., Mark, R.G., Mietus, J.E., Moody, G.B., Peng, C.-K., Stanley, H.E.: PhysioBank, Physio Toolkit, and PhysioNet: components of a new research resource for complex physiologic signals. Circulation **101**(23), e215–e220 (2000)
2. Pan, J., Tompkins, W.J.: A real-time QRS detection algorithm. IEEE Trans. Biomed. Eng. **32**(3), 230–236 (1985)
3. Pathangay, V., Rath, S.P.: Arrhythmia detection in single-lead ECG by combining beat and rhythm-level information, pp. 3236–3239 (2014)
4. McSharry, P.E., Clifford, G.D., Azuaje, F.: Advanced Methods and Tools for ECG Data Analysis. Artech House Inc., Norwood (2006)
5. Chang, C.-C., Lin, C.-J.: LIBSVM : a library for support vector machines. ACM Trans. Intell. Syst. Technol. **2**, 27: 1–27: 27 (2011). http://www.csie.ntu.edu.tw/cjlin/libsvm
6. Todd, J.W.: The only EKG book you'll ever need. Plast. Reconstr. Surg. **84**, 842 (1989)
7. Jadhav, S.M.: Artificial neural network models based cardiac arrhythmia disease diagnosis from ECG signal data. Int. J. Comput. Appl. **44**, 8–13 (2012)
8. Ethem, A.: Introduction to Machine Learning, 2nd edn. MIT Press, Cambridge (2010)
9. Mondal, P.: Cardiac arrhythmias classification using decision tree. Int. J. Adv. Res. Comput. Sci. Softw. Eng. **5**(1), 540–542 (2015)
10. Kaur, N., Manna, M.S., Dewan, R.: Int. J. Adv. Res. Comput. Sci. Softw. Eng. vol. 3(1), pp. 332–338 (2013)
11. Kohli, N., Verma, N.: Arrhythmia classification using SVM with selected features. Int. J. Eng. Sci. Technol. **3**(8), 122–131 (2012)
12. L.W. and Wilkins.: ECG Interpretation Made Incredibly Easy
13. Mohamed, M.A.: An approach for ECG feature extraction using daubechies 4 (DB4) wavelet. Int. J. Comput. Appl. **96**(12), 36–41 (2014)

14. De Chazal, P.D.C.P., ODwyer, M., Reilly, R.B.: Automatic classification of heart-beats using ECG morphology and heartbeat interval features. IEEE Trans. Biomed. Eng. **51**(7), 1196–1206 (2004)
15. Tsipouras, M.G., Fotiadis, D.I.: Automatic arrhythmia detection based on time and time-frequency analysis of heart rate variability. Comput. Meth. Programs Biomed. **74**, 95–108 (2004)

Health Data Analysis and Management

Skin Resistance as a Physiological Indicator for Quadriplegics with Spinal Cord Injuries During Activities of Daily Living

Shruthi Suresh[1(✉)], Han Duerstock[2,3], and Bradley Duerstock[1,2]

[1] Weldon School of Biomedical Engineering, Purdue University,
West Lafayette, IN, USA
{suresh9, bsd}@purdue.edu
[2] School of Industrial Engineering, Purdue University, West Lafayette, IN, USA
[3] Arizona State University, Tempe, AZ, USA
hduersto@asu.edu

Abstract. Approximately 30–50 % of all persons with a spinal cord injury (SCI) are rehospitalized every year due to secondary health complications. One of the more common post-SCI health conditions is Autonomic Dysreflexia (AD). Key physiological indicators in the detection of AD are paroxysmal increase of blood pressure and sweating above the spinal cord injury level. In this paper we developed a system to measure galvanic skin resistance and use it to study the changes in skin perspiration and pulse in nine individuals with cervical SCIs while they were performing activities of daily living (ADL). A significantly lower skin resistance was detected above the injury site compared to areas below the injury site. As the subjects performed activities of different exertion levels, there was a significant decrease in the skin resistance above the injury site. Additionally, as anxiety levels increased during activities, skin resistance decreased. The application of skin resistance sensors has been shown to be a reliable detection method of naturally-occurring anomalous variations in the skin resistance among quadriplegics due to SCI in order to identify the onset of AD during typical ADL. A possible implication of this study is to provide long-term physiological monitoring of quadriplegics to alert them and their caregivers of the occurrence of AD.

Keywords: Cervical spinal cord injury · Autonomic dysreflexia · Skin resistance · Wearable · Telemetry · Galvanic skin response

1 Introduction

There are currently 276,000 Americans with spinal cord injury (SCI) and it is estimated that there are approximately 12,500 new cases of SCI every year in the United States alone. Approximately 30–50 % of all persons with a SCI are rehospitalized every year due to secondary health complications [24]. One of the more common post-SCI health conditions is Autonomic Dysreflexia (AD). AD is caused by hyperreflexia of the sympathetic nervous system due to an irritation to the body below the injury site. If the irritation is not removed, then AD will escalate rapidly resulting in hypertension, which

© Springer International Publishing Switzerland 2016
X. Zheng et al. (Eds.): ICSH 2015, LNCS 9545, pp. 157–168, 2016.
DOI: 10.1007/978-3-319-29175-8_14

can lead to seizures, stroke or even death [21]. Key indicators of AD include a sudden increase in blood pressure, altered heart rate, sweating, flushing, cold and clammy skin, and headaches [5, 13, 16]. Typical irritations that result in AD include an extended bladder, full bowel, injuries to the body below the level of SCI, and sexual activity [15]. In some individuals and instances, it is difficult to identify or rectify what has triggered the acute elevation in blood pressure, and immediate pharmaceutical medical attention is required [18]. In cases where AD is not managed properly, it can be life threatening. Several papers discussed the monitoring of heart rate and blood pressure as ways to study AD and the effects of drugs to control AD in persons with SCI [1, 14, 17, 30]. Another common symptom to identify the onset of AD is sweating, which can be detected by changes in skin resistance. Galvanic Skin Response (GSR) is a change in skin resistance due to the activation of sweat glands to stimuli and it is usually measured by the resistance between a pair of externally placed electrodes attached or adhered to the skin [23]. GSR has been used in previous studies to reliably and conveniently monitor various SCI related health conditions [27] and is often used to study conditions such as erectile dysfunction, urinary bladder dysfunction and other autonomic disorders [6, 7, 28, 30].

In this paper we aim to determine baseline skin resistance (SR) values and pulse data in persons with cervical SCI (C3-C7) while performing typical Activities of Daily Living (ADL) such as typing, using a computer, and wheelchair operation. This information is essential in the conception of a physiological monitoring system that could continuously detect anomalous skin resistance (sweating), which could be symptomatic of AD. Such a monitoring system would be beneficial to newly spinal cord injured quadriplegics to better understand when AD has occurred in order to prevent escalation of this health condition. Current systems which detect the galvanic skin resistance of individuals with SCI may reduce the users' mobility and is typically confined to a fixed location either being performed at home or institutional setting. The most common age of sustaining a SCI is 19 years old, when a young adult is typically seeking greater independence [24]. A smart telemetry system paired with automatic mobile telephone messaging that detects the onset of AD would provide a level of emergency oversight by caregivers to quadriplegics wherever they go - work, school, grocery shopping etc. This would promote greater independence and community reentry for persons with SCIs, an important part of recovering from this condition, while providing a critical safeguard.

2   Materials and Methods

2.1   Subjects

For this study we recruited nine quadriplegic subjects with SCI (C3-C7). 3 subjects had complete SCI and 6 had incomplete SCI based on subjects' response. Each subject was assigned a unique identification code (baseline (BL) followed by a subject number) to ensure anonymity. The volunteers had a mean age of 38 years and each volunteer had sustained the injury at least 3 years prior to this study (Table 1).

Table 1. Subject description

Subject	Level of injury	Completeness of injury (complete (C)/incomplete (I))	Age	Gender (Male (M)/Female (F))	Time post-injury (years)
BL01	C4/C5	C	44	M	25
BL02	C6	I	44	M	19
BL03	C5/C6	C	25	M	3
BL04	C6/C7	C	41	M	18
BL05	C5/C6	I	27	M	11
BL06	C5/C6	I	43	F	19
BL07	C6/C7	I	44	M	26
BL08	C5	I	55	M	4
BL09	C5/C6	I	18	F	3

The volunteers were recruited through flyers sent out to students at Purdue University and through letters sent out to outpatients at the Rehabilitation Hospital of Indiana (RHI) as approved by the Purdue Institutional Review Board. Exclusion criteria included the inability to type and move any one arm. All subjects had at some level of motor ability in their dominant arm, although none had hand or finger function.

2.2 Galvanic Skin Resistance Sensor

In order to detect changes in the skin resistance, a microcontroller (Arduino®) based system (Fig. 1a) was developed to record a continuous stream of skin resistance values. This system consists of a four electrode-pair sensor array worn by the user on areas above and below the injury site, an Arduino Mini microcontroller, and a Bluetooth transmitter that wirelessly sends data to a Serial terminal on a Bluetooth-enabled computer. The data is transmitted at a sampling rate of 50 samples per second. The electrodes are placed on the Left and Right shoulders (above injury site) and on the Left and Right calves (below injury site). The system was placed on the wheelchair of the user.

To detect pulse, we used the Delsys® Trigno™ EKG Biofeedback Sensor which was attached to the chest of the subjects. The sensor was wirelessly connected to the Trigno™ Lab base receiver and pulse data was captured in real time using the EMGWorks® software at a sampling rate of 50 samples per second. Figure 1b shows the typical configuration of the system worn by subjects.

2.3 Procedure

Quadriplegic subjects due to SCI were asked to perform four tasks of daily life (resting, typing on a computer keyboard, using a mouse and travelling in their wheelchair) [9, 26, 29]. The subjects were requested to rest for a duration of 2 min, type four lines of preset text (82 words), play 5 games of Tic-Tac-Toe against the computer on

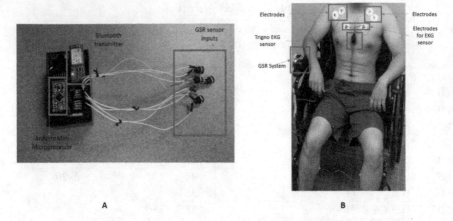

Fig. 1. A) GSR system B) subject wearing the physiological sensing system

'Easy mode' [11, 32] and lastly continuously travel for 5 min in their wheelchair. Subjects were allowed to take a break if they felt overexerted.

Prior to the commencement of activities, the subjects were asked to answer questions about their level of injury and duration since injury as well as their standard comfort level, judged through the use of the ASHRAE temperature scale [12]. The subjects were also asked to report the level of stress measured on the 5 point anxiety scale [3] ranging from 1–5 (1 being the most relaxed, 5 being the most stressful) and physical comfort they felt after each activity and also if they felt autonomic dysreflexic at any point of the activity. Figure 2 shows a subject performing an activity.

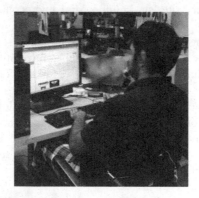

Fig. 2. Subject performing the task of typing while system records data in real time.

2.4   Data Analysis

The data was captured in Volts (V_{GSR}) and translated into Skin Resistance (SR_{sig}) in Mega Ohms (MΩ) using Eq. 1

$$SR_{sig} = \frac{-0.607 \times V_{GSR}}{V_{GSR} - 5} \tag{1}$$

Skin resistance data usually was recorded in the 0.08–0.2 Hz range. In order to reduce noise, the raw data was pre-processed with a second order Butterworth Low Pass Filter with a cut-off of 0.3 Hz [15] followed by a moving average filter. These filter out the local disturbances while maintaining the natural peaks of the signal itself, allowing the development of a clear understanding of the variations in the SR above and below the injury site of the individuals. Figure 3 shows the SR signals from a subject before and after the pre-processing of the digital signal is performed.

The pulse data was analyzed by the EMGWorks® Analysis software. The raw pulse data is processed through the native EKG Rate function which identifies the rising and falling edges of the data series, passes it through a band pass filter and produces a value for the rate in Beats per Minute (BPM) with respect to time. Figure 4 shows the pulse data before and after the EKG Rate function is used.

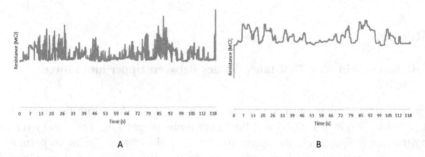

Fig. 3. Quality of raw skin resistance signal before pre-processing filters are applied (A), and after filters are applied (B)

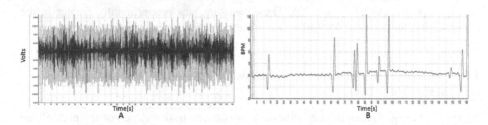

Fig. 4. Raw pulse data (A), data after processing by EKG rate function (B)

2.5 Data Normalization

Due to differences in the absolute values of the Skin resistance amongst the various subjects as a result of varying skin types, the data was normalized through the min-max normalization method [19, 20] This technique of normalization identifies the SR data in a range of [0,1], allowing for a more convenient comparison of the data in the various limbs from which the SR data was collected. The Skin resistance data for each subject SR_{sig} is normalized to SR_{norm} by subtracting the minimum SR_{min} and scaling it against the difference of maximum, SR_{max} and $SR\text{-}_{min}$ as shown in Eq. (2).

$$SR_{norm} = \frac{SR_{sig} - SR_{min}}{SR_{max} - SR_{min}} \tag{2}$$

2.6 Statistical Analysis

Statistical significance in the values of the skin resistance above and below the injury site was performed using a one way ANOVA test, $\alpha = 0.05$ for the various activities performed by the subjects. In order to identify the correlation between the pulse and the resistance data, we performed a Pearson correlation analysis between the normalized average skin resistance data with the pulse data. Statistical analysis was performed using IBM® SPSS® Statistics Software.

3 Results

3.1 Differences in Skin Resistance Values Between Upper and Lower Limbs

Figure 5 is a representation of the normalized average SR data from the upper limbs (Left Shoulder, Right Shoulder) and the lower limbs (Right Leg, Left Leg) over time during the four different activities performed by a single subject. The mean normalized SR values in the Right and Left Legs were statistically significantly larger than the mean normalized SR values in the Right and Left Shoulders during all activities, independent of the level of injury of the subject (ANOVA, $p = 0.015$). In Fig. 5, the mean SR values in the upper limbs were significantly different from the lower limb SR values for each activity ($p < 0.05$). Thus, sweating was proportionally greater in the upper limbs compared to the lower limbs during activities including rest.

3.2 Differences in Normalized Skin Resistance Based on Activity and Anxiety Level

As shown in Fig. 6, a significant difference was noted in the values of the normalized average skin resistance above and below the injury site, as compared to the relaxed state, when different activities were performed. There was a significant difference in SR during the rest state of the individuals compared to when performing the activities. (ANOVA, $p = 0.018$ for upper limbs and p = 0.042 for lower limbs).

Table 2 shows the average reported anxiety/exertion experienced by the subjects when performing each activity. On average the subjects reported the highest level of anxiety after they performed the typing activity (1.89). A corresponding decrease in normalized SR was observed with an increasing state of anxiety when the subjects performed the various activities in the upper limbs (above injury site). However, this correspondence was not exhibited between the normalized SR of the lower limbs and anxiety level reported by the subjects. Thus, the upper limbs demonstrate a much higher negative correlation coefficient with the reported anxiety levels (R = −0.91) as compared to the lower limbs (R = −0.27).

Table 2. Average values of reported anxiety experienced by the subjects during each activity. Anxiety levels are measured on a scale of 1–5 where 1 is experiencing the least stress.

Activity	Reported anxiety levels
Relax	1
Typing	1.89
TTT	1.22
Travelling	1.33

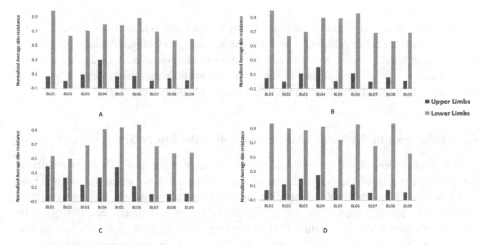

Fig. 5. Comparison of normalized average SR data above and below the injury site during (A) relaxation ($p = 0.021$) (B) typing ($p = 0.035$) (C) playing Tic-Tac-Toe ($p = 0.038$) (D) wheelchair travelling ($p = 0.043$). One way ANOVA test was performed.

3.3   Correlation Between Pulse and SR Data

There was no significant difference in the values in the pulse data collected from the subjects while performing different activities ($p = 0.36$). There was no statistically significant correlation between pulse values and the normalized skin resistance data for all activities However, the strongest correlation coefficients were observed between pulse and SR during the typing activity, which had the highest anxiety level.

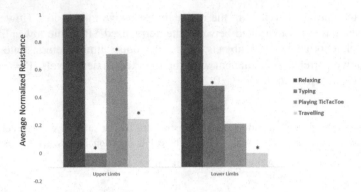

Fig. 6. Normalized subject SR values for different activities above and below injury site (*indicates statistical difference)

4 Discussion

Through this study we aimed to identify the relevance and reliability of galvanic skin resistance sensors on developing a baseline value for a physiological telemetry system (PTS) which would be able to detect any anomalous autonomic activity. In this section, we discuss the results identified in the previous section and how they help in the validation of our skin resistance detection system during typical ADL.

4.1 Difference in SR Values Above and Below the Injury Site

A high level lesion of the spinal cord as in the case of a cervical SCI often results in complete paralysis of the lower limbs of the individual with some spared level of movement in the upper limbs depending on the level of the injury. Most supraspinal control of sweat excretion is located in regions of the hypothalamus and amygdala in order to regulate body temperature [34]. A cervical level SCI prevents this supraspinal control to the individual's body below the injury site. In the sympathetic nervous system the preganglionic nerve fibers from the spinal cord began at approximately the thoracic 1 neurologic level.

Additionally, a study by Yaggie et al. [35] found that the upper limbs of subjects with SCI have a greater ability to produce sweat when compared with lower limbs and often results in a decrease in the sympathetic stimulation of sweat glands and a reduction in sweating in the lower limbs. Moreover, a cervical SCI often affects the circulation of blood to the paralyzed lower limbs [10], which may affect skin resistance in the lower limbs.

Since sweating causes a decrease in skin resistance, a reduced ability to sweat causes a generally higher absolute value of SR values [31]. Our observation of a higher level of normalized SR values in the lower limbs as compared to the upper limbs demonstrated a relatively low adapting sweating response in the lower limbs. This observation is likely due to a lack of supraspinal control of the sympathetic system as well as supports that the sweat glands in the upper limbs are more active than those in the lower limbs even at rest. We observed a strong relationship between decreasing SR in the upper limbs when engaging in more active or stressful ADL.

The significant difference in the skin resistance values in the upper and lower limbs helps in validating the use of the lower body below the SCI level of neurologic activity as a GSR reference in determining an accurate baseline for normal ADL for a specific individual.

4.2 Difference in SR Values Based on Activity

Activity and exertion have been known to affect the values of skin resistances in individuals with and without SCI [8, 33]. Exertion in cases of individuals with SCI often causes a decrease in skin resistance as discussed by Bhambani [2], although there is very limited previous work which discusses the impact of exertion on the skin resistance above and below the injury site of persons with cervical SCI. Our results show that although there is a general decrease in the normalized average SR values in the lower limbs (below the injury site), it is not impacted by the level of anxiety reported by the subjects. However, in the upper limbs, the lowest value of normalized average SR is identified during the task in which subjects reported the highest anxiety; the activity of typing. This is in agreement with the findings of other researchers in the field wherein they identified a reduction in SR in activities that cause higher stress [4, 22]. We propose that the general decrease in the normalized SR values in the lower limbs is a time-dependent change that does not correlate with varying anxiety levels of the subjects but rather progresses with the extended testing time. We would expect that SR would return to values measured during relaxation if subjects were given longer periods to rest.

Through the identification of the reduction of SR values in the upper values when engaging in more stressful activities, we validated that the system is able to successfully identify an ADL-based increase in the sweating or exertion of the individual. This is useful in contrasting exertion due to activity from an onset of an episode of AD, which is characterized by sweating above the injury site.

4.3 Correlation Between Pulse and SR Values

From our results, we observed no statistically significant change in pulse when subjects were performing different ADL. Additionally, no notable correlation between the pulse and SR values were observed based on the level of SCI, type of activity, or body location of SR measurement above or below the injury site. In non-spinal cord injured persons when there is an increase in the level of pulse, there is a concomitant decrease in the skin resistance [25]. The lack of distinction in correlation coefficient values between the upper and lower limbs and pulse in persons with SCI show that even though there is a marked difference in the trends and values of SR, the pulse of the individual is not drastically affected.

4.4   Limitations

One of the key limitations during the experiment was the presence of motion artifacts during PTS recording. Patients with SCI often needed to perform pressure reliefs on a frequent basis. This pressure relief can take the form of physically moving in the wheelchair or adjusting the position of the wheelchair (e.g. tilting and reclining). This movement introduced motion artifacts into the sensor data which was reduced by usage of a band pass filter.

5   Future Work

Future work will involve using the PTS to determine a known baseline for the SR values of individuals with SCI to detect abnormal autonomic function, such as auto-nomic dysreflexia. We would also use various sensors to monitor other physiological activity such as pulse detectors, blood pressure monitors, temperature sensors, and identify flushing using computer vision. The integration of these sensors would allow the development of a telemetry system which can be used to detect any physiological dysfunction from the pre-determined baseline. The physiological state of the user or health can then be reported to a family member, caregiver, or healthcare professional or the users themselves to allow for better care and adopt healthier practices. We will also examine the effects of the differences in the injury levels and neurologic completeness on the baseline values of the various sensors. We will also improve methods to reduce the noise detected by the system and in a timely manner in order to provide real-time sensing. More subjects will be recruited and more vigorous activities will be performed in order to develop a more comprehensive representation of the physiological parameters to ensure an accurate and reliable telemetry system.

6   Conclusion

From the results described in the paper, we identified that a wearable PTS is able to accurately detect variations in SR when performing different ADL with varying levels of exertion as well as accommodating identify individual differences in skin resistance above and below the injury site. Our objective is to substantiate the relevance of galvanic skin resistance data in the determination of a baseline for monitoring the sweating response in persons with SCI. The significantly lower normalized SR in the upper limbs of individuals with SCI as compared to the lower limbs provides insight into validating the lesser sweating response in the lower limbs. Moreover, the variation of SR during activities with different anxiety levels provides validation of the accurate and reliable detection of skin resistance by the system during different ADL that was developed for this study.

Acknowledgments. This project was supported by the Indiana Spinal Cord and Brain Injury Research Fund through the Indiana State Department of Health (awarded to B.S.D.). We would like to thank Dr. James Malec and Dr. Elena Gillespie from the Rehabilitation Hospital of Indiana for all their help and support in this study. We are grateful to the subjects that have participated in the study. We would also like to thank the Purdue Discovery Park for making this research possible and Dr. Thomas Kuczek and Evidence Matangi from the Purdue Department of Statistics for their advice on the statistical analysis of the data presented in this paper. We would also like to thank Microsoft Research and Dr. Arjmand Samuel for the use of their technologies during the conduct of this project.

References

1. Arnold, J., Feng, Q.-P., Delaney, G., et al.: Autonomic dysreflexia in tetraplegic patients: evidence for α-adrenoceptor hyper-responsiveness. Clin. Auton. Res. **5**, 267–270 (1995)
2. Bhambhani, Y.: Physiology of wheelchair racing in athletes with spinal cord injury. Sports Med. **32**, 23–51 (2002)
3. Buron, K.D., Curtis, M.: The incredible 5-point scale. Shawnee Mission (2003)
4. Chanel, G., Rebetez, C., Bétrancourt, M., et al.: Boredom, engagement and anxiety as indicators for adaptation to difficulty in games. In: Proceedings of the 12th International Conference on Entertainment and Media in the Ubiquitous Era, pp. 13–17. ACM (2008)
5. Cragg, J., Krassioukov, A.: Autonomic dysreflexia. Can. Med. Assoc. J. **184**, 66 (2012)
6. Dettmers, C., Van Ahlen, H., Faust, H., et al.: Evaluation of erectile dysfunction with the sympathetic skin response in comparison to bulbocavernosus reflex and somatosensory evoked potentials of the pudendal nerve. Electromyogr. Clin. Neurophysiol. **34**, 437–444 (1993)
7. Ertekin, C., Almis, S., Ertekin, N.: Sympathetic skin potentials and bulbocavernosus reflex in patients with chronic alcoholism and impotence. Eur. Neurol. **30**, 334–337 (1990)
8. Freeman, G., Simpson, R.: The effect of experimentally induced muscular tension upon palmar skin resistance. J. Gen. Psychol. **18**, 319–326 (1938)
9. Hoffmann, T., Russell, T., Thompson, L., et al.: Using the Internet to assess activities of daily living and hand function in people with Parkinson's disease. NeuroRehabilitation **23**, 253–261 (2007)
10. Hopman, M.T., Groothuis, J.T., Flendrie, M., et al.: Increased vascular resistance in paralyzed legs after spinal cord injury is reversible by training. J. Appl. Physiol. **93**, 1966–1972 (2002)
11. http://10fastfingers.Com/Text/119-a-Simple-Paragraph-to-Practice-Simple-Typing. Fast Fingers Improve your typing speed
12. Humphreys, M.A., Hancock, M.: Do people like to feel 'neutral'?: exploring the variation of the desired thermal sensation on the ASHRAE scale. Energy Build. **39**, 867–874 (2007)
13. Karlsson, A.: Autonomic dysreflexia. Spinal Cord **37**, 383–391 (1999)
14. Kirshblum, S.C., House, J.G., O'connor, K.C.: Silent autonomic dysreflexia during a routine bowel program in persons with traumatic spinal cord injury: a preliminary study. Arch. Phys. Med. Rehabil. **83**, 1774–1776 (2002)
15. Krassioukov, A., Warburton, D.E., Teasell, R., et al.: A systematic review of the management of autonomic dysreflexia after spinal cord injury. Arch. Phys. Med. Rehabil. **90**, 682–695 (2009)
16. Krassioukov, A.V., Furlan, J.C., Fehlings, M.G.: Autonomic dysreflexia in acute spinal cord injury: an under-recognized clinical entity. J. Neurotrauma **20**, 707–716 (2003)
17. Krassioukov, A.V., Weaver, L.C.: Episodic hypertension due to autonomic dysreflexia in acute and chronic spinal cord-injured rats. Am. J. Physiol. Heart Circ. Physiol. **268**, H2077–H2083 (1995)

18. Kwon, B.K., Okon, E., Hillyer, J., et al.: A systematic review of non-invasive pharmacologic neuroprotective treatments for acute spinal cord injury. J. Neurotrauma **28**, 1545–1588 (2011)

19. Liu, F., Liu, G., Lai, X., et al.: The model about the affection regulation based on partial least regression in the human-computer interaction. In: 2012 Eighth International Conference on Natural Computation (ICNC), pp. 1060–1063. IEEE (2012)

20. Lykken, D.: Range correction applied to heart rate and to GSR data. Psychophysiology **9**, 373–379 (1972)

21. Mcgillivray, C.F., Hitzig, S.L., Craven, B.C., et al.: Evaluating knowledge of autonomic dysreflexia among individuals with spinal cord injury and their families. J. Spinal Cord Med. **32**, 54 (2009)

22. Meyerbröker, K., Emmelkamp, P.M.: Virtual reality exposure therapy in anxiety disorders: a systematic review of process-and-outcome studies. Depress. Anxiety **27**, 933–944 (2010)

23. Montagu, J., Coles, E.: Mechanism and measurement of the galvanic skin response. Psychol. Bull. **65**, 261 (1966)

24. NSCISC. Spinal cord injury (SCI): facts and figures at a glance. In: Center, T.N.S.S. (ed.) University of Alabama at Birmingham (2015)

25. Obrist, P.A.: Cardiovascular differentiation of sensory stimuli. Psychosom. Med. **25**, 450–459 (1963)

26. Pentland, W., Twomey, L.: Upper limb function in persons with long term paraplegia and implications for independence: part I. Spinal Cord **32**, 211–218 (1994)

27. Previnaire, J., Soler, J., Hanson, P.: Skin potential recordings during cystometry in spinal cord injured patients. Spinal Cord **31**, 13–21 (1993)

28. Reitz, A., Schmid, D.M., Curt, A., et al.: Sympathetic sudomotor skin activity in human after complete spinal cord injury. Auton. Neurosci. **102**, 78–84 (2002)

29. Rogante, M., Grigioni, M., Cordella, D., et al.: Ten years of telerehabilitation: a literature overview of technologies and clinical applications. NeuroRehabilitation **27**, 287–304 (2009)

30. Sheel, A.W., Krassioukov, A.V., Inglis, J.T., et al.: Autonomic dysreflexia during sperm retrieval in spinal cord injury: influence of lesion level and sildenafil citrate. J. Appl. Physiol. **99**, 53–58 (2005)

31. Takagi, K., Ogawa, T., Terada, E., et al.: Sweating and the electric resistance of the skin. Acta Neurovegetativa **24**, 404–412 (1962)

32. Tictactoe, A.: http://www.agame.com/game/tic-tac-toe

33. Van Dooren, M., Janssen, J.H.: Emotional sweating across the body: comparing 16 different skin conductance measurement locations. Physiol. Behav. **106**, 298–304 (2012)

34. Wallin, B., Karlsson, T., Pegenius, G., et al.: Sympathetic single axonal discharge after spinal cord injury in humans: activity at rest and after bladder stimulation. Spinal Cord **52**, 434–438 (2014)

35. Yaggie, J.A., Niemi, T.J., Buono, M.J.: Adaptive sweat gland response after spinal cord injury. Arch. Phys. Med. Rehabil. **83**, 802–805 (2002)

Monitoring and Estimating Medication Abuse

Upkar Varshney[✉]

Georgia State University, Atlanta, GA 30302-4015, USA
uvarshney@gsu.edu

Abstract. Prescription medication abuse is a major healthcare problem and can lead to addiction syndrome, higher healthcare cost, and serious harm to patients. Smart health can play a major role in addressing medication abuse by monitoring patient's health conditions and medication consumption, and, by connecting with healthcare professionals and utilizing suitable interventions. More specifically, medication behavior can be analyzed using information from smart medication systems, specialized wearable sensors and/or mobile devices with patient-entered consumption data. In this paper, we study monitoring systems to predict current abuse and near-future addiction and provide interventions to reduce medication abuse. The future work involves development and evaluation of Ab-Med mobile app for monitoring medication consumption and comprehensive cost effectiveness of interventions for medication abuse.

Keywords: Smart health · Medication abuse · Interventions · Patterns of consumption · Mobile app · Performance evaluation

1 Introduction

Prescription medication abuse is any intentional use of a medication with intoxicating properties outside of a physician's prescription for a bona fide medical condition, excluding accidental misuse [3]. Addiction is defined as compulsive use of a substance for psychic effects and to satisfy a craving for the drugs [2]. Medication abuse can result in addiction leading to increased healthcare cost and injury to patients [5]. According to NIH, 20 % of all prescription medications have been used in medication abuse [7], while other studies estimate prescription abuse at 4.5 % of the population [1] and 36–56 % among chronic pain patients [6]. Prescription abuse has been linked to more deaths than automobile accidents and is estimated to cost $8.6 Billion in health and legal expenses and loss of productivity in US alone [4].

Proactive monitoring and detection of abuse can reduce the need for expensive treatment [5]. More specifically, the medication adherence and consumption of certain medications can be monitored anytime anywhere and analyzed for abuse and near-future addiction. The goal is to have an "advance warning system" to alert family members and healthcare professionals. This will allow them to intervene before the patient becomes addicted. In this paper, we present monitoring and interventions (Sect. 2), model and results for medication abuse (Sect. 3), and work in progress (Sect. 4).

© Springer International Publishing Switzerland 2016
X. Zheng et al. (Eds.): ICSH 2015, LNCS 9545, pp. 169–174, 2016.
DOI: 10.1007/978-3-319-29175-8_15

2   The Abuse Monitoring and Interventions

The following requirements for abuse monitoring are derived [1, 2, 3, 4, 5, and 6]: to monitor both average medication adherence 0 as well as the patterns of adherence, to monitor for long-term use as abuse and addiction appear to be a chronic condition, to include past history, patient's characteristics, and abuse potential of medications in analyzing medication data for current abuse and future addiction, to handle missing and/ or incorrect information by extrapolating based on past history and current consumption, and to analyze the pattern of medication adherence to detect probabilities of multi-dosing and/or frequent dosing in determining current abuse and future addiction.

Smart medication systems include monitoring and dispensing of doses, reminders to patients, and communications with healthcare professionals [8]. One such system is shown in Fig. 1, where information on medication consumption is collected from multiple sources. Figure 1 also includes monitoring and analysis of consumption information, the roles of patient and healthcare professional, and three possible interventions.

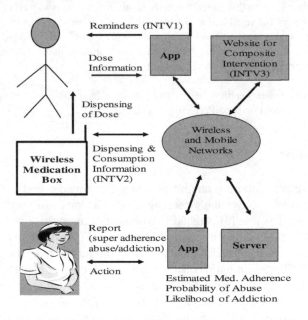

Fig. 1. Architecture of the abuse monitoring system (AMS)

Medication consumption data is analyzed to match various known patterns for both current abuse and near-future addiction based on thresholds and criteria supplied by healthcare professionals (Fig. 2). More specifically, some of the patterns are (a) certain number of doses in certain time period (such as $>=V$ doses in N hours), (b) certain number of events where patients exceed the dose limits, (c) medication holidays followed by catch-up periods, (d) excess filling or average adherence >100 for M days, and (e) patients using more doses than filled from a known pharmacy. We assume that the data on doses can be collected from monitoring of patients, mobile applications, from pharmacy, and/or smart medication dispensers. To address reliability challenges, data analysis should compensate for errors in collected data to avoid excessive false positive or inaccurate prediction of events. With consumption information, the system can process how doses are consumed by the patient and then reported to healthcare professionals for suitable interventions.

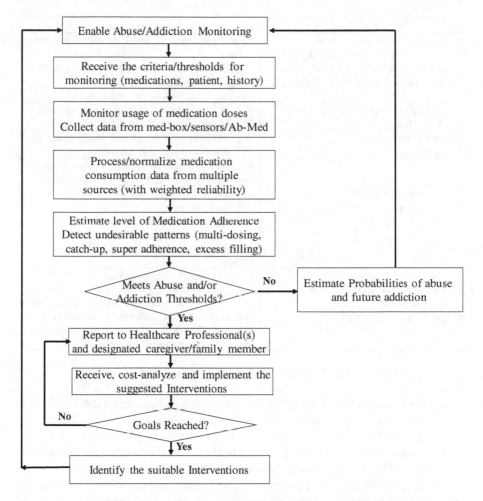

Fig. 2. Abuse monitoring and decision support (AMDS) system

3   A Model and Results for Abuse and Addiction

The analytical model implements the AMDS by taking multiple inputs including (a) the pattern of medication consumption from smart box or mobile app using patient's consent, (b) patient's history, co-morbidity, family and social influence, and vulnerability as part of the context of use, (c) probabilities of poly-pharmacy and prescription sharing among patients, and (d) information on the addiction possibilities of the medications. The predictive model processes and analyzes both average and pattern of consumption of different medications for patients. The computation includes numerous probabilities and weights of a range of values, which will improve as more data become available (Fig. 3).

Key Equations	Explanation
Estimated Medication Adherence $P_{EST} = Max(P_S \times P_C \times P_{TRUE}, P_S \times P_C \times P_{TRUE} + (1- P_S \times P_C), P_S \times P_C \times P_{TRUE} + (1- P_S \times P_C)* (0.5 \times P_{TRUE}), F_{RECALL} \times P_{TRUE})$	P_S = Probability of SMS detecting a dosing event P_C = Probability of detecting the correct event P_{TRUE} = True Medication Adherence F_{RECALL} = Patient's dosing recall factor
Probability of Multi Dosing (I=1 to M) $P_{MD} = (1/M) \Sigma (I \times P_{MD-I})$	P_{MD-I} = Probability of multi-dosing for I doses M = Max number of doses a patient can take
The probability of abuse $P_{ABUSE} = P_{MD} - P_{AD}$	P_{AD} = Probability of accidental dosing (using the frequency of dosing and past behavior)
The likelihood of addiction $P_{ADD} = W_{PAT} \times P_{PAT} + W_{MED} \times P_{MED} + W_{ABUSE} \times P_{ABUSE}$	P_{PAT} = Patient related factors, P_{MED} = Medication related factors, P_{ABUSE} = Patient behavior (monitored by smart medication boxes or mobile applications). The values of Ws to be improved, as more information becomes available, to get better personalization of monitoring and intervention system.
ROI for an intervention $= ((S_{IN} + S_{OP} + S_M + S_{MISC}))/ (C_{FIX}/(T*NP) + C_{VAR}/NP)$	S_{IN} = Savings in inpatient cost, S_{OP} = Savings in outpatient cost, S_M = Savings in medication cost, S_{MISC} = Misc savings (quality of life, job), NP = Number of patients, T = Intervention duration, C_{FIX} = Fix cost of intervention, and C_{VAR} = Variable cost of intervention

Fig. 3. High-level description of the model

The model generates (a) probability of multi-dosing and accidental dosing, (b) likelihood of current abuse and addiction, and (c) cost effectiveness of "personalized" interventions. The likelihood of abuse is non-linear with changes in adherence level. Further the abuse is higher for lower multi-dose thresholds, supplied by healthcare professional for specific medication and, if available, patient's history of abuse (Fig. 4). The difference between healthcare cost of patients with abuse and patients with desirable adherence (80–100 %) increases non-linearly with cost of medications, hospital cost/day, and the degree of abuse. Using the adherence and abuse data in our model, we derived the ROI for different interventions for different level of abuse (Fig. 5). The ROI is lower than 1 (not cost effective) for light abuse (100–120 % adherence). However, the ROI rises rapidly (although not in the same proportion for all three interventions) as the level of abuse increases to moderate (150 %) to high (200 %). We are working on results using different outpatient frequency, scenarios involving polypharmacy and excess fillers, and other interventions and their cost effectiveness.

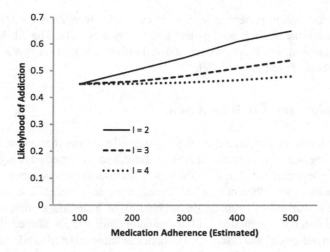

Fig. 4. The likelihood of addiction for different thresholds

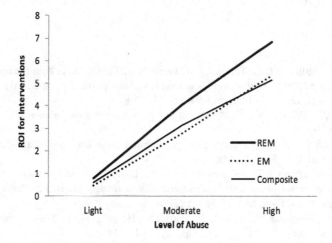

Fig. 5. ROI for three interventions based on the level of abuse

The limitations of the model include the reliance on limited and/or unreliable adherence data from patients and approximations of various parameters. In future, being able to populate the model with better parameter values and weights to derive the probabilities will improve the accuracy of prediction.

4   Work in Progress

In addition to analyzing patterns of medication consumption, we are expanding the model to predict abuse using the probabilities and weights of patterns for a patient, condition and medications. We are also working with healthcare professionals in substance abuse. The development of a mobile app, termed Ab-Med, is underway for monitoring consumption pattern as well as integrating information, of different reliability levels, from medication box, patient and family members. The Ab-Med will be part of implementing interventions for abuse. Further, we plan to test Ab-Med app against the validated predictive model.

5   Conclusion and Further Research

We addressed medication related challenges, designed a system to monitor and analyze the patterns of medication use to detect current abuse, and presented an analytical model to evaluate the performance. The probabilities of multi-dosing is observed to be rising non-linearly with super adherence (>100 % medication adherence). The probability of current abuse is utilized to estimate the probability of near-future addiction. We are aware that additional work, such as field study and/or clinical trials, is needed to improve the accuracy of our model and results. Additional challenges related to HIPAA, patient's agreement for monitoring, and having strong controls for privacy and non-disclosure need to be addressed.

References

1. Becker, W.C., Sullivan, L.E., Tetrault, J.M., Desai, R.A., Fiellin, D.A.: Non-medical use, abuse and dependence on prescription opioids among US adults: psychiatric, medical and substance use correlates. Drug Alcohol Depend. **94**, 38–47 (2008)
2. Benedict, D.G.: Walking the tightrope: chronic pain and substance abuse. J. Nurse Pract. **4**, 604–609 (2008)
3. Compton, W.S., Volkow, N.D.: Abuse of prescription drugs and the risk of addiction. Drug Alcohol Depend. **83S**, S4–S7 (2006)
4. Davis, J.M., Severtson, S.G., Bucher-Bartelson, B., Dart, R.C.: Using poison center exposure calls to predict prescription Opioid abuse and misuse-related emergency department visits. Pharmacoepidemiol. Drug Saf. **23**, 18–25 (2014)
5. Garland, E.L., Froeliger, B., Zeidan, F., Partin, K., Howard, M.O.: The downward spiral of chronic pain, prescription opioid misuse, and addiction: cognitive, affective and neuropsychopharmacologic pathways. Neurosci. Biobehav. Rev. **37**, 2597–2607 (2013)
6. Martell, B.A., O'Connor, P.G., Kerns, R.D., Becker, W.C., Morales, K.H., Kosten, T.R., Fiellin, D.A.: Systematic review: opioid treatment for chronic back pain: prevalence, efficacy, and association with addiction. Ann. Intern. Med. **146**, 116–127 (2007)
7. NIH website for prescription drug abuse. http://www.nlm.nih.gov/medlineplus/prescriptiondrugabuse.html. Accessed 15 March 2014
8. Varshney, U.: Smart medication management system and multiple interventions for medication adherence. Decis. Support Syst. **55**(2), 538–551 (2013)

Real-Time Prediction of Blood Alcohol Content Using Smartwatch Sensor Data

Mario A. Gutierrez$^{(\boxtimes)}$, Michelle L. Fast, Anne H. Ngu,
and Byron J. Gao

Department of Computer Science, Texas State University,
San Marcos, TX, USA
{mag262,mlf96,angu,bgao}@txstate.edu

Abstract. This paper proposes an application that collects sensor data
from a smartwatch in order to predict drunkenness in real-time, dis-
creetly, and non-invasively via a machine learning approach. This system
could prevent drunk driving or other dangers related to the consumption of alcohol by giving users a way to determine personal intoxication
level without the use of intrusive breathalyzers or guess work. Using
smartwatch data collected from several volunteers, we trained a machine
learning model that may work with a smartphone application to predict
the user's intoxication level in real-time.

1 Introduction

Internet of Things (IoT) is a domain that represents the next most exciting technological revolution since the Internet. IoT will bring endless opportunities and
impact every corner of our planet. In the healthcare domain, IoT promises to
bring personalized health tracking and monitoring ever closer to the consumers.
This phenomena is discussed in a recent Wall Street Journal article, "Why Connected Medicine Is Becoming Vital to Health Care" [8]. Modern smartphones
and smartwatches now contain a more diverse collection of sensors than ever
before, and people are warming up to them. In January 2014, approximately
46 million US smartphone owners were reported to have used health and fitness applications [9]. Currently, sports and fitness are the predominant foci of
IoT-based health applications. However, applications in disease management and
health care are becoming increasingly prevalent. For example, detecting falling
of elderly patients [13].

Drunk driving is a dangerous, worldwide problem. This problem is not only
a hazard to the drunk drivers, but also to pedestrians and other drivers. It is
reported by the Bureau of Transportation Statistics that in 2010, 47.2 % of pedes-
trian fatalities and 39.9 % of vehicle occupant fatalities were caused by drunk
driving [4]. The Centers for Disease Control and Prevention (CDC) reported that
between the years 2008 and 2010, roughly two-thirds of adults were drinkers, with
adults between the ages 18 and 24 having the greatest association with heavy
drinking [11].

© Springer International Publishing Switzerland 2016
X. Zheng et al. (Eds.): ICSH 2015, LNCS 9545, pp. 175–186, 2016.
DOI: 10.1007/978-3-319-29175-8_16

At dangerous levels of intoxication, it can be difficult to judge ones own drunkenness. Instead it would be better to get a definitive measurement of the BAC, or simply a binary response: "drunk" or "not drunk." Compact breathalyzers are probably the best option at the moment, but these are not discreet and require deliberate action by the user. The other option is to use a smartphone application to manually calculate BAC, but these demand a greater deal of involvement from the user. To be practical, it would be useful to have some sort of non-invasive and accurate monitoring system that will warn its user if they become too intoxicated. It has been shown that electronic intervention programs are more successful at reducing college student drinking than a general alcohol awareness program [14]. This system can also be used to warn friends and family, or prevent the operation of the user's car.

In this paper, we investigate the prediction of intoxication level from smartwatch sensor data via machine learning. We also briefly discuss a general Android-based gateway system which can collect data from any type of physical or virtual sensor accessible by the host smartphone.

2 Related Work

There are a few ways of approaching the problem of determining a person's blood alcohol content. One approach is to devise a mathematical model of the elimination of ethanol in the human body. In this case, the Widmark equation, published in 1932 by E.M.P. Widmark, is a very popular one;

$$C = \frac{A}{rW} - (\beta t), \tag{1}$$

where C is the BAC, r and β are empirically determined constants, A is the mass of the consumed alcohol, and W is the body weight of the person. These days, there have been several improvements and variants. Douglas Posey and Ashraf Mozayani published an excellent article comparing this model using parameters determined by different researchers and discussing different models [10]. They found that the Widmark equation tends to overestimate, and that there can be significant discrepancy between the results of the different models. Despite that, they do provide a rough estimate. The problem is that these models also require a good deal of information that prohibit their use in a non-intrusive, drunkenness warning system.

Another approach to the problem is simply to measure the BAC directly. Transdermal ethanol sensors have been a recent option for this approach. These can provide a discreet way to measure intoxication, but they are accompanied by the problem of a significant time lag between the sensed alcohol concentration and actual blood alcohol concentration. Gregory D. Webster and Hampton C. Gabler closely investigated this problem. They found that the lag is predictable, but not constant, and requires additional information about the number of drinks taken by the user to accurately predict it [15].

Similar to our project, James A. Baldwin has a patent on a system involving a wearable transdermal ethanol sensor and a mobile device to capture the information [3]. Baldwin describes his system as using a mathematical model to predict the user's BAC given the transdermal sensor data and information about the drinks the user plans to consume. A benefit of our system is that it involves no input by the user about the drinks taken, and the user need not buy a special sensor dedicated to this task alone.

Aside from measuring BAC directly, or developing a biologically-based mathematical model, machine learning is another good approach. Georgia Koukiou and Vassilis Anastassopoulos published research this year in using a neural network to identify drunkenness from thermal infrared images of peoples' faces [7]. Neural networks were trained on different parts of the face in order to determine which areas can be used to classify drunkenness. They found the forehead was the most significant facial location to observe for determining the drunkenness of a person. Their study takes advantage of the effect of alcohol making blood vessels dilate allowing warm blood to come closer to the skin; which is also an important effect for our research. Such a system may be good for ignition interlock systems, or drunk surveillance.

Outside of BAC studies, there has been plenty of research into detecting other activities using smartphone and smartwatch sensor data. In [6], John J. Guiry, Pepijin van de Ven, John Nelson, attempt using the sensor data to identify various daily activities, such as: walking, running, cycling, and sitting. In their study, they use several machine learning algorithms for their approach: C4.5, CART, Naïve Bayes, ANN, and SVM. Their results showed some promise for better future models, with their model for classifying whether a user is indoors or outdoors being the most impressive. Successful models for predicting daily activities will certainly be important in a practical implementation of our system. This is because the body's response to alcohol consumption may share significant similarity to exercise, dance, or other activities.

Using smartphones and smartwatches, there is an active desire to create monitoring applications for serious health problems. Such as in [12], where Vinod Sharma, Kunal Mankodiya, Fernando De La Torre, et al., developed a smartwatch-smartphone system for the monitoring and analysis of data from patients with Parkinson Disease. This system, named SPARK, includes the analysis of speech and detection of: facial tremors, dyskinesia, and freezing of gait. Their system is intended to provide useful recommendations to physicians based on the collected information. They concluded noting some potential problems of a full implementation of their system, the most relevant problem being misplacement of the sensors. This may also be a problem for us considering the potential importance of the motion-based accelerometer and gyroscope data.

3   System Architecture

A huge end-goal of ours is to have a public system where participating users' phones transmit sensor information to a central database through a REST-based web service. The service stores this information in the database and another data processing system. Other users who are not contributing information can connect to our system to access other related services, like a choropleth map of the sensor data; BAC prediction data in our case, but the system would not be limited to it. The particular protocols and setup used should be designed to protect the privacy of the sensor data contributors (Fig. 1).

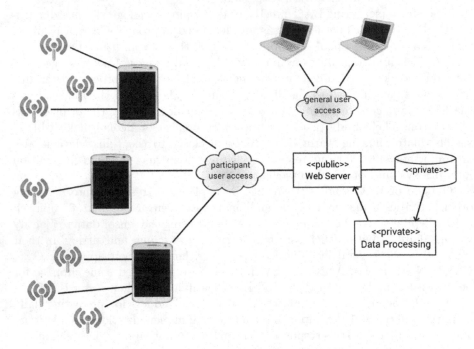

Fig. 1. Example general system for large-scale sensor data collection

3.1   Smartphone Sensor Gateway

Each of the smartphones in this system are behaving as a type of sensor gateway. In order to collect our data, we built such a system on the Android platform. Though we used primarily a Microsoft Band, our system allows the easy addition of any sensor that can be connected to from the Android smartphone. In Fig. 2, we show an overview of the classes used in this system.

4   Methodology

In this section, we will describe how we collected the data, we will present an analysis of the data, and then lead into the discussion of the machine learning models used.

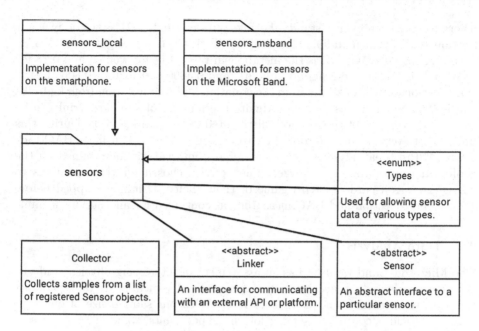

Fig. 2. Gateway implementation for our data collection application

4.1   Collection

Our collection began with the development of an Android application that can connect to and store data from available sensors on the Microsoft Band smartwatch. Next, we developed a general procedure for our volunteers to follow during the collection of data. Our volunteers were eager to freely contribute the anonymous data used in this paper. The data collected by the system was stored into a .csv file on the Android smartphone and also transmitted to a central database server.

We used Android platform version 5.0 (kernel 3.4.0-4432708) running on a Samsung S5 smartphone. The Microsoft Band had Build Version 10.2.2818.0 09 R. Samples of the sensor data were collected every three seconds, based on the update speed of the Band's heart rate sensor. Each sample used the most recent sensor value if available, otherwise it would use the last value; or in the case of the accelerometer and gyroscope sensors, the three most recent values were averaged with linear weighting (the most recent having highest importance). There may be a better weighting, but this weighting was suitable for our purposes.

The procedure followed by the volunteers during data collection lasted two-hours. First, we established some necessary information about the subject in order to estimate the amount of alcohol necessary to reach 0.08 BAC in a 1.5 h period using the Widmark equation (1). The particular formulation of it we used is the following:

$$SD = BW \cdot Wt \cdot (EBAC + (MR \cdot DP)) \cdot 0.4690, \qquad (2)$$

where SD is the number of standard drinks (10 g ethanol), BW is the body water contant (0.58 for men and 0.49 for women), Wt is the body weight in lbs, EBAC is the estimated BAC, MR is the metabolism rate (0.17 for women and 0.18 for men), DP is the drinking period in hours, and $0.4690 = 0.4536 \div (0.806 \cdot 1.2)$, a combination of two constants from the equation and a converstion from kg to lbs [1,16]. This amount was used to estimate the number of standard drinks to be consumed over the set time period, distributed over equal intervals. During this process, at every 25 min we took a measurement of the BAC using a BACtrack Trace[TM] Pro breathalyzer. This measurement interval was determined by the cooldown rate of the breathalyzer. The activity chosen for the volunteers to engage in was a card or board game of their choice. Drinking stopped before 1.5 h while collection and BAC measurement continued for another 30–45 min.

4.2 Data Analysis

The Microsoft Band we used has an assortment of interesting physical and virtual sensors, including: accelerometer, gyroscope, distance, heart rate, pedometer, skin temperature, and ultraviolet level. With our sample size of only five volunteers and a controlled setting for the experiments, some of these sensors will not be very useful for this study, such as the: distance, pedometer, and ultraviolet level, sensors. In fact their usefulness may be limited even with larger datasets.

We begin our analysis with the heart rate (HR) data by normalizing the heart rates and BACs per subject. This way we can plot and compare the HR values over the BAC and see if there are any obvious patterns. Doing this we get the plots shown in Fig. 3.

The heart rate increases over time for three of the subjects (0, 2, 3) at different rates, decreases for one (4), and stays level for one (1). These observations are consistent with data in [2]; a study where the authors relate low and high

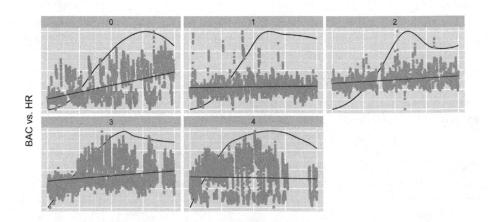

Fig. 3. Heart Rate and BAC per subject (normalized)

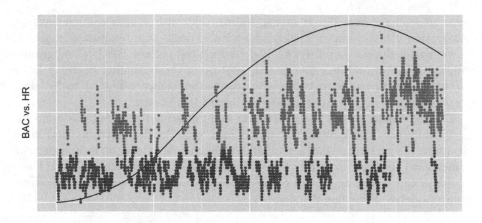

Fig. 4. Heart rate split into baseline and excited states

HR responses to behavioral traits. Interestingly, most of the subjects seem to show two patterns of HR activity. One is the baseline HR activity, and another is an excitied HR activity that seems to have better correlation with BAC. This is most clearly seen in the plot for subject 0, shown in Fig. 4. It's not a consistent pattern, however. Subject 1 had a very level heart rate with spikes at the regular drinking intervals, and subject 2 had relatively little variance throughout. Overall, it seems that experiencing excitement while intoxicated results in a more exaggerated HR response than while sober. This may be useful information for determining drunkenness.

Next, we plotted the normalized skin temperature over time on top of the normalized BAC values; this is shown in Fig. 5. Visually, we see that the correlation of skin temperature and BAC is highly significant. This is because of the well known vasodilation effect of alcohol causing warm blood to come near

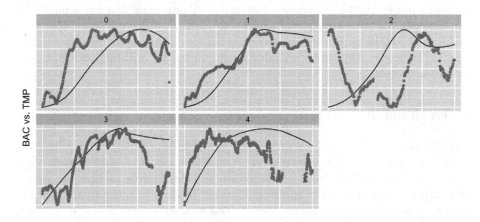

Fig. 5. Skin Temperature and BAC per subject (normalized)

the surface of the skin [5]. It is also known that with a high enough level of intoxication it behaves as a vasoconstrictor and drops skin temperature, which we see with subjects 3 and 4 who had reached the highest BAC of the group. Subject 2 had a rapid decrease in temperature at the beginning (we may have started collection too soon before the smartwatch sensor adjusted to his skin temperature), it may be appropriate to discard this portion.

The movement sensors (accelerometer and gyroscope) were not too interesting visually or statistically. They might have some hidden patterns that contribute to the performance of a modeling technique. We think its usefulness will be increased if we can use it first to predict whether a user is taking a drink, then provide a time-based aggregate of the estimated number of drinks as a feature in our model to determine drunkenness.

4.3   Features Setup

Skin temperature and heart rate will have different ranges of values unique to each subject, so per-subject normalization must be performed to put them on the same scale. A simple unity-based normalization (min-max) is used to put the feature values in the range 0 to 1. No transformations are applied to the movement data.

4.4   Models and Tools

We will be taking a look at BAC prediction as both a classification and regression problem. As a classification problem, we will threshold the BAC values at a point where we may want to warn the user. This allows the data to be used as a binary classification problem. For this we will use logistic regression and SVM.

As a regression problem, we will be attempting to predict the observed BAC directly. To do this, we will use linear regression and artificial neural networks (ANN). Using a regression approach, this will allow a user to select their own threshold rather than the threshold determined in a classification model. We may however want the threshold to be fixed.

All work will be performed in R version 3.2.1 using the additional 'nnet' and 'kernlab' packages. Any necessary additional information will be provided in the evaluation section.

5   Evaluation

Overall, our data set contains 233,538 samples that were collected from five volunteers. Each sample was collected every three seconds from a Microsoft Band smartwatch by our Android data collection system. In this section, we evaluate the performance of a few machine learning models on our dataset. We use some standard performance measures for our evaluation: precision, recall, and F1-score, for the classification models; RMSE and R^2 for the regression models. All reported performance values are determined via 5-fold cross-validation.

5.1   Classification

We want to warn a person if they are close to reaching the legal limit of 0.08 BAC. A good time to warn a user is at about 0.065 BAC. Using this threshold, the classes are split into 64 % is *DRUNK*, and 36 % *SOBER*.

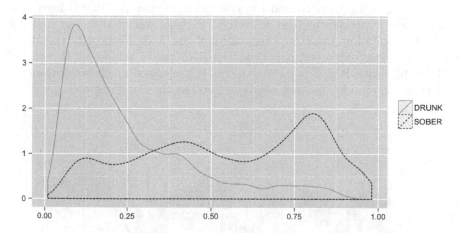

Fig. 6. Logistic regression output frequency with actual labels

To get a baseline, we first trained a logistic regression model. This model outputs values from 0.0 to 1.0, so we need to determine where to best split this output into each class. In Fig. 6, we show a plot of the predictions of the model on the test data, using the actual labels to distinguish the output. In this plot, we see that the best threshold value for the logistic model predictions is around 0.32; above that we classify *SOBER* and below that *DRUNK*. Using this, we achieved a precision of 0.855 ± 0.002, recall of 0.730 ± 0.004, and F1-score of 0.787 ± 0.003.

Moving forward, we trained a SVM model using the Gaussian Radial Basis Function (RBF) kernel. For time constraints, the dataset was reduced by half using a uniform subsample. Even so, we found the SVM was able to achieve great performance with a precision of 0.886 ± 0.002, recall of 0.930 ± 0.002, and overall F1-score of 0.907 ± 0.001. Ideally we do not want to warn our users that they are drunk when they are not actually drunk, so we want to try and optimize the model to be as precise as possible. By modifying the error weighting to train against false positive errors, the SVM model achieved a precision of 0.970 ± 0.002, with recall of 0.729 ± 0.003, and F1-score of 0.832 ± 0.002. Our recall dropped for a higher precision, which is a well-known tradeoff for this kind of tuning, but this is fine. We can set a threshold on our smartphone warning system that if at least a recall fraction of the samples from our smartwatch are classified as *DRUNK*, then there is a precision chance that the user is actually at 0.065 BAC.

5.2   Regression

So how does this do as a regression problem? We first considered the most basic: a linear regression model. This did not perform well at all. We next trained a neural network (ANN) model on the data. The best performing ANN had a structure with twenty nodes in one hidden layer. This was determined by doubling and then reducing node count to find the best performance. Additional layers did not show any improvement (the 'neuralnet' package was used to test multiple layers). Figure 7 plots the BAC predictions of the ANN along with the actual values using data from a test partition. The ANN model achieved a R^2 value of 0.524 ± 0.015, with RMSE of 0.026 ± 0.000. It performed much better than the linear regression model, but not nearly as good as the classification models.

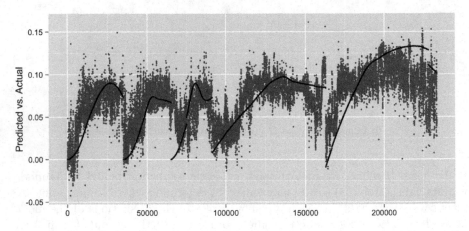

Fig. 7. ANN predictions (blue) with actual BAC data (black) on test partition (Color figure online)

6   Conclusions

We investigated the design of a general system that could be used for many applications, whether it be a BAC warning system, or a geographical mapping service that displays the smartwatch data of users on a choropleth map. Part of this system was a general Android-based gateway that can be used to collect data from a variety of sensors connected to an Android smartphone.

We then designed an experiment to collect labeled data consistently from volunteers. After this, we analyzed the data to discover if there were any interesting patterns that were immediately obvious. We found that skin temperature was a good indicator of drunkenness (in our controlled setting). We also discovered that excited heart rate looks to also be a good indicator of intoxication level.

Following the overview analysis, we dove into training some regression and classification models. Achieving good performance as a regression problem was difficult. We found that the problem was much better tackled as a classification problem. This worked better because our classification models could ignore a good deal of the variance in the straight BAC predictions. In the end, we found SVM to perform the best on our data.

There are still many other factors to consider in forming a better models. From this research, we found that the accurate prediction of drunkenness in a real application looks possible in theory. There are still many obstacles surrounding the collection of a larger and better data set. Ideally, we would want a data set from a thousand volunteers in candid situations over several days. The two biggest problems are, how do we label the data with the alcohol levels in this scenario, and how can we model this enormous amount of data in reasonable time? Also, will we need to first determine the activity of the user, or will the other sensors provide sufficient information? And if the former, how can we consistently tag these activities in the data? The answers to this may be simple, or infeasible. In any case, it would be worth it to try and find out.

Acknowledgement. We thank the National Science Foundation for funding the research under the Research Experiences for Undergraduates Program (CNS-1358939) at Texas State University to perform this piece of work and the infrastructure provided by a NSF-CRI 1305302 award.

References

1. Andersson, A., Wiréhn, A.B., Ölvander, C., Ekman, D.S., Bendtsen, P.: Alcohol use among university students in Sweden measured by an electronic screening instrument. BMC Public Health **9**, 229 (2009)
2. Assaad, J.M., Pihl, R.O., Séguin, J.R., Nagin, D.S., Vitaro, F., Tremblay, R.E.: Intoxicated behavioral disinhibition and the heart rate response to alcohol. Exp. Clin. Psychopharmacol. **14**(3), 377 (2006)
3. Baldwin, J.: Wearable blood alcohol measuring device, US Patent App. 14/298,847 (2014). http://www.google.com/patents/US20140365142
4. Chambers, M., Liu, M., Moore, C.: Drunk driving by the numbers
5. Dekker, D.O.A.: What are the effects of alcohol on the brain? July 1999. http://www.scientificamerican.com/article/what-are-the-effects-of-a/. Accessed 16 August 2015
6. Guiry, J.J., van de Ven, P., Nelson, J.: Multi-sensor fusion for enhanced contextual awareness of everyday activities with ubiquitous devices. Sensors **14**(3), 5687–5701 (2014)
7. Koukiou, G., Anastassopoulos, V.: Neural networks for identifying drunk persons using thermal infrared imagery. Forensic Sci. Int. **252**, 69–76 (2015). http://www.sciencedirect.com/science/article/pii/S0379073815001681
8. Landro, L.: Why connected medicine is becoming vital to health care, June 2015. http://www.wsj.com/articles/why-connected-medicine-is-becoming-vital-to-health-care-1435243250
9. Hacking health: How consumers use smartphones and wearable tech to track their health, April 2014. http://www.nielsen.com/us/en/insights/news/2014/hacking-health-how-consumers-use-smartphones-and-wearable-tech-to-track-their-health.html

10. Posey, D., Mozayani, A.: The estimation of blood alcohol concentration. Forensic Sci. Med. Pathol. **3**(1), 33–39 (2007)
11. Schoenborn, C.A., Adams, P.F., Peregoy, J.A.: Health behaviors of adults: United states, 2008–2010. Vital Health Stat. **257**, 14–29 (2013). Data from the National Health Survey
12. Sharma, V., Mankodiya, K., De La Torre, F., Zhang, A., Ryan, A., Ton, T.G.N., Gandhi, R., Jain, S.: SPARK: personalized parkinson disease interventions through synergy between a smartphone and a smartwatch. In: Marcus, A. (ed.) DUXU 2014, Part III. LNCS, vol. 8519, pp. 103–114. Springer, Heidelberg (2014)
13. Tacconi, C., Mellone, S., Chiari, L.: Smartphone-based applications for investigating falls and mobility. In: 2011 5th International Conference on Pervasive Computing Technologies for Healthcare (PervasiveHealth), pp. 258–261, May 2011
14. Ward, L.: How to cut student drinking. Wall Street J., p. R5 (2015)
15. Webster, G.D., Gabler, H.C.: Feasibility of transdermal ethanol sensing for the detection of intoxicated drivers. Associating Adv. Automot. Med. **51**, 449–464 (2007)
16. Wikipedia, : Blood alcohol content – wikipedia, the free encyclopedia (2015). https://en.wikipedia.org/w/index.php?title=Blood_alcohol_content&oldid=674051485. Accessed 13 July 2015

Time and Economic Burden of Comorbidities Among COPD Inpatients

Jiaqi Liu[1], James Ma[3], Jiaojiao Wang[1], Daniel Zeng[1],
Hongbin Song[4], Ligui Wang[4], and Zhidong Cao[1,2(✉)]

[1] The State Key Laboratory of Management and Control for Complex Systems,
Institute of Automation, Chinese Academy of Sciences, Beijing, China
{jiaqi.liu,Zhidong.cao}@ia.ac.cn
[2] Cloud Computing Center, Chinese Academy of Sciences, Dongguan, China
[3] College of Business, University of Colorado, Colorado Springs, USA
[4] Institute of Disease Control and Prevention, Academy of Military
Medical Sciences, Beijing, China

Abstract. Chronic obstructive pulmonary disease (COPD) is a major public health problem and usually associated with various comorbidities. Base on electronic health records of inpatients, aged 40 to 80 years old, from 169 hospitals located across China between 2013 and 2014, this paper summarized 27 comorbidities of COPD and compared the time and economic burdens of COPD patients to non-COPD patients. The 17 comorbidities included in Charlson Comorbidity Index (CCI) and 10 additional comorbidities were employed while odds ratios were considered to compare differences. The results disclosed that COPD patients had higher comorbidity burdens than non-COPD patients did. Moreover, COPD patients had 6.40 % more hospital stay and 12.96 % lower medical cost. Seven morbidities had positive correlations with hospital stay and medical cost, which indicated that COPD patients should be paid more attention to those comprehensive comorbidities when making therapeutic plans.

Keywords: COPD · Comorbidity · Time burden · Economic burden · Inpatient · CCI · Population study

1 Introduction

Chronic obstructive pulmonary disease (COPD) is a preventable and treatable disease state characterized by airflow limitation that is not fully reversible [1]. Depending on World Health Organization (WHO), COPD is the third major killers during the past decade, which resulted in 3.1 million deaths in 2012 [2]. Furthermore, COPD places heavy economic burdens on patients. In 2010, the cost of COPD in the USA was projected to be approximately US $50 billion, which includes $20 billion in indirect costs and $30 billion in direct health care expenditures [3].

A variety of comorbidities are associated with COPD, which markedly affect health outcomes in COPD [4]. COPD can no longer be considered a disease only of the lungs, as it is often associated with a wide variety of systemic consequences [5]. For example, researchers found that patients with COPD are in an increased risk of developing type 2

X. Zheng et al. (Eds.): ICSH 2015, LNCS 9545, pp. 187–195, 2016.
DOI: 10.1007/978-3-319-29175-8_17

diabetes, because some aspects of inflammation can predict the development of diabetes and glucose disorders [6]. Charlson Comorbidity Index (CCI) and its modified comorbidity index were used widely to measure patients' comorbidity conditions [11]. In addition, researchers disclosed that Medicaid COPD patients had higher comorbidity burdens, more medical claims, and more medical cost than did patients without COPD [8]. However, existing research works related to this issue were based on small data sets, normally thousands of patients. Health big data analysis may find more interesting results.

In this paper, we evaluated the comorbidity burdens of COPD patients through mining a large Electronic Health Records data set. The time and economic burdens of inpatients with COPD were analyzed and compared with non-COPD inpatients. The object of this study is to analyze the degrees of time and economic impact among COPD inpatients with different comorbidities.

The rest of this paper is organized as follows. Section 2 provided a description to our data set and methods utilized in this study. We reported our statistical results in Sect. 3. In Sect. 4, we discussed and concluded the paper.

2   Data and Methods

2.1   Data Set

The Electronic Health Records (EHRs) being analyzed in this study were provided by the Chinese National Surveillance System. This surveillance system had been adopted by 192 hospitals located across China. In order to maintain a high data quality, EHRs from 169 hospitals for 2013 to 2014 were used in this research. The patient's personal and medical information was collected by clinical doctors while the patient was hospitalized. The data was then summarized by trained staff and checked by certified agencies before the data was submitted to the surveillance system. Thus the information included in the EHRs should be highly reliable and objective.

The study population was limited to inpatients aged 40 to 80 years old. Patients younger than 40 years were excluded because they usually have a low risk for COPD. Patients older than 80 years were also excluded due to the limited number of data records.

Only patient's sex, age, time, cost, and clinical diagnostic information were utilized to perform our analysis. Patient's identity-related information was masked automatically by the system before we started our study.

2.2   Measures of Comorbidity Burden

Comorbidity burden of inpatients with COPD was mainly evaluated by the CCI with the Sundararajan modification [9, 10]. The CCI was a useful tool for health researchers to measure comorbid disease status in health databases. It defined 17 comorbidities through reviewing hospital charts and assessed their relevancies in the prediction of 1-year mortality. A weighted score was assigned to each comorbidities, and the sum of the score (defined as CCI score) is identified as an indicator of disease burden, and a robust estimator of mortality [9]. Because COPD is a kind of chronic pulmonary disease (CPD), we excluded COPD patients from CPD and considered CPD without COPD as a unique class of diseases. Moreover, 10 additional conditions, including 6 conditions according to Lin [11] and 4 commonly observed comorbidities among patients with COPD in our data set, were also taken into account in our study.

All 27 comorbidities were identified through International Classification of Diseases, 10th Revision, Clinical Modification (ICD-10-CM), which is the statistical classification of disease published by the WHO.

Four measures were employed to evaluate the comorbidity burden: (1) mean CCI score; (2) prevalence of each morbidity and odds ratio (OR), which described the ratio of the odds for a patient with COPD and a specific comorbidity to the odds for a patient without COPD and with that same comorbidity; (3) mean number of comorbidities; and (4) total number of comorbidities (categorized as 0, 1, 2, 3, and ≥4).

2.3 Measures of Time and Economic Burdens

In evaluating the time burden of inpatients with COPD, we use the duration of hospital stays, which defined as the total number of nights staying in a hospital. In our research design, if the admission date is the same as the discharge date in one EHR, we defined the hospital stay of this patient as 0.

In order to assess the economic burden, total medical cost, which obtained directly from EHRs, was used. Total medical cost contained the out-of-pocket expenses that an inpatient was required to pay in hospital.

2.4 Analysis

Independent-samples t-test was used to compare mean CCI score, mean number of comorbidities, mean hospital stay, and mean medical cost for patients with COPD and patients without COPD. Odds ratio (OR) of each comorbidity was predicted by binary logistic regression while Wald chi-square statistic tested the unique contribution of each comorbidity. Incremental hospital stay of each comorbidity was calculated by taking the difference of mean hospital stay between COPD and non-COPD patients; the same process was repeated for obtaining the incremental medical cost.

3 Results

3.1 Characteristics of the Study Population

EMRs from 196,388 COPD and 4,332,068 non-COPD patients were employed in our study. The demographic characteristics of the study population are summarized in Table 1. Compared with non-COPD patients, COPD patients have a significantly higher mean age (66.76 vs. 57.29), higher male hospitalization rate (68.92 % vs. 54.44 %), and prefer medical insurance to cover their hospitalization cost (68.40 % vs.

Table 1. Characteristics of the study population

	Original sample (n = 4,528,456)	
	COPD (n = 196,388)	N-COPD (n = 4,332,068)
Mean age, years (s.d.)	66.76 (8.923)	57.29 (10.474)
Male, %	68.92	54.44
Level of hospital, %		
Grade 3-A	70.48	76.79
Grade 3-B	12.48	10.78
Grade 3-C	0.97	1.11
Grade 2	16.07	11.33
Payment method, %		
Medical insurance	68.40	56.52
Out-of-pocket expenses	24.91	34.89
Other	6.69	8.58

COPD: chronic obstructive pulmonary disease; s.d.: standard deviation.

56.52 %). Moreover, different level of the hospital was of comparable admission rate between COPD patients and non-COPD patients.

3.2 Comorbidity Burden

The comorbidity prevalence for COPD and non-COPD patients was summarized in Table 2. In overall, the comorbidity burden is significantly higher in COPD patients than non-COPD patients (mean CCI score: 1.35 vs. 1.13; mean number of comorbidities: 1.73 vs. 1.11).

For comorbidities included in the CCI, the prevalence rates of congestive heart failure (19.23 %), cerebrovascular disease (16.11 %), any malignancy (13.41 %), diabetes (12.61 %), and chronic pulmonary disease (12.15 %) were high in patients with COPD. Although some of them were also prevalent in patients without COPD, patients with COPD were significantly more likely to have chronic pulmonary disease (OR: 12.095), congestive heart failure (OR: 5.468), myocardial infarction (OR: 1.521), and cerebrovascular disease (OR: 1.391). The prevalence rates of other comorbidities included in CCI were either too low to report or almost similar for patients with and without COPD.

Among the 10 additional comorbidities, 6 comorbidities had high prevalence rates. Patients with COPD were more likely to have pulmonary heart disease (18.51 %, OR: 54.464), atherosclerosis (5.44 %, OR: 2.000), hypertension (34.66 %, OR: 1.569), and gastritis and duodenitis (18.51 %, OR: 1.468). Cholelithiasis (5.29 %, OR: 1.258) and disorders of lipoprotein metabolism (7.14, OR: 1.116) did not have a big difference between COPD patients and non-COPD patients. Because of different data acquisition methods, prevalence rates of 4 comorbidities proposed by Lin [11] were very low. Therefore, we removed those 4 comorbidities and comorbidities with low prevalence rates in CCI from our study.

Table 2. Comorbidity prevalence for COPD and non-COPD patients

Comorbidity	COPD (n = 196388)	N-COPD (n = 4332068)	Odds ratio (95 % CI)	p-value
Mean CCI score (s.d.)	1.35(1.788)	1.13(1.839)	-	<0.001
Comorbidities included in the CCI				
Myocardial infarction	2.17 %	1.43 %	1.521 (1.474, 1.570)	<0.001
Congestive heart failure	19.23 %	4.17 %	5.468 (5.402, 5.535)	<0.001
Peripheral vascular disease	0.28 %	0.20 %	-[a]	-
Cerebrovascular disease	16.11 %	12.13 %	1.391 (1.374, 1.409)	<0.001
Dementia	0.35 %	0.16 %	-[a]	-
Chronic pulmonary disease[b]	12.15 %	1.13 %	12.095 (11.900, 12.292)	<0.001
Rheumatologic disease	1.15 %	0.98 %	1.169 (1.120, 1.220)	<0.001
Peptic ulcer disease	2.03 %	1.62 %	1.254 (1.214, 1.295)	<0.001
Mild liver disease	1.97 %	4.08 %	0.472 (0.457, 0.487)	<0.001
Diabetes	12.61 %	12.66 %	0.995 (0.982, 1.009)	0.4681
Diabetes with chronic complications	1.79 %	2.62 %	0.676 (0.654, 0.699)	<0.001
Hemiplegia or paraplegia	0.12 %	0.18 %	-[a]	-
Renal disease	3.98 %	3.61 %	1.109 (1.084, 1.135)	<0.001
Any malignancy, including leukemia and lymphoma	13.41 %	15.08 %	0.872 (0.860, 0.883)	<0.001
Moderate or severe liver disease	0.89 %	0.86 %	-[a]	-
Metastatic solid tumor	4.26 %	4.81 %	0.881 (0.862, 0.901)	<0.001
AIDS	0.04 %	0.03 %	-[a]	-
Comorbidities not included in the CCI				
Hypertension	34.66 %	25.26 %	1.569 (1.554, 1.584)	<0.001
Depression	0.25 %	0.28 %	-[a]	-
Sleep apnea	0.54 %	0.21 %	-[a]	-
Tobacco use	0.00 %	0.00 %	-[a]	-
Edema	0.24 %	0.11 %	-[a]	-
Pulmonary heart disease	18.51 %	0.42 %	54.464 (53.463, 55.484)	<0.001
Gastritis and duodenitis	8.27 %	5.79 %	1.468 (1.444, 1.492)	<0.001
Disorders of lipoprotein metabolism	7.14 %	6.44 %	1.116 (1.097, 1.136)	<0.001
Atherosclerosis	5.44 %	2.80 %	2.000 (1.960, 2.041)	<0.001

(Continued)

Table 2. (*Continued*)

Comorbidity	COPD (n = 196388)	N-COPD (n = 4332068)	Odds ratio (95 % CI)	p-value
Cholelithiasis	5.29 %	4.25 %	1.258 (1.232, 1.283)	<0.001
Mean number of comorbidities (s.d.)				
	1.73(1.306)	1.11(1.209)	-	<0.001
Total number of comorbidities				
0	18.05 %	40.12 %	0.329 (0.325, 0.333)	<0.001
1	29.64 %	27.94 %	1.087 (1.076, 1.097)	<0.001
2	27.22 %	18.74 %	1.622 (1.605, 1.638)	<0.001
3	15.56 %	8.56 %	1.968 (1.943, 1.993)	<0.001
≥4	9.53 %	4.64 %	2.166 (2.132, 2.200)	<0.001

AIDS: acquired immune deficiency syndrome; CCI: Charlson Comorbidity Index; CI: confidence interval; COPD: chronic obstructive pulmonary disease.
[a]Odds ratio was not reported because too few patients had this comorbidity. [b]Excluding COPD.

Table 3. Incremental stay and cost for COPD and non-COPD cohorts by comorbidity

Comorbidity[a]	Mean stay		Δ day	p-value	Mean Cost, $		Δ cost	p-value
	COPD	N-COPD			COPD	N-COPD		
Overall	11.97	11.25	0.72	<0.001	2610.97	2999.84	−388.87	<0.001
Comorbidities included in the CCI								
Myocardial infarction	11.34	10.35	0.99	<0.001	3638.20	5378.96	−1740.77	<0.001
Congestive heart failure	11.79	11.52	0.27	<0.001	2511.15	3991.01	−1479.87	<0.001
Cerebrovascular disease	13.35	12.98	0.37	<0.001	2808.08	3200.67	−392.59	<0.001
Chronic pulmonary disease[b]	11.78	11.52	0.26	0.001	2250.20	2318.70	−68.50	0.008
Rheumatologic disease	12.70	11.79	0.91	<0.001	2523.94	2274.80	249.14	0.001
Peptic ulcer disease	12.45	11.47	0.98	<0.001	2967.86	2901.89	65.97	0.316
Mild liver disease	13.08	12.00	1.08	<0.001	4112.35	3921.73	190.62	0.042
Diabetes	12.78	12.37	0.41	<0.001	2869.38	2997.34	−127.96	<0.001
Diabetes with chronic complications	13.19	12.80	0.39	0.023	2569.23	2172.60	396.63	<0.001
Renal disease	13.88	14.72	-0.84	<0.001	3394.73	3167.55	227.18	<0.001
Any malignancy, including leukemia and lymphoma	14.08	13.16	0.92	<0.001	4182.19	4374.48	−192.28	<0.001
Metastatic solid tumor	13.07	12.03	1.04	<0.001	3939.17	3814.40	124.76	0.010
Comorbidities not included in the CCI								
Hypertension	12.38	11.83	0.55	<0.001	2642.71	3016.78	−374.06	<0.001
Pulmonary heart disease	11.86	13.69	-1.83	<0.001	2290.90	4821.00	−2530.10	<0.001
Gastritis and duodenitis	11.62	10.32	1.30	<0.001	2296.59	2156.12	140.47	<0.001
Disorders of lipoprotein metabolism	11.50	10.87	0.63	<0.001	2257.23	2296.38	−39.15	0.106

(*Continued*)

Table 3. (*Continued*)

Comorbidity[a]	Mean stay		Δ day	p-value	Mean Cost, $		Δ cost	p-value
	COPD	N-COPD			COPD	N-COPD		
Atherosclerosis	12.07	11.45	0.62	<0.001	2566.75	2469.75	97.00	0.001
Cholelithiasis	12.14	11.11	1.03	<0.001	2805.84	3100.36	−294.53	<0.001

AIDS: Acquired Immune Deficiency Syndrome; CCI: Charlson Comorbidity Index; COPD: Chronic Obstructive Pulmonary Disease;
[a]8 comorbidities with <1 % of prevalence were excluded. These comorbidities were peripheral vascular disease, dementia, hemiplegia or paraplegia, moderate or severe liver disease, AIDS, depression, sleep apnea, edema.
[b]Excluding COPD.

As for the total number of comorbidities, the rates of patients with and without COPD had 1 comorbidity were comparable (29.64 % vs. 27.94 %). However, 27.22 %, 15.56 %, and 9.53 % of COPD patients had 2, 3 and ≥4 comorbidities, respectively, compared to 18.74 %, 8.56 %, and 4.64 % in patients without COPD. In terms of 27 comorbidities proposed, only 18.05 % COPD patients had none comorbidity compared to 40.12 % in non-COPD patients.

3.3 Incremental Hospital Stay and Medical Cost by Comorbidity

Incremental hospital stay and medical cost were calculated for 18 remaining comorbidities and summarized in Table 3. In general, patients with COPD had 6.40 % higher hospital stay than non-COPD patients (11.97 vs. 11.25, $p < 0.001$). Gastritis and duodenitis (11.62 vs. 10.32), mild liver disease (13.08 vs. 12.00), metastatic solid tumor (13.07 vs. 12.03), and cholelithiasis (12.14 vs. 11.11) had the biggest incremental hospital stay. An overwhelming majority of comorbidities, except renal disease and pulmonary heart disease, had positive incremental hospital stay.

However, the medical cost of COPD patients was 12.96 % lower than non-COPD patients ($2610.97 vs. $2999.84, $p < 0.001$). Compared with non-COPD patients, COPD patients who had pulmonary heart disease ($2290.90 vs. $4821.00), myocardial infarction ($3638.20 vs. $5378.96), and congestive heart failure ($2511.15 vs. $3991.01) had the biggest decline in medical cost. Among comorbidities with significantly difference ($p < 0.05$), only 7 of 16 comorbidities had positive medical cost. COPD patients who had diabetes with chronic complications ($2569.23 vs. $2172.60), rheumatologic disease ($2523.94 vs. $2274.80), and renal disease ($3394.73 vs. $3167.55) had higher medical cost than non-COPD patients. In addition, the medical cost of patients with peptic ulcer disease and disorders of lipoprotein metabolism did not show significant differences.

4 Discussion and Conclusion

In our research, prevalence rates of 27 comorbidities as well as their time and economic implications had been investigated among inpatients with and without COPD. With higher mean CCI score, higher ORs for 13 out of the 18 comorbidities examined, higher mean number of comorbidities, and higher total number of comorbidities, we found that COPD patients had bigger comorbidity burden. We also found that COPD patients with most of the proposed comorbidities had incremental medical time, measured by hospital stay, compared with non-COPD patients, which indicated the patients with COPD should be paid more attention to comprehensive comorbidity risk when making therapeutic plans. In addition, although our study disclosed the reduced medical cost among COPD patients with 18 comorbidities, there were still 7 comorbidities with considerably incremental medical cost which should be focused on.

The results of this study showed that CCI was an effective way to measure comorbidity burden. Even though it was initially put forward for mortality analysis, CCI gave a clear and concise list of the most important comorbidities. The weight score of comorbidities in CCI and the simple calculation method were useful in measuring comorbidities burden in our case study as well. Besides, prevalent comorbidities for the specific disease were as important as comorbidities in CCI. In our study, gastritis and duodenitis together with atherosclerosis was two important comorbidities which prevalent in COPD patients.

There were a few limitations in this study. First, although our inpatients data had been examined by professional inspectors before being submitted to the surveillance system, some comorbidities (e.g. depression) or conditions (e.g. tobacco use), which were easy to be neglected, may escape medical staffs notice. Second, CCI is a common approach to evaluate patient's mortality. However, it may not be the best index in evaluating patient's comorbidity burden. The Comorbidity-Poly pharmacy Score [12] and the Elixhauser Comorbidity Measure [13] are both potentially useful measures. Third, the measures, which proposed evaluating time and economic implications, were somewhat simple and preliminary. More systematic and comprehensive evaluation system would give a more accurate description of the time and economic burdens among patients.

Acknowledgments. This study was funded by National Natural Science Foundation of China (Nos. 91024030, 71025001, 91224008, 91324007) and National Science and Technology Major Project of China (Nos. 2012ZX10004801, 2013ZX10004218).

References

1. Celli, B.R., MacNee, W., Agusti, A., et al.: Standards for the diagnosis and treatment of patients with COPD: a summary of the ATS/ERS position paper. Eur. Respir. J. **23**, 932–946 (2004)
2. Top 10 causes of death. http://www.who.int/mediacentre/factsheets/fs310/en/
3. Guarascio, A.J., Ray, S.M., Finch, C.K., Self, T.H.: The clinical and economic burden of chronic obstructive pulmonary disease in the USA. ClinicoEconomics and Outcomes Res.: CEOR **5**, 235–245 (2013)
4. Sin, D.D., Anthonisen, N.R., Soriano, J.B., Agusti, A.G.: Mortality in COPD: role of comorbidities. Eur. Respir. J. **28**, 1245–1257 (2006)
5. Fabbri, L.M., Luppi, F., Beghe, B., Rabe, K.F.: Complex chronic comorbidities of COPD. Eur. Respir. J. **31**, 204–212 (2008)

6. Rana, J.S., Mittleman, M.A., Sheikh, J., et al.: Chronic obstructive pulmonary disease, asthma, and risk of type 2 diabetes in women. Diabetes Care **27**, 2478–2484 (2004)
7. Schmidt, M.I., Duncan, B.B., Sharrett, A.R., et al.: Markers of inammation and prediction of diabetes mellitus in adults (atherosclerosis risk in communities study): a cohort study. Lancet **353**, 1649–1652 (1999)
8. Sharabiani, M.T.A., Aylin, P., Bottle, A.: Systematic review of comorbidity indices for administrative data. Med. Care **50**, 1109–1118 (2012)
9. Charlson, M.E., Pompei, P., Ales, K.L., Mackenzie, C.R.: A new method of classifying prognostic co-morbidity in longitudinal-studies - development and validation. J. Chron. Dis. **40**, 373–383 (1987)
10. Sundararajan, V., Henderson, T., Perry, C., et al.: New ICD-10 version of the Charlson comorbidity index predicted in-hospital mortality. J. Clin. Epidemiol. **57**, 1288–1294 (2004)
11. Lin, P.J., Shaya, F.T., Scharf, S.M.: Economic implications of comorbid conditions among Medicaid beneficiaries with COPD. Resp. Med. **104**, 697–704 (2010)
12. Evans, D.C., Cook, C.H., Christy, J.M., et al.: Comorbidity-polypharmacy scoring facilitates outcome prediction in older trauma patients. J. Am. Geriatr. Soc. **60**, 1465–1470 (2012)
13. Van Walraven, C., Austin, P.C., Jennings, A., et al.: A modification of the elixhauser comorbidity measures into a point system for hospital death using administrative data. Med. Care **47**, 626–633 (2009)

How Price Affect Online Purchase Behavior in Online Healthcare Consulting? Perceived Quality as a Mediator

Jianwei Liu[✉] and Qiang Ye

School of Management, Harbin Institute of Technology, Harbin, China
{liujianwei.email@gmail.com,yeqiang@hit.edu.cn}

Abstract. Price has a major influence on online health consulting purchases; however, healthcare customers regard perceived quality based on the exposed information about physicians' abilities as an important basis for decision-making. This research examined the influencing mechanism of price on purchase behavior in the e-health context using a data set of 1,785 physicians from one largest online healthcare consulting platform. The results show that perceived quality has an incomplete mediating effect on the impact of price on purchase behavior. It means that the online healthcare counseling price not only has a direct positive effect but also indirect effect mediated by perceived quality on purchase behavior.

Keywords: Online healthcare · Counseling price · Perceived quality · Mediating effect · Purchase behavior

1 Introduction

E-health services developed rapidly towards more convenient and wieldy direction, and people gradually begin to accept, try and be used to this technology in recent years. With the growing availability of online professional doctors, as well as the consideration of taking less time and costs, an increasing number of people are using online medical sources to solve their healthcare problems. Recent surveys of online healthcare estimate that 59 % of American adults use Internet to help find medical information sources and support their treatment [1]. In addition, there are has been significant increased e-health consulting platform for customers to obtain useful information includes symptoms information, advice from professional doctors and treatment options.

Online healthcare distinguished from traditional offline healthcare as the following advantages: cost and time savings, more reliable privacy protection, avoiding embarrassment, convenient retrieval of information, and the ability to make an appointment of commutation with a specific doctor [2, 3]. Obviously, communicating with professional doctors by telephone counseling will lead a better effect on patients' conditions compared to waiting doctors' replies on their web page slowly. However, telephone counseling is paid-per-time, unlike leaving a message on doctors' websites is free in HaoDF which is one of the largest online healthcare consulting community in China. Moreover, the former just needs to upload the necessary information about patient' condition and make an appointment time to communicate by telephone, the latter is

© Springer International Publishing Switzerland 2016
X. Zheng et al. (Eds.): ICSH 2015, LNCS 9545, pp. 196–203, 2016.
DOI: 10.1007/978-3-319-29175-8_18

almost overwhelmed by the seekers and not sufficiently meet the seekers' expectations [4].

Although an increasing number of papers on online healthcare counseling have recently been published in the information system (IS) field, a large proportion of existing researches focus on the adoption and impact of e-health technology from the perspective of healthcare provider and vindicator. Literature studying online healthcare purchase behavior from a patient's perceptive is scanty. Most of studies demonstrated that quality is a main barrier on the Internet [5]. Facing such various information of plausible quality on the online health consulting platform, it is so hard for health customers to choose the most appropriate doctor. Relatively little is found about the impact of health customers' perceived quality on online healthcare service purchase behavior. In addition, researchers had investigated the influence of price on customers' perceived in e-commerce context, while this function is not yet confirmed in e-health.

The aim of this study is to examine how consulting price influence health customers' online healthcare purchase behaviors. More specifically, how perceived quality has a mediating effect between price and online healthcare purchase behavior.

2   Literature Review and Hypotheses

2.1   Quality Perceived by Customers

Perceived quality of online service by customers has been of increasing interest of e-commerce researchers, while they don't reach a consensus in online healthcare counseling field. However it is general agreed that perceived quality is primarily driven by an attractive and professional design [5, 6], visual anchors, and other prominent features related to quality [7]. Despite the importance of perception of online service, most related studies have focused on the aspects of web design included the code of conduct, a quality label, a user guidance system, and filtering tools [8]. Perceived quality of online service means the ability to meet customers' external and internal requirements [9]. In the online healthcare counseling context, consumers form perception about the overall quality of a specific doctor based on the website information they have been exposed to [8]. And evidence-based information is particularly important for customers within a healthcare context [10].

2.2   The Relationship Among Price, Perceived Quality and Online Purchase Behavior

The Relationship Between Price and Perceived Quality. There are a large number of researches studying the relationship between price and perceived quality both online and offline. Most researchers agreed that this relationship is significant and moderated by product type in traditional offline markets [11], while studies on e-commerce generally hold the same idea and indicate that price is positively related to perceived quality [12]. Oh demonstrates that online asymmetric information affects positive or genitive price deviation, then misleads buyers' judgements of quality [13]. So it can be assumed that health customers will take price into account when evaluating the targeted doctors' perceived quality directly and when making feedbacks that can influence their perception of service quality indirectly. So the first hypothesis is proposed as follow:

Hypothesis 1: The online healthcare counseling price has a positive effect on perceived quality.

The Relationship Between Perceived Quality and Online Purchase Behavior. Numerous researches have focused on the relationship among perceived quality, patient satisfaction, and behavioral intentions [14–16], and indicates that perceived quality has a direct and positive impact on customer satisfaction and trust [17]. Based on the Theory of Reasoned Action (TRA) [18] which implies belief → attitude → intention → behavior, we can deduce that perceived quality enhances belief and attitude of satisfaction and trust, then induces purchase intentions and lead to a purchase behavior finally. So we get the second hypothesis:

Hypothesis 2: The online healthcare perceived quality has a positive effect on purchase behavior.

The Relationship Between Price and Online Purchase Behavior. The customer online healthcare counseling behavior is both similar and different from the traditional e-commerce such as taobao.com. On the one hand, healthcare customers have higher privacy and security concerns who will require a higher cognitive and affective-based trust from sellers (physicians) [19]. On the other hand, these customers are confronted with various degrees of information asymmetry during online healthcare counseling purchase [20]. "Trust can mitigate information asymmetry by reducing transaction-specific risks, generating therefore price premiums [21]." Based on the above analysis, we can assume that facing higher privacy and security concerns and various degrees of information asymmetry online healthcare counseling customers need higher cognitive trust, which will generate price premiums for the sellers to mitigate information asymmetry and meet higher privacy and security concerns. In other words, healthcare customers are willing to pay more for the final purchase behavior, hence:

Hypothesis 3: The online healthcare counseling price has a positive effect on purchase behavior.

In addition, based on the above analysis, we can assume that the online healthcare counseling price not only has a direct positive effect but also indirect effect mediated by perceived quality on purchase behavior, hence:

Hypothesis 4: The online healthcare perceived quality has a mediated effect on the relationship between counseling price and purchase behavior.

3   Empirical Analysis

3.1   Data Description

The data used in this empirical study were collected from one of the largest online healthcare counseling platform (http://www.haodf.com) in China.

We obtained all the doctors' data possessed telephone consulting function which is a paid-per-time service on Nov 11 2014 by LocoySpider (a data collection software). To avoid the impact of different level of hospital, we just selected all the available physicians of the highest level hospitals from Beijing, Shanghai, Guangzhou and Shenzhen which are the four undoubted first-tier cities in China mainland. Ultimately, a data set of 1,785 physicians was applied in this empirical research. Table 1 provides the data description for this sample. In addition, to satisfy the classical linear model more closely, all the variables are calculated using a natural logarithm analysis [22].

Table 1. Description of variables

Variables	Description
Physician ID	Physician's ID
Purchase	Number of physician's times to be telephone consulted
Price	Price of physician's telephone counseling at a time
Perceived quality	Calculation by factor analysis extracted from the following six variables
N_Visit	Number of physician's online visitors
N_Patient	Number of physician's online patients
N_Gift	Number of physician's gifts that patients need to take extra money to buy from the website
N_Love	A comprehensive indicator measuring physician's active degree online provided by the website
N_Contibution	A indicator measuring physician's contribution to patients and website provided by the website
N_Letter	Number of thanks letters physician has received
OtherCon	Control variables as the following seven variables
Title	Physician's professional title
Positive_Rating	Percentage of positive evaluation
Mid_Rating	Percentage of middle evaluation
Time	Start time when physician joined in the website
N_Paper	Number of paper physician has written online
N_Abstract	Number of characters in personal introduction physician has written online
N_Speciality	Number of characters in personal speciality physician has written online

3.2 Empirical Models

In line with previous researches, we extracted perceived quality from related variables including N_Visit, N_Patient, N_Gift, N_Love, N_Contibution and N_Letter. We firstly conducted a factor analysis to extract a factor as a measure of perceived quality explaining most of the variance in the six components. Table 2 shows the Factor Analysis confirmed the existence of Factor I with eigenvalue (4.7630) greater than 1.0 that accounted for 79.38 % of the total variance.

Table 2. Results of factor analysis

	Mean	Standard deviation	Factor I extraction matrix	Factor I score coefficient
N_Visit	11.9075	2.1047	0.8250	0.4275
N_Patient	2.0552	1.8177	0.8031	0.4299
N_love	3.8464	1.7068	0.7824	0.4177
N_Gift	7.0315	3.1845	0.7813	0.3942
N_Contibution	5.3242	2.1732	0.8778	0.4296
N_Letter	1.8401	1.3233	0.8898	0.3434
Extraction sum of square loadings: 79.38 % (Eigenvalue: 4.7630)				
KMO measure of sampling adequacy: 0.8186				
Bartlett's test: Significance .000				

Based on the Table 2 and the following Eq. 1, perceived quality can be measured.

$$Perceived\ Quality = \sum_{i=1}^{6} Factor\ I\ Score\ Coefficient_i * \frac{Component_i - Mean_i}{Standard\ Deviation_i} \quad (1)$$

To highlight the primary ideas and variables in this empirical study, we use *OtherCon* as a comprehensive variable to represent all possible control variables including Title, Positive_Rating, Mid_Rating, Time, N_Paper, N_Abstract and N_Speciality. According to the above hypotheses, the following regression model can be constructed and examined.

$$Perceived\ Quality = \alpha_0 + \alpha_1 Price + \alpha_2 OtherCon + \varepsilon_1 \quad (2)$$

$$Purchase = \beta_0 + \beta_1 Perceived\ Quality + \beta_2 OtherCon + \varepsilon_2 \quad (3)$$

$$Purchase = \gamma_0 + \gamma_1 Price + \gamma_3 OtherCon + \varepsilon_3 \quad (4)$$

$$Purchase = \delta_0 + \delta_1 Price + \delta_2 Perceived\ Quality + \delta_3 OtherCon + \varepsilon_4 \quad (5)$$

4 Empirical Results

All the results of the regression analysis including robust check of Model 2–5 are presented in Table 3. The coefficient of price is positive and significant indicated by the regression result of model 2. Thus, Hypothesis 1 is supported demonstrating that online healthcare counseling price has a positive effect on customers' perceived quality.

The results of model 3 show that the coefficient of perceived quality is positive and significant, which supports Hypothesis 2 indicating that online healthcare perceived quality has a positive effect on purchase behavior.

Table 3. Results of regression analysis of model 2–5

	Model 2	Model 3	Model 4	Model 5
Price	0.4903*** (0.1060)		1.2320*** (0.0893)	0.4727*** (0.0201)
Perceived Quality		0.5059*** (0.0210)		1.2896*** (0.1012)
Title	0.0099 (0.1312)	0.7645*** (0.1093)	0.15184 (0.0894)	0.2173** (0.1049)
Positive_rating	1.6600*** (0.1061)	2.7491*** (0.0937)	3.1770*** (0.0707)	2.5623*** (0.0923)
Mid_rating	7.0186 (4.7989)	5.2563 (6.0355)	7.6344 (5.6239)	2.4666 (5.2467)
Time	0.8722*** (0.1340)	−0.1998*** (0.0506)	0.2961*** (0.0372)	−0.1377** (0.0467)
N_Paper	0.5492*** (0.0255)	−.1277*** (0.0240)	0.1941*** (0.0201)	−0.0994 (0.0225)
N_Abstract	−.0384 (0.0285)	−.0418** (0.0221)	−0.0473** (0.0187)	−0.0607*** (0.0209)
N_Speciality	0.0859** (0.0397)	−0.0929*** (0.0359)	−0.0099 (0.0314)	−0.0630 (0.0349)
Constant	−10.1544 (0.9985)	1.9026*** (0.3818)	−7.5955*** (0.4639)	−3.9218*** (0.5907)
N	1785	1785	1785	1785
Adjust R^2	0.4337	0.5567	0.5326	0.6041

Robust standard errors in parentheses-***$p < 0.01$, **$p < 0.05$, *$p < 0.1$

The results of model 4 indicates that the coefficient of price is positive and significant. Hence, Hypothesis 3 is also supported showing that online healthcare counseling price has a directly positive effect on purchase behavior.

Moreover, based on the regression results of model 5 with both positive and significant coefficients of price and perceived quality, we find an incomplete mediation of perceived quality on the relationship between price and purchase behavior in the online healthcare counseling context. It means that the online healthcare counseling price not only has a direct positive effect but also indirect effect mediated by perceived quality on purchase behavior.

5   Conclusion

The research problems of this study are generally solved by the empirical analysis using a data set of HaoDF. This study has deeply investigated the influencing mechanism of price on purchase behavior with an incomplete mediation of perceived quality in the online healthcare counseling context. As a result, healthcare customers' perceived quality based on the exposed information from the website contributes to a better understanding of the significantly positive impact of price on purchase behavior by a mediation function. The results suggest that the online healthcare consulting price has both direct and indirect effect on the final purchase behavior for customers.

From a theoretical perspective, our findings imply that perceived quality has a significant impact on the influencing mechanism of price on purchase behavior, which is an important implement for price-purchase theory in e-health. Simultaneously, this empirical study provides a vital reference for the online physicians to perform better for more purchase though increasing customers' perceptions of quality in a practical aspect.

We must note that our findings have limitations such as data collection only from a single online healthcare consulting website and four major cities in China.

Future research may be conducted from various aspects of information asymmetry, type of patients and price premium to research online healthcare consulting purchase behavior.

References

1. Fox, S., Duggan, M.: Health Online 2013. Pew Internet and American Life Project, Washington (2013)
2. Xiao, N., Sharman, R., Rao, H.R., et al.: Factors influencing online health information search: an empirical analysis of a national cancer-related survey. Decis. Support Syst. **57**, 417–427 (2014)
3. Ybarra, M., Suman, M.: Reasons, assessments and actions taken: sex and age differences in uses of Internet health information. Health Educ. Res. **23**, 512–521 (2008)
4. Nie, L., Li, T., Akbari, M., et al.: Wenzher: comprehensive vertical search for healthcare domain. In: Proceedings of the 37th International ACM SIGIR Conference on Research and Development in Information Retrieval, pp. 1245–1246. ACM (2014)
5. Papanikolaou, V., Zygiaris, S.: Service quality perceptions in primary health care centers in Greece. Health Expect. **17**(2), 197–207 (2014)

6. Ye, Q., Li, H., Wang, Z., et al.: The influence of hotel price on perceived service quality and value in e-tourism an empirical investigation based on online traveler reviews. J. Hospitality Tourism Res. **38**(1), 23–39 (2014)
7. Jones, J., Cassie, S., Thompson, M., et al.: Delivering healthcare information via the Internet: cardiac patients' access, usage, perceptions of usefulness, and web site content preferences. Telemed. e-Health **20**(3), 223–228 (2014)
8. Goetzinger, L., Park, J., Jung Lee, Y., et al.: Value-driven consumer e-health information search behavior. Int. J. Pharm. Healthc. Mark. **1**(2), 128–142 (2007)
9. Lin, Y., Su, H.: Strategic analysis of customer relationship management – a field study on hotel enterprises. Total Qual. Manag. Bus. Excellence **14**, 715–731 (2003)
10. Maloney, S., Ilic, D., Green, S.: Accessibility, nature and quality of health information on the internet: a survey on osteoarthritis. Rheumatology **44**(33), 382–385 (2005)
11. Lichtenstein, D.R., Burton, S.: The relationship between perceived and objective price-quality. J. Mark. Res. **26**, 429–443 (1989)
12. Cui, L., Yang, H.X., Hou, H.P.: A study of perceived quality and price: customer value-based pricing strategy. Paper presented at ICVE&VM 2009: Proceedings of the 2nd International Conference on Value Engineering and Value Management, Beijing, China (2009)
13. Oh, H.: Price fairness and its asymmetric effects on overall price, quality, and value judgments: the case of an upscale hotel. Tour. Manag. **24**, 387–399 (2003)
14. Sweeney, J.C., Danaher, T.S., McColl-Kennedy, J.R.: Customer effort in value cocreation activities improving quality of life and behavioral intentions of health care customers. J. Serv. Res. (2015). doi:10.1177/1094670515572128
15. Murti, A., Deshpande, A., Srivastava, N.: Service quality, customer (patient) satisfaction and behavioural intention in health care services: exploring the Indian perspective. J. Health Manag. **15**(1), 29–44 (2013)
16. Choi, K.S., Cho, W.H., Lee, S., et al.: The relationships among quality, value, satisfaction and behavioral intention in health care provider choice: a South Korean study. J. Bus. Res. **57**(8), 913–921 (2004)
17. Moliner, M.A.: Loyalty, perceived value and relationship quality in healthcare services. J. Serv. Manag. **20**(1), 76–97 (2009)
18. Fishbein, M., Ajzen, I.: Belief, Attitude, Intention, and Behavior: an Introduction to Theory and Research. Addison-Wesley, Reading (1975)
19. McCole, P., Ramsey, E., Williams, J.: Trust considerations on attitudes towards online purchasing: The moderating effect of privacy and security concerns. J. Bus. Res. **63**(9), 1018–1024 (2010)
20. Chiu, C.M., Chang, C.C., Cheng, H.L., et al.: Determinants of customer repurchase intention in online shopping. Online Inf. Rev. **33**(4), 761–784 (2009)
21. Ba, S., Pavlou, P.A.: Evidence of the effect of trust building technology in electronic markets: price premiums and buyer behavior. MIS Q. **26**, 243–268 (2002)
22. Wooldridge, J.M.: Introductory Econometrics: A Modern Approach, 4th edn. South Western Cengage Learning, Mason (2009)

Stress Quantification Using a Wearable Device for Daily Feedback to Improve Stress Management

Jesus Garcia-Mancilla[(✉)] and Victor M. Gonzalez

Usability and Interactive Systems Lab, Department of Computer Science,
Instituto Tecnológico Autónomo de México, Mexico City, Mexico
{jgarc293,victor.gonzalez}@itam.mx

Abstract. Stress is becoming a major problem in our society and most people do not know how to cope with it. We propose a novel approach to quantify the stress level using psychophysiological measures. Using an automatic stress detector that can be implemented in a mobile application, we managed to create an alternative to automatically detect stress using sensors from a wearable device, and once it is detected, a score is calculated for each one of the records. By identifying the stress during the day and giving a numeric value from biological signals to it, a visualization could be produced to facilitate the analysis information by users.

Keywords: Stress · Stress management · Wearables · Heart rate · Skin temperature · Galvanic skin response

1 Introduction

Stress can be defined as the state of psychological response to stimulus (either external or internal) that generates changes in several systems of the body. Stress is usually visible by observable behavior like perspiration, mouth dryness, breathing difficulties, or an increase in speech speed [1]. The correct management of stress, on the other hand, could help to reduce reported health problems like flu, sore throat, headaches, or backaches that occur when stress is present several times a day [2]; and to attenuate more challenging problems like immune system impairment, sleep difficulties, and the rise of the glucose level [3, 4].

Given the great variety of stress reactions, predicting behavior by only describing a particular situation becomes an impossible task, mainly because someone could tremble, sweat, and experience discomfort, but in the same situation, another person might not show the same level of subjective discomfort [5], or visible changes in behavior like facial expressions [6]. Given this scenario, for long time people have been used psychological measurements, starting with the formal description of a polygraph in 1881 [7], and later on, with the first efforts to measure emotions in 1925 with the use of galvanic skin response [8]. However, it was until the works of Schwartz [9] and Ekman [10] when this information was measured more accurately, and a better understanding was achieved on how emotions produce body responses.

© Springer International Publishing Switzerland 2016
X. Zheng et al. (Eds.): ICSH 2015, LNCS 9545, pp. 204–209, 2016.
DOI: 10.1007/978-3-319-29175-8_19

For this work, based on the work done by [10–12], we are characterizing stress by the rise of heart rate (HR), due to the effect of the cortisol hormone, which also decreases the blood flow to the limbs, causing a decrease in skin temperature (ST) and a rise of GSR; this last change is caused by increase in the limbs perspiration.

2   Formulas to Characterize Stress

Traditional ways to assess stress and anxiety are self-reported; one good example in this area is the Beck Anxiety Inventory [13]. Here we propose a non-subjective characterization of stress and anxiety.

2.1   Development

The sympathetic autonomous nervous system reacts when a stress episode occurs, and based on that, we created the next formula using the product of HR, ST, and GSR. The final value is squared to avoid negative numbers:

$$Stress = \left(\alpha_1 \varphi_{\alpha_1} (HR) \cdot \alpha_1 \varphi_{\alpha_1} (100 - ST) \cdot \alpha_2 \varphi_{\alpha_2} (GSR) \right)^2, \tag{1}$$

where $\phi \alpha_i (x)$ is defined as a sigmoid by:

$$\varphi_{\alpha_i} (x) = \frac{e^{\alpha_i x}}{1 - e^{\alpha_i x}}, \tag{2}$$

and x to the value of HR, ST, and GSR in the same period of time. The equations were created to give a positive value in which a higher value means a higher level of stress. In this particular case, the low raw value of ST is interpreted as a higher level of stress; that is why the inverse value has to be calculated, to match the logic of the equation. To do this, we select the maximum possible value that a wrist in normal condition could rise.

A parameter α was added to the formula to balance and to give more importance to the GSR value. Previous research shows that this metric is strongly related to the activation of the sympathetic autonomous nervous system. This activation increases perspiration in the limbs and is correlated to emotional activity [12, 14–16]. For that reason, the value of α_2 is higher (0.5) than that of α_1 (0.25) and the sum of the three values equals one, giving the 50 % of the weight to calculate the stress to the GSR. Finally, with the purpose of helping in the visualization and making easier understanding of the values, the next formula was used to normalize the values between 1 and 100.

$$StressNorm = \frac{Stress_i - min(Stress)}{max(Stress) - min(Stress)} \cdot 100 \tag{3}$$

3   Testing

To test the stress formula, we used a filtering algorithm[1] that receives the HR, ST, and GSR values and detects when the persons have a stress episode; after the detection, the formula is used to measure the stress intensity. The main reason to have this distinction was for minimum and maximum values of the normalization formula, if it was applied to all the data, these values could not reflect the real parameters.

In the present work, one person used a Basis PeakI® for 28 different days between January and April of 2015. The days were randomly selected and the participant had to keep a diary of stressful events. After data collection, we ran a filtering algorithm to detect stressful events and then, the stress formula to get minimum and maximum values for this particular user to do the normalization in the next step. The values were: min(Stress) = 283.61 and max(Stress) = 1, 397.79.

We plot a visualization of the normalized stress level to help a user to understand the changes during a day. All graphics presented in this work starts at 7 a.m. and finish at midnight. On Fig. 2 we can see how stress episodes can be visualized; one between 8:48 to 8:56 h. with score of 726.097, other between 17:24 to 17:45 h. with a score of 1540.76 and the third one at 22:38 until midnight with a score of 5,611.59. With a final score for March 18th was 7,878.45 (Fig. 1).

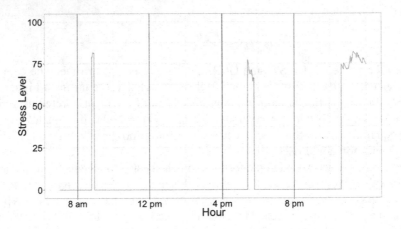

Fig. 1. March 18th.

4   Application

A possible application for this new approach is in a cognitive-behavioral program aimed to help people with a degenerative disease like diabetes or high blood pressure. In both cases stress management is important, because stress can compromise

---

[1] The algorithm will be publish on a future work by the same authors.

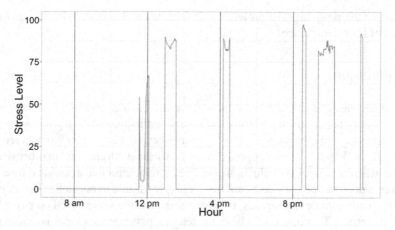

Fig. 2. January 21st.

treatment adherence and metabolic control, increase glucose levels in people with diabetes, and even accelerate the appearance of complications [17, 18].

Evidence-based decision making, as part of this approach, can use this information to help a patient to take better decisions to improve his/her health [19, 20]. This information could help to take healthier choices, facilitating change in patient's life style. This will improve quality of life and avoid health complications [21].

As can be seen in Fig. 2, it has the highest values from all the figures, the total score of that day was 12,283.46. This could be one day before a stress management program starts, the patient could wear a device for a week and the information collected could be the baseline. At the end of the program, a post-evaluation can be done to see how the patient improved, and as seen as in Fig. 3, a visual difference can be seen on stress intensity. Even though the stress episode lasted longer on April 1st, now the patient can handle it in a healthier way and the day's score is 4,462.759 (64 % lower than January 21st). An ongoing evaluation could be helpful if the patient can have the wearable device

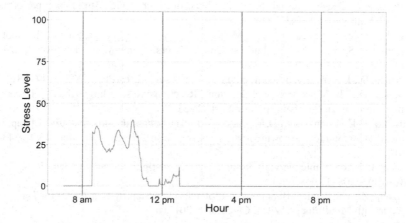

Fig. 3. January 21st.

every day of the program. The patient could take better decisions with this additional evidence of his performance.

5 Conclusion

With new technologies available and new wearable devices with several sensors that used to be big and uncomfortable to use, the new scenario presents as a great opportunity to create new ways to assess emotional responses like stress 24/7. The formula proposed in this work, could lead to novel approaches, not only in health care, but in other stressful scenarios where an ongoing evaluation could be more helpful that a post-test inventory.

Future work must be to collect data from a bigger sample to normalize the values on people with different demographics, to have a standardized scale based on psychophysiological metrics. This data could be collected in a psychoeducational program and it can help to test if this new approach can improve stress management.

Acknowledgments. This work has been supported by Asociación Mexicana de Cultura A.C. and the Consejo Nacional of Ciencia and Tecnología of México (CONACyT).

References

1. The APA Dictionary of Psychology (1st edn.). American Psychological Association, Washington, DC (2006)
2. DeLongis, A., Folkman, S., Lazarus, R.S.: The impact of daily stress on health and mood: psychological and social resources as mediators. J. Pers. Soc. Psychol. **54**(3), 486 (1988)
3. Alipour, A., Zare, H., Poursharifi, H., Sheibani, K.A., Ardekani, M.A.: The intermediary role of self-efficacy in relation with stress, glycosylated haemoglobin and health-related quality of life in patients with type2 diabetes. Iran. J. Public Health **41**(12), 76 (2012)
4. A.D. Association, American Diabetes Association Complete Guide to Diabetes: the Ultimate Home Reference from the Diabetes Experts, 5th edn. American Diabetes Association, Alexandria (2011)
5. Lazarus, R.S., Deese, J., Osler, S.F.: The effects of psychological stress upon performance. Psychol. Bull. **49**(4), 293–317 (1952)
6. Tsai, J.L., Pole, N., Levenson, R.W., Muñoz, R.F.: The effects of depression on the emotional responses of Spanish-speaking Latinas. Cultur. Divers. Ethnic Minor. Psychol. **9**(1), 49–63 (2003)
7. Newman, D.: Description of a polygraph. J. Anat. Psychol. **15**(Pt. 2), 235–237 (1881)
8. Wechsler, D.: The Measurement of Emotional Reactions: Researches on the Psycho-galvanic Reflex. Archives of Psychology, New York (1925)
9. Schwartz, G.E., Weinberger, D.A., Singer, J.A.: Cardiovascular differentiation of happiness, sadness, anger, and fear following imagery and exercise1. Psychosom. Med. **43**(4), 343–364 (1981)
10. Ekman, P.: Autonomic nervous system activity distiguishes among emotions. Science **221**(4616), 1208–1210 (1983)
11. Khazan, I.Z.: The Clinical Handbook of Biofeedback: a Step-by-Step Guide for Training and Practice with Mindfulness. Wiley, Chichester (2013)

12. Westerink, J.H., Van Den Broek, E.L., Schut, M.H., Van Herk, J., Tuinenbreijer, K.: Computing emotion awareness through galvanic skin response and facial electromyography. In: Westerink, J.H., Ouwerkerk, M., Overbeek, T.J.M., Pasveer, W.F., de Ruyter, B. (eds.) Probing experience, pp. 149–162. Springer, The Netherlands (2008)
13. Beck, A.T., Epstein, N., Brown, G., Steer, R.A.: An inventory for measuring clinical anxiety: psychometric properties. J. Consult. Clin. Psychol. 56(6), 893 (1988)
14. Ayzenberg, Y., Hernandez Rivera, J., Picard, R.: FEEL: frequent EDA and event logging–a mobile social interaction stress monitoring system. In: CHI 2012 Extended Abstracts on Human Factors in Computing Systems, pp. 2357–2362 (2012)
15. Nourbakhsh, N., Wang, Y., Chen, F., Calvo, R.A.: Using galvanic skin response for cognitive load measurement in arithmetic and reading tasks. In: Proceedings of the 24th Australian Computer-Human Interaction Conference, pp. 420–423 (2012)
16. Setz, C., Arnrich, B., Schumm, J., La Marca, R., Troster, G., Ehlert, U.: Discriminating stress from cognitive load using a wearable EDA device. IEEE Trans. Inf. Technol. Biomed. 14(2), 410–417 (2010)
17. Casillas-Mendoza, A.D., González-Pérez, O.P., Montes-Delgado, R.: Influence of progressive relaxation in old age adults who suffer type 2 diabetes - pilot study.pdf. Int. J. Hisp. Psychol. 3(2), 293–301 (2011)
18. Florentino, M.T.: Conductas de la Salud. Psicologia de la salud y calidad de vida, pp. 57–82. Cengage Learning, Mexico (2010)
19. Funnell, M.: New roles in diabetes care. Diab. Voice 46, 11–13 (2001)
20. Henrichs, H.R., Diabetes, G.: The need for knowledge of self. Diab. Voice 54, 3 (2009)
21. Lawn, S.J.: A behavioural therapy approach to self-management: the flinders program (2009)

Relationship Between Multiple Joint Movements Using Fitts Law

Neeraj K. Gupta[1(✉)], Siva Dantu[2], and Arvind Nana[3]

[1] Department of Computer Science Medicine, University of Texas at Dallas, Richardson, USA
ngupta94@yahoo.com
[2] School of Medicine, University of Texas Medical Branch, Galveston, Texas, USA
svdantu@utmb.edu
[3] Department of Orthopedic Surgery, UNT Health Science Center, Fortworth, Texas, USA
Arvind.Nana@unthsc.edu

Abstract. Fitts Law predicts the time required to move to an object given the distance to the object's center and its size. Over the years, Fitts law has been tested on various body parts/joints such as the elbow, wrist, fingers and even tongues. In this paper, we extend Fitts law to model movement by multiple joints. To accomplish this, we first establish a relationship between the performances of different joints, using the concept of *atomic movement*. We define the *atomic movement* as the movement of the fastest joint from amongst the joints under consideration. We propose that every other joint movement is a multiple of this *atomic movement*.

Keywords: Fitts law · Prosthetic limb controller · Human robot interface · Atomic movement

1 Introduction

Human movement science, the study of human body movements, has applications in several fields. In medicine, studying psychological impairment and impairment of body limb functionality enables development of new therapies, the creation of better treatments, and design of more effective artificial limbs. Researchers in Computer Science also benefit from these studies of human movement as they create applications that focus on human-robot interaction or human-computer interaction (HCI) when designing human-machine interfaces. The results of human movement studies allow designers to consider what body movements are efficient and, accordingly, design devices so that untrained people can also use them. For example, to our knowledge, there is not a accepted method to quantitatively evaluate prosthesis and prosthesis control performance.

Fitts Law predicts the time required to move to an object given the distance to that object's center and size. For example, if a hand is moving a mouse cursor towards a specific point on the screen, Fitts Law predicts that the time it takes to reach the target is a logarithmic function of the width of the target and the distance to the target. The original Fitts law was applicable to the one-dimensional movement of the arm [1].

© Springer International Publishing Switzerland 2016
X. Zheng et al. (Eds.): ICSH 2015, LNCS 9545, pp. 210–216, 2016.
DOI: 10.1007/978-3-319-29175-8_20

Subsequent extensions of this law have studied movements in two dimensions [2], three dimensions [3] or even cyclical [4] movements.

In this paper, we present the results of experiments to study the applicability of Fitts law for task-control using upper and lower limbs. We also present experiments to model Fitts law for different joint movements and multiple joint movements. Based on the results of these experiments, we extend Fitts law. An important application of such a modified Fitts law is in the design prosthetic controllers and human-robot-interaction.

2 Fitts Law and Task Activities

In this section, we present an introduction to Fitts Law and a brief description of the problem we attempt to solve. Our study relates to tasks involving multiple joints and a mathematical model to compare them.

2.1 Fitts Law and Current Literature

In 1954, Paul Fitts proposed the original Fitts law that describes an aimed, rapid type of motion [1]. Since then, Fitts Law has been used to design efficient Computer interfaces and layouts of the computer display screens, as a part of Human-Computer Interaction applications. Over the years, several studies have been done on various movements of different body parts.

The application of the Fitts Law has opened new areas of research and application. For example, Fitts Law can be used when designing computer games requiring not only one-direction hand movements but also movements of other body parts in several directions.

Following discussion of these studies of the arm and head movements, we propose that we can apply Fitts law to the motion of other joints. During the rehabilitation, the physiotherapist may give instructions to a patient for exercises based on limb movements. Such instructions may be explicit steps to move human joints. Equation 1 shows Fitts law equation as modified by Shannon's [6]

$$T = a + b * \log_2\left(\frac{D}{W} + 1\right) \tag{1}$$

Where T = the time, it takes to complete a movement, D = the distance of the movement to the center of a target object, W = width of the target object; a, b = constants.

Index of Difficulty (*ID*) is defined as in Eq. 2:

$$ID = \log_2\left(\frac{D}{W} + 1\right) \tag{2}$$

2.2 Problem Definition

In many physiotherapy situations, more than one joint needs to be considered. Our ultimate goal is to develop an application that uses Fitts Law to analyze accurately such multiple-joint movement. To date, researchers have used Fitts law to model the motion of human body parts, particularly one-dimension arm movement. *In this research, our goal was to study the comparison between the movements of different joints to determine how this relationship would affect Fitts Law. For example, we wanted to evaluate whether a mathematical relationship existed between one wrist-joint movement and one elbow-joint movement.* An attempt at such a comparison made in a previous study [5]. But in that study no mathematical formulation was made. Based on the mathematical formulations arrived at in our study, we propose to enhance Fitts Law so that the equation reflects the mathematical relationship between multiple-joint movements.

3   Components of Modified Fitts Law

3.1   Motion Activity

The current Fitts Law equation does not distinguish between movements of one body part as compared to another. For example, walking to an object (moving legs) will have a different difficulty level than moving an arm or a hand. Also, a task may involve a complex movement such as moving several joints in multiple directions to complete the task successfully. Our objective is to extend Fitts law to account for different joints having differing IDs.

To acceptably extend Fitts Law, we first need to resolve whether we can compare movement of two or more joints. That is, can we define a Difficulty Index for each joint so that we can compare the ID of one joint with the ID of another joint? To compare different joints' IDs, we introduce the concept of *atomic movement*. We define atomic movement to be the speed of the joint that moves the fastest unit distance. We consider every other joint movement as a multiple of this atomic movement. If we denote α as a factor whose value depends on the joint that is moved, we write the modified Eq. 2 for Difficulty Index for *atomic joint* as follows:

$$ID_{atomic} = \alpha_{atomic} * \log_2\left(\frac{D}{W} + 1\right) \tag{3}$$

Where α_{atomic} = α value of the atomic joint, the joint used to define the atomic movement.
Similarly, we rewrite Eq. 3 for any joint, joint₁ as follows:

$$ID_{joint1} = \alpha_{joint1} * \log_2\left(\frac{D}{W} + 1\right) \tag{4}$$

Using Eqs. 3 and 4, we express the relationship of one joint to another as follows:

$$\alpha_{joint1} = \lambda_{joint1} * \alpha_{atomic} \tag{5}$$

Where λ_{joint1} is the ratio of atomic movement between the atomic joint and joint1, we can rewrite Eq. 5 for index of difficulty for joint1 as in Eq. 6:

$$ID_{joint1} = \lambda_{joint1} * \alpha_{atomic} * \log_2\left(\frac{D}{W} + 1\right) \tag{6}$$

Equation 6 represents a relationship between the atomic joint and the index of difficulty for any joint.

In the following subsections we present results of our experiments and validate our concept of atomic movement by showing that bigger joints move faster than smaller joints. In other words, the time required to move smaller joints is a multiple of the time required to move bigger joints.

A motor motion takes a few seconds to complete. An arm or a leg's full, free movement takes approximately 4 to 5 s. This short duration makes our study error prone. Careful planning was needed to complete the experiments successfully. Error also can be introduced not only from the measurement of the time but due to the variable nature of a body's joint movement. Each repetition of a joint movement can give a different timing. Given each measurement is of the order of 2–3 s, a small error in measurement can contribute to an accumulation of inaccurate results. To reduce this error, we conducted the experiments with repeated motions several times and averaged the measurements.

3.2 Methodology for the Set of Experiments

A set of experiments was carried out to confirm further the following hypothesis:

- Bigger joints move faster than a smaller joint.
- Slower moving joints are multiple of the faster-moving joint.

  These experiments involve motion of four joints.

- Hip joint (walking)
- Shoulder joint–moving the arm all the way up,
- Elbow joint–full elbow joint movement
- Wrist joint movement.

In this study, 20 males and females of different heights and weights participated. Volunteers were unaware of the experiment's purpose.

Joint movements are angular in nature. Therefore, to calculate the distance moved, we measured the total distance that the extremity of the body part moved. We asked the volunteers to move at their normal speed. We used the stop watch in a Google phone (which had an accuracy of milliseconds) to measure the time the subject required to complete a motion. To collect hip joint data, we asked each participant to walk a fixed distance once. But, to gather data on the movement of the shoulder, elbow, and wrist, we asked volunteers to complete five repetitions. This repetition prevented skewing results as would occur if volunteers moved the joint only once. This method reduced the error margin because we determined the average distance moved.

3.3 Results

Figure 1 shows the relative speeds of four joints for each participant. The bar graph shows the time per inch of movement for each joint. For all participants, the Hip joint movement had the smallest time. The shoulder joint movement had the next smallest time, and so on. This confirms our first hypothesis that the larger joint is consistently faster than the smaller joint.

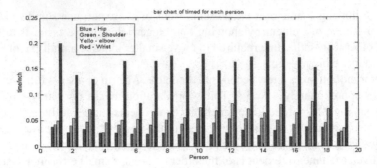

Fig. 1. Bar graph showing relative speeds of joints for each subject (Color figure online).

To compare the performance of each joint, X, we calculated the ratio of movement time for X to the hip joint movement. The time of hip joint was given a value of 1. Figure 2, shows the relative speed of joints as a ratio of time to move the hip joint. We can observe that the ratios are consistent with our hypothesis that the movement of all joints is multiple of the fastest joint, and this observation is consistent across all subjects.

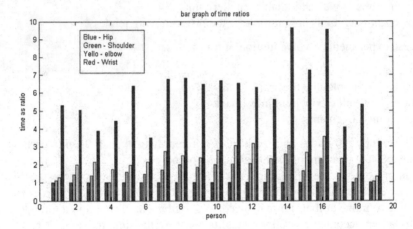

Fig. 2. Comparison of Ratio of Speed for Each Joint for Each Subject, hip joint is given a value of 1 (Color figure online).

Figure 3 shows a comparison of the speed of each joint with respect to the index of difficulty for each subject. The times are based on an average of the subject's speed for each of four joints. The X-axis provides the range of the Index of Difficulty from 0 to 4. The Y-axis shows the time per inch of movement. Each plot line represents a participant in the experiment. This confirms our assumption that as the difficulty increases the time necessary to move joints increases.

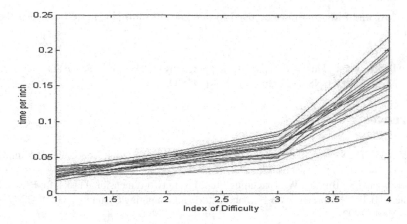

Fig. 3. The plot of Index of Difficulty for each person showing the increase of time.

3.4 Conclusions

Our analysis of the data collected supports the following conclusions. Several studies have been done to confirm the validity of Fitts law for analyzing the movement of joints. We wanted to apply Fitts law to establish a correlation between joint movements. Our goal was to define a mathematical relationship between different joint movements. Our experiments confirmed that larger joints move more quickly than smaller joints. When we calculated the ratio of speeds of any two joints, our results indicated that the ratio for same joints was consistent across all participants. Based on these results, we have formulated a mathematical model of joint movements and have extended Fitts Law as given in Eq. 6.

3.5 Applications of This Study

The design of Physiotherapeutic Exercises: Physiotherapists design instructions consider the patient's sensory and cognitive states, as well as their physical capabilities. The extension of Fitts law facilitates the design and control of the effective exercises in a clinical setting.

The design of Prosthetics Devices: Our extended Fitts Law permits researchers to investigate multiple-joint movements in both unimpaired and impaired individuals. Using this comparative data, researchers can design effective prosthetics and prosthesis controllers for upper and lower limbs.

3.6 Future Work

Future work should first focus on studying more subjects to gather more data on multiple-joint movement, sensory indicators, and cognitive indicators. Future studies should evaluate the effect of impairment by analyzing EEG waves. A model that combines

Hook's law and Fitts law may be used to design optimum HRH, HCI and prosthetics design.

Acknowledgements. This work is partially supported by the National Science Foundation under grants CNS-0751205, CNS-0821736 and CNS-1545599.

References

1. Fitts, P.M.: The information capacity of the human motor system in controlling the amplitude of movement. J. Exp. Psychol. **47**, 381–391 (1954)
2. MacKenzie, I.S., Buxton, W.: Extending Fitts' law to two-dimensional tasks. In: Proceedings of the CHI 1992 Conference on Human Factors in Computing Systems, pp. 219–226. ACM, New York (1992)
3. Murata, A., Iwase, H.: Extending Fitts' law to a three-dimensional pointing task. Hum. Mov. Sci. **20**, 791–805 (2001)
4. Guiard, Y.: Fitts' law in the discrete vs. cyclical paradigm. Hum. Mov. Sci. **16**, 97–131 (1997)
5. Balakrishnan, R., MacKenzie, I.S.: Performance differences in the fingers, wrist, and forearm in computer input control. In: Proceedings of the ACM Conference on Human Factors in Computing Systems - CHI 1997, pp. 303–310. ACM, New York (1997)
6. Shannon, C.E., Weaver, W.: The Mathematical Theory of Communication. University of Illinois Press, Urbana (1949)

Big Data and Smart Health

Electronic Health Records and Patient Activation – Their Interactive Role in Medication Adherence

Yunfeng Shi[1(✉)], Veronica Fuentes-Caceres[1], Megan McHugh[2],
Jessica Greene[3], Nina Verevkina[1], Lawrence Casalino[4],
and Stephen Shortell[5]

[1] Pennsylvania State University, University Park, USA
yus16@psu.edu
[2] Northwestern University, Evanston, USA
[3] George Washington University, Washington, DC, USA
[4] Weill Cornell Medical College, New York, USA
[5] University of California, Berkeley, USA

Abstract. We investigate the association between the use of Electronic Health Records (EHR) core functions in physician practices and medication adherence among chronically ill adults, as well as how patient activation moderates this relationship. Cross-sectional logistic regressions are conducted using data from the Aligning Forces for Quality Consumer Survey and the National Study of Small and Medium Physician Practices (2007–2009). Only 43 % of the practices have a basic EHR. The use of electronic communication and connectivity is positively associated with medication adherence for patients who are highly activated, but the association is negative for less activated patients. EHR based interventions may need to be customized based on patient activation and other factors.

Keywords: Electronic health records · Medication adherence · Patient behavior · Consumer engagement · Patient activation · Physician practice · Chronic illness

1 Introduction

1.1 Background

Approximately 133 million individuals in the United States are affected by chronic conditions [1]. It is estimated that 75 % of the U.S. health care expenditures are spent on care related to chronic conditions [2], and the cost may reach $1.07 trillion by 2020 [3]. An essential component in managing chronic conditions is medication adherence, which refers to the extent to which patients follow the medication regimen recommended by their health care providers [4, 5]. Previous studies have shown that better adherence decreases hospitalizations and disease related costs [6], increases duration and quality of life [7], and reduces absenteeism at the workplace [8].

© Springer International Publishing Switzerland 2016
X. Zheng et al. (Eds.): ICSH 2015, LNCS 9545, pp. 219–230, 2016.
DOI: 10.1007/978-3-319-29175-8_21

Electronic Health Records (EHR) has the potential of improving care delivery and lowering costs, although empirical evidence for its impact has been so far inconclusive [9–13]. In particular, to our knowledge, no studies examined whether medication adherence among chronically ill adults is associated with the use of EHR in physician practices. We explore this important link using data from two unique national surveys conducted between 2006 and 2008. Our study contributes to the literature in several aspects. First, we measure the adoption and use of core EHR functions at the physician practice level. Second, we focus on small and median sized physician practices, which are still the predominant sources of primary care provision in the United States [14]. Finally, we examine the potential interaction between the core EHR functions and patients' different levels of engagement in self-managing their health [15].

1.2   EHR, Patient Self-engagement, and Medication Adherence

According to the definitions by the Institute of Medicine (Committee on Identifying Priority Areas for Quality Improvement, 2003), there are five core EHR functions: (1) health information and data, (2) decision support management, (3) order entry and management, (4) electronic communication and connectivity, and (5) quality reporting. We hypothesize that the above functions influence medication adherence through four mechanisms: (1) prevention of negative drug interactions, (2) patient counseling and reinforcement of medication regimen, (3) better patient self-monitoring, and (4) better internal quality monitoring by practices. In addition, we further hypothesize that the core EHR functions may have different influences on medication adherences depending on the patients' different levels of self-engagement.

Prevention of negative drug interactions. Poor medication adherence can result from patients' concerns or experiences with adverse effects and negative drug interactions [16]. Better recorded patient health information, decision support system, electronic order entry and management potentially help physicians avoid prescribe drugs that may lead to such problems. Electronic communication (e.g. email exchanges between patient and physician) may help patients obtain timely clarifications and hence avoid taking their medications incorrectly.

Patient counseling and reinforcement of medication regimen. Many patients with chronic condition(s) need to take different medicines at different times throughout a day. This often results in failure to follow the prescribed medical regimen [16]. Patient health data, decision support (e.g. progress notes), and electronic communication may help physicians better understand challenges faced by patients in meeting their specific medication needs. As a result, physicians may provide specific counseling to patients and reinforce their medication regimen.

Better patient self-monitoring. Electronic communication (e.g. online patient records and test results) enables patients to better monitor their own conditions and more promptly understand potential consequences from non-adherence. It may also facilitate patient-physician interactions outside office visits (e.g. through e-mail communication via web portals) and help resolve unexpected medication issues in a timely manner.

Better internal quality monitoring. Data on the quality of care are better documented, more detailed, and more convenient when collected using EHR [17–19]. As a result, this may improve efficiency and transparency in both internal quality monitoring by practices and external monitoring by other agencies (e.g. regional organizations sponsoring public reporting). Better quality monitoring potentially facilitates and incentivizes physicians in their efforts to improve patients' medication adherence.

Patient Self-Engagement. Previous research in patient engagement has developed the Patient Activation Measure (PAM): a set of 13 questions designed to measure patients' overall "activation" level, namely their ability and willingness in self-managing their health [15]. PAM has been validated and used in previous studies [20]. More specifically, in this study, we hypothesize that the core EHR functions may have more positive influence on medication adherence when patients have higher level of PAM.

2 Methods

2.1 Data and Sample

We merged information from two surveys: the Aligning Forces for Quality Consumer Survey (AF4QCS) and the National Study of Small and Medium Physician Practices (NSSMPP).

AF4QCS was a random-digit-dial survey initially conducted between June 2007 and June 2008 for chronically ill adults (18 or older) in 14 communities in the AF4Q project funded by the Robert Wood Johnson Foundation (RWJF). The survey also included a comparison sample of respondents from the rest of the U.S. Overall, 8140 respondents completed the survey. The response rate is 45.8 % based on the method of Council of American Survey Research Organizations (CASRO) and 27.6 % based on the method of American Association of Public Opinion Research (AAPOR). To be included in the survey, a respondent must have visited a doctor or health care professional during the previous two years for the care of one or more of the following five conditions: diabetes, hypertension asthma, chronic heart disease and depression. AF4QCS has been used and discussed in previous studies [21, 22]. NSSMPP, conducted between July 2007 and March 2009, was also funded by RWJF. The survey used a nationally representative sample of small and medium physician practices with 19 or fewer physicians. 1,809 practices completed the survey and the response rate was 63.9 %. NSSMPP has also been used in previous studies [22, 23].

The two data sets were merged using providers' names and locations collected in both surveys [22]. Since the AF4QCS and the NSSMPP were designed with random sampling, practices reported by AF4QCS respondents as their primary sources of care were not necessarily included in NSSMPP. Our study sample consists of 915 patients from AF4QCS matched to 384 practices from NSSMPP.

2.2   Key Variables

Dependent Variable. Many patients in our sample have multiple chronic conditions and have medication(s) for each condition. The outcome measure is an indicator for perfect adherence to *all* recommend medications, self-reported by respondents in the AF4QCS. Medication adherence is commonly measured by electronic monitoring, pill count, pharmacy fill rates, and self-reported information [24]. Self-reported adherence has been shown to be correlated with other measures [25] and predictive of outcomes [26]. Nevertheless, information reported by survey respondents may overestimate adherence [27, 28].

Key Independent Variables. The explanatory variables of interest are five composites corresponding to the five core functions of EHR identified using the IOM definitions and the Patient Activation Measure (PAM). The EHR composites are calculated using responses by physician practices to a series of questions in NSSMPP, as shown in Table 1. These variables measure the availability and intensity of use of the core EHR functions in each physician practice. In this study, PAM is a binary indicator based on the different stages of activation calculated using responses by consumers in AF4QCS [15, 20].

Table 1. Measuring core EHR functions

EHR core functions	Question(s) in NSSMPP	Value
Health information and data Sum of the responses to 6 NSSMPP questions Scale: 0–6	Does your practice make available an electronic medical record that includes the patient's medications?	Yes = 1 No = 0
	Percentage of physicians who are using the electronic medical record for the patient's problem list?	Number of physicians using this feature divided by the total number of physicians in the practice. 0–100 %
	For a majority of the patients in your practice with asthma, does your practice maintain an electronic registry?	Yes = 1 No = 0 If the patient does not have asthma, the final value is 0
	For a majority of the patients in your practice with CHF, does your practice maintain an electronic registry?	Yes = 1 No = 0 If the patient does not have CHF, the final value is 0
	For a majority of the patients in your practice with depression, does your practice maintain an electronic registry?	Yes = 1 No = 0 If the patient does not have depression, the final value is 0
	For a majority of the patients in your practice with diabetes, does your practice maintain an electronic registry?	Yes = 1 No = 0

(Continued)

Table 1. (*Continued*)

EHR core functions	Question(s) in NSSMPP	Value
Decision support management Sum of the responses to 4 NSSMPP questions Scale: 0–4	Percentage of physicians who are using the electronic medical record for progress notes?	Number of physicians using the feature divided by the total number of physicians in the practice
	Percentage of physicians who are using the electronic medical record for potential drug interactions?	
	Percentage of physicians who are using the electronic medical record for prompts and reminders?	
	Percentage of physicians who are using the electronic medical record for alerts on abnormal test results?	
Order entry and management Response to a single NSSMPP question Scale: 0–1	Percentage of physicians who transmit prescriptions electronically DIRECTLY TO PHARMACIES via computer or PDA (personal digital assistant)?'	Number of physicians using this feature divided by the total number of physicians in the practice
Electronic communication and connectivity Sum of the responses to 3 NSSMPP questions Scale: 0–3	Does your practice allow patients to view their medical record online?	Yes = 1 No = 0
	Is the PHARMACY RECORD of prescriptions filled by your patients accessible within an individual patient's electronic medical record at your practices office?	Yes = 1 No = 0
	Percentage of physicians who communicate with patients via e-mail?	Number of physicians using this feature divided by the total number of physicians in the practice. This value goes from 0 to 1
Quality Reporting Response to a single NSSMPP question Scale: 0–1	Does your practice use its electronic medical record to collect data for quality measures?	Yes = 1 No = 0

Other covariates. Various patient-related (e.g. patient demographic characteristics) and provider-related (e.g. patient-provider relationship) factors have been shown to have influence on medication adherence [29, 30]. Our analysis controls for the following patient level covariates: age, minority status, college education, type and number of chronic conditions, and having switched physicians within the past year. In addition, three covariates at the physician practice level are also included: the number of physicians, the type of the practice, and an index reflecting the extent to which the practice uses care management processes for chronically ill patients [31].

2.3 Analytical Approach

The outcome is binary and we use multivariate logistic regression models to estimate the association between patient medication adherence and physician practices' use of the five core functions of EHR. In addition, we interact PAM with EHR functions to explore the differential impact of EHR due to patients' different level of commitment to self-managing. We also cluster standard errors at the practice level, as multiple patients may go to the same practice. Two different specifications are estimated. The baseline model includes all the independent variables, without any interaction terms. Then, we include interaction terms between the EHR functions and PAM in the full model.

3 Results

The characteristics of the study sample are summarized in Table 2. Less than half (43 %) practices in this study have a basic EHR and a much smaller proportion (27 %) manages all their procedures electronically. The average scores for decision support management, electronic communication and connectivity and health information and data are 1.19 (out of 4), 0.27 (out of 3), and 0.96 (out of 5). 38 % of the practices have order entry/management and 32 % have quality reporting. Among the patients in our study sample, about 75 % report that they always take all the recommended medications.

Table 2. Sample characteristics

Practice-level variables	Mean/proportion (SD)
Use of Electronic Health Record	
Do not possess a basic EHR	57.06 %
Some procedures embedded in the EHR	16.18 %
All procedures embedded in the EHR	26.76 %
Electronic Health Record functions	
Decision support management (DSM)	1.19 (1.62)
Electronic communication and connectivity (ECC)	0.27 (0.51)
Health information and data (HID)	0.96 (1.13)

(Continued)

Table 2. (*Continued*)

Practice-level variables	Mean/proportion (SD)
Order entry and management (OEM)	37.85 %
Quality reporting (QR)	32.06 %
Care Management Processes	1.29 (1.02)
Practice Size	
1 to 4 physicians	60.59 %
5 to 19 physicians	39.41 %
Practice Composition	
Non-primary care	3.82 %
Primary care	82.06 %
Patient-level variables	
Always take medication as prescribed	74.71 %
Socio-demographics	
White Non-Hispanic	76.28 %
Minorities	
Black Non-Hispanic	15.99 %
Hispanic	4.46 %
Other	3.28 %
Age	58.42 (13.71)
College Education	33.55 %
Income (in thousands)	48.88 (33.44)
High Patient Activation	75.36 %
Health status	
Poor and fair	27.92 %
Good	43.25 %
Very good and excellent	28.83 %
Chronic conditions (not mutually exclusive)	
Hypertension	73.26 %
Diabetes	32.63 %
Asthma	20.31 %
Heart Disease	17.56 %
Depression	32.37 %
Switched provider within the last 12 months	11.66 %

The odds ratios (OR) from the logistic regressions are presented in Table 3. We do not find significant association between medication adherence and the five EHR functions in the base model. The analysis with the interaction terms shows that the association with electronic communication and connectivity (ECC) depends on the level of activation of the patient. When practices have more advanced function of electronic communication and connectivity, patients with high activation are more likely to always take all recommended medications. However, this relationship is reversed for patients with low activation. In addition, with or without interactions, more activated patients consistently show better adherence.

Among other covariates, being minority, being younger, having asthma, having depression, and having switched to a different provider within the past 12 months are associated with poorer adherence.

Table 3. Odds ratios from logistic regressions

	Base model		Model with interactions	
	OR	95 % CI	OR	95 % CI
HER functions				
DSM	1.06	0.83–1.35	0.92	0.60–1.43
ECC	1.08	0.72–1.62	0.44*	0.17–1.14
HID	0.83	0.56–1.21	1.07	0.51–2.23
OEM	0.85	0.52–1.39	0.57	0.23–1.42
QR	0.86	0.50–1.47	1.31	0.47–3.68
Interactions				
PAM-DSM	–	–	1.27	0.81–2.01
PAM-ECC	–	–	3.80**	1.34–10.79
PAM-HID	–	–	0.68	0.33–1.42
PAM-OEM	–	–	1.76	0.63–4.91
PAM-QR	–	–	0.47	0.15–1.45
Care management	0.96	0.78–1.19	0.96	0.78–1.19
Practice size				
1 to 4 physicians	Ref	–	Ref	–
5 to 19 physicians	0.84	0.56–1.27	0.86	0.57–1.29
Practice composition				
Primary care	Ref	–	Ref	–
Non-primary care	1.14	0.32–4.05	0.97	0.29–3.29
Socio-demographics				
Minorities	0.48***	0.32–0.71	0.45***	0.30–0.68
Age	1.01*	1.00–1.03	1.01*	1.00–1.03
College Education	0.81	0.55–1.19	0.80	0.54–1.19
Income	1.00	0.99–1.00	1.00	0.99–1.00
High Activation	2.06***	1.41–3.03	1.62*	0.96–2.73
Health status				
Poor and fair	Ref	–	Ref	–
Good	1.00	0.64–1.56	1.00	0.63–1.59
Very good and excellent	1.11	0.66–1.87	1.12	0.65–1.93
Chronic conditions				
Hypertension	0.89	0.57–1.37	0.90	0.57–1.41
Diabetes	1.27	0.85–1.88	1.24	0.83–1.85

(Continued)

Table 3. (*Continued*)

	Base model		Model with interactions	
	OR	95 % CI	OR	95 % CI
Asthma	0.59**	0.39–0.89	0.58**	0.38–0.89
Heart disease	0.68	0.42–1.10	0.66*	0.40–1.07
Depression	0.53***	0.34–0.83	0.54***	0.34–0.84
Switched providers	0.53**	0.32–0.89	0.55**	0.33–0.92

* $p < .1$; ** $p < .05$; *** $p < .01$

4   Discussion

Overall, the use of EHR among small and medium sized physician practices is low. This is true in terms of both the basic EHR system and the individual core functions. Those practices, although being the major source of primary care in the U.S., may face significant resource barrier to adopting and use EHR [32]. Our logistic regressions show that four of the five EHR core functions used in physician practices are not associated with medication adherence among chronically ill adults. There are several possible reasons for this finding. First, the adoption and use of EHR among small and medium sized physician practices might still be at an early stage when the data were collected, and it often took considerable time for the new technology to be fully incorporated into the daily operations of those practices. Moreover, implementing electronic health records can be disruptive and may even result in lost productivity for an extended period of time. Second, the lack of interconnectivity among providers is still a significant barrier to information sharing. For patients with multiple chronic conditions who often seek care and receive medications from different providers, EHR may not be effective without interconnectivity among providers. Finally, changes in physician practices alone may not have discernible effects, unless they also induce sustainable changes in patient behaviors. Ultimately, patients have an essential role in managing their own health, including adhering to medication.

We found that the use of one EHR function, electronic communication and connectivity, is positively associated with medication adherence for highly activated patients. This function may be particularly sensitive to patient activation, as electronic communication (e.g. patient-physician interactions via web portals) can potentially replace some of the conventional patient-physician interactions (e.g. communications and instructions during office visit). Highly activated patients are more likely to take advantage of new technologies (e.g. view medical records online) and obtain important feedback more efficiently. On the other hand, less activated patients may suffer from this, as they potentially face more challenges in adapting to new modes of communications. We also notice that patient activation on its own is positively associated with adherence. This finding suggests that future studies investigating EHR based interventions may target patients with low activation.

Various patient related factors (age, minority status, provider switching, having asthma and depression) are associated with medication adherence, whereas none of the practice characteristics are. These results are consistent with previous findings in the literature [15, 20, 33–35]. Considering the lower adherence rate among minorities and the elderly, policies may need to target those groups (e.g. customized design of EHR functions).

To our knowledge, this is the first study exploring the link between medication adherence and physician practice level EHR, explicitly using patient engagement as a moderating factor. However, there are several important limitations in this study and the findings need to be interpreted with caution. First our analysis is cross-sectional and the findings may not be causal. Second, our survey based measurement of practice level use of EHR functions is limited by the data. Additional specificity on the usage (e.g. the exact information system being used and the specific way it is used) can significantly enhance our understanding of the relationship in question. Finally, health information technology is an area of constant and fast development. There have been great advancements in the use of EHR since our study period. Although we provide an important perspective of patient engagement in exploring the impact of EHR, to better understand the moderating effects of PAM, there need to be future studies using more current data with longitudinal design.

References

1. Wu, S., Green, A.: Projection of Chronic Illness Prevalence and Cost Inflation. RAND Health, Santa Monica (2000)
2. Dentzer, S.: Reform chronic illness care? Yes, We Can. Health Aff. **28**(1), 12–13 (2009)
3. National Research Council. http://www.nap.edu/catalog.php?record_id=10593
4. Brown, M.T., Bussell, J.K.: Medication adherence: WHO cares? Mayo Clin. Proc. **86**(4), 304–314 (2011)
5. Osterberg, L., Blaschke, T.: Adherence to medication. New Engl. J. Med. **353**(5), 487–497 (2005)
6. Sokol, M.C., McGuigan, K.A., Verbrugge, R.R., Epstein, R.S.: Impact of medication adherence on hospitalization risk and healthcare cost. Med. Care **43**(6), 521–530 (2005)
7. Cutler, D.M., Long, G., Berndt, E.R., Royer, J., Fournier, A.A., Sasser, A., Cremieux, P.: The value of antihypertensive drugs: a perspective on medical innovation. Health Aff. **26**(1), 97–110 (2007)
8. Loeppke, R., Haufle, V., Jinnett, K., Parry, T., Zhu, J., Hymel, P., Konicki, D.: Medication adherence, comorbidities, and health risk impacts on workforce absence and job performance. J. Occup. Environ. Med. **53**(6), 595–604 (2011)
9. Bhattacherjee, A., Hikmet, N., Menachemi, N., Kayhan, V.O., Brooks, R.G.: The differential performance effects of healthcare information technology adoption. Inf. Sys. Manage. **24**(1), 5–14 (2007)
10. Chaudhry, B., Wang, J., Wu, S., Maglione, M., Mojica, W., Roth, E., Shekelle, P.G.: Systematic review: impact of health information technology on quality, efficiency, and costs of medical care. Ann. Intern. Med. **144**(10), 742–752 (2006)
11. Miller, A.R., Tucker, C.: Can health care information technology save babies? J. Polit. Econ. **119**(2), 289–324 (2011)
12. Parente, S.T., McCullough, J.S.: Health information technology and patient safety: evidence from panel data. Health Aff. **28**(2), 357–360 (2009)

13. Rollman, B.L., Hanusa, B.H., Lowe, H.J., Gilbert, T., Kapoor, W.N., Schulberg, H.C.: A randomized trial using computerized decision support to improve treatment of major depression in primary care. J. Gen. Intern. Med. **17**(7), 493–503 (2002)
14. Alexander, J.A., Maeng, D., Casalino, L.P., Rittenhouse, D.: Use of care management practices in small- and medium-sized physician groups: do public reporting of physician quality and financial incentives matter? Health Serv. Res. **48**(2pt1), 376–397 (2013)
15. Hibbard, J.H., Stockard, J., Mahoney, E.R., Tusler, M.: Development of the patient activation measure (PAM): conceptualizing and measuring activation in patients and consumers. Health Serv. Res. **39**(4Pt1), 1005–1026 (2004)
16. Williams, A., Manias, E., Walker, R.: Interventions to improve medication adherence in people with multiple chronic conditions: a systematic review. J. Adv. Nurs. **63**(2), 132–143 (2008)
17. Cebul, R.D., Love, T.E., Jain, A.K., Hebert, C.J.: Electronic health records and quality of diabetes care. New Engl. J. Med. **365**(9), 825–833 (2011)
18. Davis, A.M., Cannon, M., Ables, A.Z., Bendyk, H.: Using the electronic medical record to improve asthma severity documentation and treatment among family medicine residents. Fam. Med. **42**(5), 334–337 (2010)
19. Fielstein, E.M., Brown, S.H., McBrine, C.S., Clark, T.K., Hardenbrook, S.P., Sperff, T.: The effect of standardized, computer-guided templates on quality of VA disability exams. In: AMIA Annual Symposium Proceedings 2006, pp. 249–253 (2006)
20. Hibbard, J.H., Mahoney, E.R., Stock, R., Tusler, M.: Do increases in patient activation result in improved self-management behaviors? Health Serv. Res. **42**(4), 1443–1463 (2007)
21. Maeng, D.D., Martsolf, G.R., Scanlon, D.P., Christianson, J.B.: Care coordination for the chronically Ill: understanding the patient's perspective. Health Serv. Res. (2007)
22. Martsolf, G.R., Alexander, J.A, Shi, Y., Casalino, L.P., Rittenhouse, D.R., Scanlon, D.P., Shortell, S.M.: The patient-centered medical home and patient experience. Health Serv. Res. 1–23 (2012)
23. Rittenhouse, D.R., Casalino, L.P., Shortell, S.M., Sean, R., Gillies, R.R., Alexander, J.A., Drum, M.L.: Small and medium-size physician practices use few patient-centered medical home processes. Health Aff. **30**(8), 1575–2219 (2011)
24. Morisky, D.E., Ang, A., Krousel-Wood, M., Ward, H.J.: Predictive validity of a medication adherence measure in an outpatient setting. J. Clin. Hypertens. **10**(5), 348–354 (2008)
25. Cohen, H.W., Shmukler, C., Ullman, R., Rivera, C.M., Walker, E.: Measurements of medication adherence in diabetic patients with poorly controlled HbA1c. Diabet. Med. **27**(2), 210–216 (2010)
26. Gehi, A.K., Ali, S., Na, B., Whooley, M.A.: Self-reported medication adherence and cardiovascular events in patients with stable coronary heart disease: the heart and soul study. Arch. Intern. Med. **167**(16), 1798–1803 (2007)
27. Nieuwenhuis, M.W., Jaarsma, T., van Veldhuisen, D.J., van der Wal, H.L.: Self-reported versus "true" adherence in heart failure patients: a study using the medication event monitoring system. Neth. Heart J. **20**(7–8), 313–319 (2012)
28. Mason, B.J., Matsuyama, J.R., Jue, S.G.: Assessment of sulfonylurea adherence and metabolic control. Diab. Educ. **21**(1), 52–57 (1995)
29. Golin, C.E., Liu, H., Hays, R.D., Miller, L.G., Beck, C.K., Wenger, N.S.: A prospective study of predictors of adherence to combination antiretroviral medication. J. Gen. Intern. Med. **17**(10), 756–765 (2002)
30. Kato, N., Kinugawa, K., Ito, N., Yao, A., Watanabe, M., Imai, Y., Kazuma, K.: Adherence to self-care behavior and factors related to this behavior among patients with heart failure in Japan. Heart Lung: J. Crit. Care **38**(5), 398–409 (2009)

31. Casalino, L., Gillies, R.R., Shortell, S.M., Schmittdiel, J.A., Bodenheimer, T., Robinson, J.C., Rundall, T., Oswald, N., Schauffler, H., Wang, M.C.: External incentives, information technology, and organized processes to improve health care quality for patients with chronic diseases. JAMA 289(4), 434–441 (2003)
32. Ajami, S., Bagheri-Tadi, T.: Barriers for adopting electronic health records (EHRs) by physicians. Acta Informatica Med. 21(2), 129–134 (2013)
33. Kripalani, S., Gatti, M.E., Jacobson, T.A.: Association of age, health literacy, and medication management strategies with cardiovascular medication adherence. Patient Educ. Couns. 81(2), 177–181 (2010)
34. Krueger, K.P., Berger, B.A., Felkey, B.: Medication adherence and persistence: a comprehensive review. Adv. Ther. 22(4), 313–356 (2005)
35. Parchman, M.L., Palmer, R.F.: Activation, medication adherence, and intermediate clinical outcomes in type 2. Ann. Family Med. 8(5), 410–417 (2010)

Chronic Knowledge Retrieval and Smart Health Services Based on Big Data

Ye Liang[1,2(✉)], Ningning Guo[1], Chunxiao Xing[2], Yong Zhang[2], and Chaoran Guo[3]

[1] Department of Computer Science, Beijing Foreign Studies University, Beijing, China
{liangye,guoningning}@bfsu.edu.cn
[2] Tsinghua National Laboratory for Information Science and Technology,
Department of Computer Science and Technology, Research Institute of Information Technology,
Tsinghua University, Beijing, China
{xingcx,zhangyong05}@tsinghua.edu.cn
[3] School of Software, Sun Yat-Sen University, Guangzhou, China
zztsabc@163.com

Abstract. According to data released by World Health Organization (WHO), chronic non-communicable diseases have become the highest mortality disease. This paper is from the perspective to secure the health of people with chronic diseases. The research achieves the health knowledge from Big Data of the chronic diseases and is applied to Smart Health Service methods. Through collecting data in social media and integrating vast amounts of electronic health records, medical research literature and wearable device in personal health data, our purpose is to build a healthy big data environment. On this basis, we achieve the related knowledge of chronic disease by extracting the symptoms, the diseases and treatment options, inferring adverse drug reactions relationship, collecting health-related emotional reactions, and digging patients' social communication information, etc., which is to provide decision support for the patients and to achieve personalized Medical Services and Community Service. This paper focuses on the contents concluding knowledge discovery technology, personalized decision support technology, community health care services and so on, which relates to the health Big Data in the social media, then proposes collecting, digging and management of chronic disease health Big Data and builds the theoretical framework of chronic disease knowledge, in order to promote the realization of the Smart Health Services.

Keywords: Chronic knowledge retrieval · Smart health services · Health big data

1 Introduction

With the continuous improvement of our living conditions, Health-related chronic diseases have become a main cause of death. According to the latest report of World Health Organization (WHO), from a worldwide perspective, currently deaths caused by chronic non-communicable diseases have been in the first place in a variety of causes of death. Typical chronic diseases include diabetes, hypertension, cancer, coronary heart disease, chronic kidney disease, stroke, heart disease, Parkinson disease, Alzheimer

© Springer International Publishing Switzerland 2016
X. Zheng et al. (Eds.): ICSH 2015, LNCS 9545, pp. 231–240, 2016.
DOI: 10.1007/978-3-319-29175-8_22

disease, etc. Take diabetes as an example, it has become a major challenge affecting human health and development of the world, and there's no curing method. It has caused millions of deaths every year. The impact of diabetes on people does not vary because of nationality, race, religion, or economic strength. According to the year 2014 Statistics on the incidence of diabetes from International Diabetes Federation (IDF), in the whole world there are more than 387 million people suffer from diabetes, 4800 thousand people die of diabetes complications annually. Related medical expenses are more than 471 billion US dollars. It is predicted that more than 592 million people will suffer from diabetes in the entire world by 2035. According to a survey of Chinese Diabetes Association, 114 million people have been diagnosed with diabetes in China in 2014, leading the whole world.

Due to the chronic non-communicable diseases having become the highest mortality disease, to avoid the development of chronic diseases and diseases produced as far as possible in order to ensure the quality of life has become an urgent problem of the Wisdom Health Services. This paper is from the point of view that secures the health of people with chronic diseases, to research in the health-related knowledge digging from the chronic big data collected in a variety of sources, to build development framework of wisdom health service technology, providing support for the protection of the public health.

2 Literature Review

In 2013, soon after the emergence of the concept of Big Data, the researchers proposed the knowledge and Wisdom Health Service based on Big Data of chronic diseases. As the big data problems gradually clear and bright, the researchers use the mobile cloud computing technology and made a lot of progress on the key issues such as the application, the privacy and the security in the medical aspects. However, due to the privacy of the medical health data sources and the information island effect, there is certain difference in the research emphasis between the chronic Big Data and traditional Big Data. In recent years the problem gradually attracts more and more attention and research rush academically. Related research topics can be summarized as follows.

2.1 Application of Mobile Cloud Computing in Medical Area

Technology innovation of wearable wireless sensor and the popularity of smart phones have greatly promoted the development of E-Health, so that any person can receive medical services at any time and any place become a possibility. Through access to cloud services, mobile end computing power and storage space will be unlimitedly expanded. Mobile cloud computing will bring a revolution to the healthcare. Sensors collect health data anywhere at any place and send it to the phone, and the phone has a variety of applications for data. Finally the data will be sent to the cloud for further analysis and processing. These data have a high value. MIT researchers found [4–6] that collecting user's location, movement trajectory and communication data through mobile phones can predict the onset of influenza and gastrointestinal diseases. This brings research in three areas:

First is the research on application of sensors and mobile terminals. sickletREMOTE [11] provides daily data monitoring for pediatric sickle cell disease, and caREMOTE [13] provides daily data monitoring for the cancer patients. William Kaiser [12] proposed a system for monitoring stroke patient health data, [14] using a special headset to monitor the heartbeat and collect the patient's heart rate data at any time, and then sent it to the iPhone, so that iPhone can decide what kind of music to play following the user's heart rate changes to adjust the user's mood. SmartMood [1] can analyze the user's voice data to monitor the user's emotional state, and then to discover whether the user has emotional disorders.

Second is the research on the application of the cloud. Unlimited cloud computing and storage resources can make us take advantage of sophisticated data mining method [7–9] analyzing the health data. [8] The use of attribute selection methods make us find ECG abnormalities, [13] the use of classification make us determine the user's mood, and EEG cloud analysis system [10] use SVM epilepsy find other brain diseases. [7–9] Multiple data mining methods have been proposed to be used to analyze the user's sensor data. In addition, you can use cloud applications provide online services anytime and anywhere, twelve-lead ECG cloud services [16] can manage the patients' electrocardiogram online from the hospital's side. The services can be accessed with any mobile device anytime and can support cross-hospital share.

Third is the research on the overall system framework. Compared to the cloud service infrastructure, what we are missing now is more mobile cloud computing framework research systems in the medical area. [3] Proposing Smart Health framework, through Smart Health framework, we can know what kind of medical services we should propose and how to provide efficient services. The European Union has launched a home-based medical services based on the trusted cloud platform [15]. This platform can monitor, diagnose and help patients those are not in the hospital. E-Home health care system [2] for cardiovascular disease surveillance and diagnosis provides daily monitor of health data, medical data for remote access, instant medical diagnostics, disease-driven data upload and synchronization, emergency management and other functions, which meet a variety of users' needs.

2.2 Problems Relates to the Medical Knowledge Base

Semantic computing has been applied maturely to many key areas, such as national security, life sciences and healthcare. The key to their success is to obtain the knowledge base containing a rich field of relations. Currently the knowledge base existing in the healthcare field contains rich classified relations, but it is the lack of non-classified and areas-related relationship. Sujan [17] and others proposed a semi-automatic technology to enrich the causality in the field of knowledge base from the electronic medical record (EMR) data, which improved the efficiency of knowledge acquisition.

2.3 Data Analysis Problem of Health Documents

With the rapid growth of electronic health documents, related professionals need to spend a lot of time to analyze these documents; therefore many researchers have begun to pay attention to the data analysis problem of health documents. Hui [18] and others outlined four health care related researches. These studies demonstrated a unique perspective, analysis methods, health care applications and technology transfer opportunity, and prove the capacity which the Big Data generated from health care transferred into the useful knowledge, to provide support for the smart healthcare decisions. Omiros [19] and others present a comprehensive information processing, knowledge discovery and simulation platform for the Big Data healthcare. The platform helps a lot to the daily routine of doctors and biomedical research. Hanna [20] and others pointed out how to dig out the potential of natural language processing technology to help healthcare professionals, researchers, patients and others improve information application effect.

3   Proposed Method

The constantly increasing accumulation of big health data through mass electronic health records, clinical tests, research findings on high throughput genome sequencing, research literature on biomedical sciences, and home collection of health data from wearable devices like smart bands, smart necklace and pedometer have made it possible to provide precise smart health service well targeted to different individuals. The basic principle of smart health service is to give targeted suggestions on how to ensure body health through health diets, daily routine timetables, exercise according to patients' life habits so as to reduce hospital readmission rate and to improve individual patients' life quality through symptom extraction, disease and therapeutic schedule extraction, and relationship inference of side effects of drugs.

Therefore, the smart health service for chronic disease patients needs to cover both professional medical services and home health care services. However, the latter part is still at the initial stage of development and there are still a lot of blank areas in relevant research.

So it it's the key area which the smart health service needs to promote. And currently the key technical problems which impede its further development include analysis, measurement, modeling approach of chronic disease data, building multi-layer knowledge maps and its evolution methods, measurement of similarity degree and the construction of chronic disease prediction models.

3.1   The Analysis, Measurement, and Modeling Methods of Chronic Disease Data

To ensure the reliability of basic data, the diagnosis and treatment information and health indicators information of chronic diseases should be extracted from the electronic medical data of the chronic patients and the real cases of the diseases, symptoms, treatment, patient care should be extracted with machine learning methods and the cases should be analyzed and measured for integrity and consistency. And the relationship between different symptoms, diseases and treatment plans of chronic diseases with diseases at the core should also be extracted so as to construct models of relationship among cases. The relationships include relationship between drugs and their side effects, relationship between health-related contents in social media networks and emotional reactions and etc.

Meanwhile, physical and emotional models of the individual patients' conditions should be established and the sequential health archives of individual patients should be set up so as to analyze the effects of positive, neutral and negative emotions and work and life pressure and other chronic factors on the disease situation of the patients and in the end to use the themed models to identify the relationship between contents, patients and group emotions and provide health advice and suggestions based on locations.

Find the impact of climatic conditions of the region, forest coverage rate of the living places, pollution situation in the work environment, components of underground water, mineral resources and other natural resources on health and find the relationship between the influencing factors and the acquisition of chronic diseases. Regions along rivers or the sea have more rheumatism patients, and dusty places have more pneumoconiosis patients. According to the links between geographic information and regional features, we can quantify and measure the regional environment data, and on this basis, we can set up models of the relevancy between chronic disease morbidity and the environment so as to provide targeted prevention and home rehabilitation service (Fig. 1).

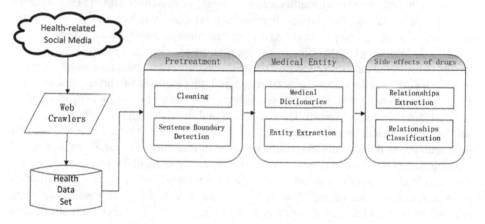

Fig. 1. Chronic knowledge retrieval flow diagram

3.2 The Establishment and Evolution Approaches of Multi-level Knowledge Maps

As the advent of the age of big data, the way people acquire knowledge has witnessed revolutionary changes. The professional knowledge based on tradition together with the experience accumulated by the general public have formed the information sources of the chronic disease knowledge maps in the age of big data. In the process of building the maps, we need to use the smallest possible number of cases to set up a professional knowledge base in the medical field to set up and sequentially evolve a medical and health knowledge map which can realize basic expansion in principle so as to realize the integration of multi-source knowledge on chronic diseases such as linkage to real cases and model reflection, identifying data updates including checks on compatibility and reduction based on knowledge so as to set up a multi-layer knowledge map based on the relationship between different chronic diseases and find the methods to update the map, check conflicts, avoid conflicts and retrieve information from the map.

In the area of application, we use complicated network model to identify key individuals, communities, development themes and information transmission mechanisms. We set up the patients relationship map through the information patients have posted on social media networks and use clustering and visualization technologies to identify "similar" contents and patients.

Through collecting and managing big health data on chronic diseases, setting up relevant knowledge maps, constructing framework of smart health services we can develop the smart question-and-answer service on chronic diseases.

3.3   Measuring Similarity Degree and Setting Up Prediction Models for Chronic Diseases

In order to better set up smart health service systems, we need to construct new similarity measurement methods for chronic diseases and on that basis to improve the current information filtering and personalized recommendation strategies. Based on the multi-layer knowledge maps with some reduction and the physical and mental indicators of the chronic disease patients groups, we set up the risk analysis model for chronic diseases based on Cox to reflect how the occurrence and development of chronic diseases are affected by various internal and external factors. The cloud computing platform is used for analyzing big data on health. The individual mobile health data collected from smart sensors and wearable devices can provide personalized analysis and advice which could help with medical decisions and realize home health services. The family members and nursing staff of the chronic patients can use websites or handheld devices to receive real-time feedback on health situation from home health service devices. The prediction on chronic diseases based on multiple health indicators with electronic medical data can serve as theoretical foundation for early warning for chronic diseases with multiple data sources.

4   Chronic Smart Health Service Framework

The core of smart health service is to construct a description framework of the occurrence and development of diseases based on the features of chronic diseases through the construction of models based on data of disease symptoms, physical indicators of patients, life habits, food habits, characteristic features and living environment. With the help of chronic disease doctors, such frameworks integrate the data collected from wearable devices, put forward early warning mechanisms and control theories, realize big data of chronic diseases and relevant calculation methods on medical knowledge construction, and provide decision support to individual patients so as to realize individualized smart medical service and community health service.

Smart health service has five parts: collecting data, building models from data, making multi-layer knowledge maps, making early warning models and individualized smart health service.

First, extracting information on health indicators (including physical and mental indicators) from patients' electronic medical data to analyze and measure data of chronic diseases. Among the data, the physical indicators information of the patients includes basic information (gender, age, smoking history, weight, HbAlc, etc.), examination results (e.g. fundus ophthalmoscope results), diagnosis results (e.g. nutrition, internal secretion), treatment indicators (e.g. the usage of insulin, anti-platelet agents), time indicators (e.g. the change trend of weight, HbAlc), and etc. The mental indicators of the chronic patients include cognition, emotion, will, actions, etc. And to establish sequential health archives of the chronic disease patients based on the physical and mental indicators.

Second, study the paths for knowledge dissemination in social media networks so as to recognize static and dynamic rules of knowledge dissemination.

Discover models and Network Patterns from medical health data on the Internet through the modification of ERGM model. The modified model focuses on how network node properties influence the sequence of internet connection generation, and testing how users' properties affect the knowledge dissemination networks in health communities.

Third, under the instructions of chronic disease doctors, study methods of extracting from big data chronic diseases cases such as the symptoms, diseases, treatment, side effects of diseases, and methods of constructing models on the correlation among difference cases.

Fourth, under the instructions of chronic disease doctors, study the methods of the construction and updating of knowledge maps of chronic disease, methods of conflicts testing and avoiding, methods of building and evolving the multi-layer knowledge maps and the quick retrieval methods in the knowledge maps based on the patients' cases in the form of natural languages and the knowledge base of organization ontology from health data Identify and discover the rules how patients use social media to make exchanges on health knowledge through checking the information posted by patients on social media communities and find groups of patients with similar symptoms, set up relationship maps among patients, so that patients can actively recommend experiences and health knowledge exchanges among patients can be realized.

At last, study the correlation and mutual influence among different chronic diseases with the multi-tasking learning method. Meanwhile, bases on the similarity measurement and chronic disease prediction models, build risk analysis model of chronic diseases based on Cox with the physical and mental indicators of the patients groups of chronic diseases to reflect how the occurrence of chronic diseases is affected by time and other factors so that we can send early warnings to susceptible population of chronic diseases and give suggestions on how to avoid or delay the acquisition of chronic diseases (Fig. 2).

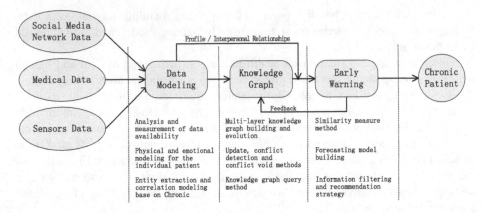

Fig. 2. Chronic smart health service framework

5   Conclusion

Currently, 85 % of Chinese who die from diseases every year die from chronic diseases. And every chronic disease patient suffers from the diseases for averagely 13 years. So effective ways to ensure life quality of chronic disease patients are to let them learn chronic disease related health knowledge and to provide them with smart health service. Particularly, as China becomes an aged society and as the need for caring old patients constantly increases year by year, the home medical health service for chronic diseases have gradually become an important area for future development in the medical health field.

The medical health field has entered the age of big data as we can see from the accumulation of electronic medical archives in health sectors, smart sensors which are widely applied in people's homes, the data collected from wearable devices, and the health-related information posted on social media such as Weibo, WeChat and etc. In order to get knowledge from such seas of big data, we need to do study on big data and through the discovery of health knowledge and the support to personalized decisions, we can help the patients and their family members fully participate in the decision making of medical treatment and such active participation in their own health management and decision making can help to improve their life quality.

The ideas of acquisition and integration of health knowledge based on big data put forward in this essay can efficiently integrate medical health big data from different areas and help to tap potential medical health knowledge. It has provided a theoretic framework for smart health service so has practical significance. In addition, the related research findings in this essay can be widely applied to the information collection from various types of networks and provide theoretic foundation for internet anti-terrorism, public opinion surveys, and follow-ups to scientific research progress.

Acknowledgments. This work was supported in part by the Young Faculty Research Fund of Beijing Foreign Studies University (2015JT008), the National High-tech R&D Program of China (Grant No. SS2015AA020102), the Scientific Research Foundation for the Returned Overseas Chinese Scholars, State Education Ministry, and Beijing Higher Education Young Elite Teacher Project (YETP0847).

References

1. Wang, X., Gui, Q., Liu, B., et al.: Enabling smart personalized healthcare: a hybrid mobile-cloud approach for ECG telemonitoring. IEEE J. Biomed. Health Inform. **18**, 739–745 (2014)
2. Ma, J.L., Dong, M.C.: R&D of versatile distributed e-home healthcare system for cardiovascular disease monitoring and diagnosis. In: 2014 IEEE-EMBS International Conference on Biomedical and Health Informatics (BHI), pp. 444–447. IEEE (2014)
3. Ng, J.K.Y., Wang, J., Lam, K.Y., et al.: Capturing and analyzing pervasive data for SmartHealth. In: 2014 IEEE 28th International Conference on Advanced Information Networking and Applications (AINA), pp. 985–992. IEEE (2014)
4. Madan, A., Cebrian, M., Lazer, D., Pentland, A.: Social sensing to model epidemiological behavior change. In: Proceedings of ACM Ubicomp, pp. 291–300 (2010)
5. Madan, A., Moturu, S.T., Lazer, D., Pentland, A.S.: Social sensing: obesity, unhealthy eating and exercise in face-to-face networks. In: ACM Conference on Wireless Health, pp. 104–110 (2010)
6. Moturu, S.T., Khayal, I., Aharony, N., Pan, W., Pentland, A.: Sleep, mood and sociability in a healthy population. In: International Conference of the IEEE Engineering in Medicine and Biology Society, pp. 5267–5270 (2011)
7. Reyes, J.T., Hernández, E.E., Garcia, J.S.: DSP-based oversampling adaptive noise canceller for background noise reduction for mobile phones. In: International Conference on Electrical Communications and Computers, pp. 327–332 (2012)
8. Sufi, F., Khalil, I.: Diagnosis of cardiovascular abnormalities from compressed ECG: a data mining-based approach. IEEE Trans. Inf. Technol. Biomed. **15**(1), 33–39 (2011)
9. Swangnetr, M., Kaber, D.: Emotional state classification in patient-robot interaction using wavelet analysis and statistics-based feature selection. IEEE Trans. Hum.-Mach. Syst. **43**(1), 63–75 (2013)
10. Shen, C.-P., Chen, W.-H., Chen, J.-M., Hsu, K.-P., Lin, J.-W., Chiu, M.-J., Chen, C.-H., Lai, F.: Bio-signal analysis system design with support vector machine based on cloud computing service architecture. In: Proceedings of the International Conference on IEEE Engineering in Medicine and Biology Society, pp. 1421–1424 (2010)
11. Cheng, C., Brown, C., New, T., Stokes, T.H., Dampier, C., Wang, M.D.: SickleREMOTE: a two-way text messaging system for pediatric sickle cell disease patients. In: Proceedings of the IEEE-EMBS International Conference on Biomedical and Health Informatics, pp. 408–411 (2012)
12. William, M.S., Kaiser, J.: Introduction to special issue on wireless health. ACM Trans. Embed. Comput. Syst. **10**(1), 10 (2010)
13. Cheng, C., Stokes, T.H., Wang, M.D.: caREMOTE: the design of a cancer reporting and monitoring telemedicine system for domestic care. In: Proceedings of the International Conference on IEEE Engineering in Medicine and Biology Society, pp. 3168–3171 (2011)
14. Poh, M.-Z., Kim, K., Goessling, A., Swenson, N., Picard, R.: Cardiovascular monitoring using earphones and a mobile device. IEEE Pervasive Comput. **11**(4), 18–26 (2012)

15. IBM: European Union consortium launches advanced cloud computing project with hospital and smart power grid provider (2010). http://www-03.ibm.com/press/us/en/pressrelease/33067.wss

16. Hsieh, J.-C., Hsu, M.-W.: A cloud computing based 12-lead ECG telemedicine service. BMC Med. Inf. Decis. Making **12**(77), 1–12 (2012)

17. Perera, S., Henson, C., Thirunarayan, K., et al.: Semantics driven approach for knowledge acquisition from EMRs. IEEE J. Biomed. Health Inf. **18**(2), 515–524 (2014)

18. Yang, H., Kundakcioglu, E., Li, J., et al.: Healthcare intelligence: turning data into knowledge. IEEE Intell. Syst. **29**(3), 54–68 (2014)

19. Metaxas, O., Dimitropoulos, H., Ioannidis, Y., et al.: AITION: a scalable KDD platform for big data healthcare. In: 2014 IEEE-EMBS International Conference on Biomedical and Health Informatics (BHI), pp. 601–604. IEEE (2014)

20. Suominen, H.: Text mining and information analysis of health documents. Artif. Intell. Med. **61**, 127–130 (2014)

When a Teen's Stress Level Comes to the Top/Bottom: A Fuzzy Candlestick Line Based Approach on Micro-Blog

Yiping Li[✉], Zhuonan Feng, and Ling Feng

Department of Computer Science and Technology,
Centre for Computational Mental Healthcare Research, Institute of Data Science,
Tsinghua University, Beijing 100084, China
liyp09@mails.tsinghua.edu.cn, fzn0302@163.com,
fengling@mail.tsinghua.edu.cn

Abstract. Recent researches on micro-blog based adolescent stress level prediction prove the feasibility of forecasting a teen's future stress level through the stress time series detected from tweets. The previous work focuses on predicting the stress level or stress level change at the next time point, and doesn't consider the problem of predicting the future stress trend in a period of time. In this paper, we employ a fuzzy candlestick line based model to address this problem on micro-blog, *i.e.*, when a teen's stress level comes to the top/bottom in the future. The candlestick line technique is a widely used stock trend analysis method in the financial domain. Experienced analysts usually use linguistic variables to describe the candlestick lines, such as *long*, *short*, and *small*. Thus we use the fuzzy set theory to represent the stress candlestick line in this paper. We define the stress patterns as a set of neighboring candlestick lines represented with fuzzy linguistic variables. Based on these fuzzy stress patterns, we make predictions using the fuzzy decision tree model. Experiments show the effectiveness of our prediction method.

Keywords: Stress · Micro-blog · Prediction · Candlestick chart · Fuzzy theory

1 Introduction

Nowadays, teenagers are feeling the stress in all areas of their lives, from school to family, friends and academic future [1,14]. Some of them choose the wrong methods to cope with the stress, such as crying, smoking, hating themselves, lack of sleep, lack of exercise, or changing appetites. These unhealthy behaviors associated with stress may continue or worsen through adulthood, and result in a variety of physical and emotional illness, such as anxiety, high blood pressure, a weakened immune system, or even depression, obesity and heart disease. Therefore, the study of teens' stress during their growth should be paid much attention. Some guidance may be provided to help teenagers manage their stress before it causes serious consequences.

© Springer International Publishing Switzerland 2016
X. Zheng et al. (Eds.): ICSH 2015, LNCS 9545, pp. 241–253, 2016.
DOI: 10.1007/978-3-319-29175-8_23

Facilitated by the convenience and constant access provided by mobile devices, 92 % of teens go online daily, and 24 % say they go online "almost constantly" [17] in a new study from Pew Research Center. More and more, teens are taking Twitter as a way to express their innermost thoughts or follow popular trends. The billions of tweets generated on the social media platforms every day give us a window in looking at the stress situations of teenagers. By analyzing the stress in teens' tweets, we can then know their stress changing patterns, and then predict the future stress trend as early warning of stress crisis. If their stress will continue and ascend rapidly to a high level, some coaching may be provided to help them release and overcome the stress.

In this paper, we predict two important values which teens' guardians and helpers may concern: *the reversal speed*, how long the current uptrend/downtrend of the adolescent stress will go on before the next stress peak/valley time; *reversal range*, how much is the changing range of stress level between the current time and the next stress peak/valley time? To address this problem, we employ the widely used stock technical analysis methods. In some way, the stock price determination mechanisms work in a similar way with the adolescent stress regulation mechanism. Firstly, in stock market, the stock price is basically determined by the business fundamentals of the company. The stress level of a teenager is also mainly determined by his/her personality. Secondly, the stock price fluctuates a lot with the change of the internal/external events from the company/environment, such as the publication of a new economic policy. The adolescent stress level is also affected by the events including his/her personal events as well as the society/environment breaking events, such as the physical health situations, exams, and social relationships. Thus, we adopt the well-studied stock analysis tools to analyze teens' stress situations. We choose the candlestick line technique, one of the most popular and effective stock technical analysis method, as our stress analysis tool. That is because this method contains the most comprehensive and rich information of the daily stress dynamics and really does well in discovering the trend continuation and reversal patterns.

There are two challenges in using candlestick theory to predict the future stress reversal speed and range. Firstly, the technical analysis and judgement of candlestick lines usually use linguistic variables, such as *long*, *short*, and *small*. For example, the hammer candlestick line which usually appears as a bullish reversal indication from downtrend to uptrend is a candlestick line with "small" black real body, "long" lower shadow, and "short" or non-existent upper shadow. In this paper, we employ the fuzzy theory to represent seven features describing a teen's stress candlestick line and the candlestick lines relationship. This symbolic representation is more intuitive and suitable for recognition of stress candlestick patterns. Secondly, the determination of membership function is an important problem in fuzzy theory, which may influence the prediction results. In this paper, we take two different methods to determine the membership function of fuzzy sets on basis of the data distribution. We then employ the fuzzy decision tree to make prediction on the stress patterns composed of neighboring candlestick lines.

2 Related Work

2.1 Fuzzy Time Series Prediction

Song and Chissom [15,16] first apply the fuzzy set theory to modeling the time series problems when historical data are defined as linguistic values. By defining the fuzzy sets on the universe of discourse, each historical value in the time series can be fuzzified according to its membership degrees of fuzzy sets assigned with linguistic labels. A fuzzy time series can then be modeled for forecasting according to the fuzzy relationships between historical data and the future values. A lot of researches are further done to deal with more complicated situations such as multi-factors and high-order fuzzy time series and improve the execution performance in various applications [3–5].

Recently, some researchers aim to combine the fuzzy time series with the candlestick charts in financial domain. Lee et al. [7] model the imprecise and vague candlestick patterns with fuzzy linguistic variables and transfer the financial time series data to fuzzy candlestick patterns for pattern recognition. The classification algorithm is used to classify candlestick patterns for forecasting the stock price and the weighted stock index. Lan et al. [6] apply the fuzzy logic theory to the Japanese candlestick theory for finding the reversal points of the stock price. They define the candlesticks before the reversal point as "symptom sequence", and use the ADTree method to identify these reversal patterns.

2.2 Stress Detection and Prediction on Micro-Blog

Park et al. [13] find the depressed and non-depressed Twitter users have different attitudes and behaviors toward online social media. Non-depressed individuals perceive Twitter as an information consuming and sharing tool, while depressed individuals perceive it as a tool for social awareness and emotional interactions. The study of individual stress detection on micro-blog has been made to analyze the stress containing in micro-blog users' tweets. Lin et al. [11] use the deep neural network model to incorporate user-scope attributes from micro-blog postings to detect users' psychological stress. [8,19] focus on teens' stress detection. They investigate a number of teens' typical tweeting behaviors that may reveal adolescent stress, and apply five classifiers to teens' stress detection.

In Li et al. [10], based on the stress time series extracted from the tweeting timeline of teenagers, the adolescent stress level at the next time is predicted through a multi-variant time series prediction model. In our earlier work [9], we bring in the candlestick line to represent the stress situation within a time interval, and define a distance function to measure the similarity between two candlestick lines. Then we use pattern matching to predict whether the stress level of a teenager is to increase, decrease, or stay steady at the next time. Different from the previous two work, we aim to predict the reversal speed and range in the next few time points in a teen's stress level time series in this paper. The fuzzy set theory is employed to represent the candlestick lines, and we use the fuzzy decision tree to make prediction on the stress patterns composed of fuzzified candlesticks.

3 Problem Statement

The stress level of a tweet published by a teenager can be detected through the tweeting content as well as a variety of tweeting/retweeing behaviors. In this paper, we apply the stress detection function in [11,19] to detect the adolescent stress level. It examines a number of tweeting features like linguistic content, number of negative emotion words, number of positive and negative emoticons, number of exclamation and question marks, emotional degree lexicons, shared music/picture genres, as well as abnormal tweeting time and frequency, and returns an adolescent stress level ranging from 0 to 5, representing the "no-stress" to "very severe" stress state. Therefore, for a tweet sequence in a time interval ordered by the tweeting time, we can obtain a corresponding tweet-based stress level sequence.

Definition 1. *Let $I_1, I_2, \cdots, I_n$ be n successive time intervals of equal temporal length $|I|$, where $|I_1|=|I_2|=\cdots=|I_n|$. Here the time interval length $|I|$ can be a day, week, month, etc. Let $L_{i,open}$, $L_{i,close}$, $L_{i,high}$, $L_{i,low}$, $L_{i,avg}$ represent the first, last, highest, lowest, average stress level separately obtained from the stress level sequence in the time interval I_i, $i = 1, \cdots, n$. A stress candlestick line K_i can be determined according to the four characteristic values in time interval I_i: ($L_{i,open}$, $L_{i,close}$, $L_{i,high}$, $L_{i,low}$). Then we get the average stress level time series $< L_{1,avg}, L_{2,avg}, \cdots, L_{n,avg} >$, as well as the stress candlestick line series $< K_1, K_2, \cdots, K_n >$.*

Definition 2. *On the average stress level time series $< L_{1,avg}, L_{2,avg}, \cdots, L_{n,avg} >$, time interval I_i can be called the **reversal time** if it satisfies $(L_{i-1,avg} < L_{i,avg}) \wedge (L_{i,avg} > L_{i+1,avg})$ or $(L_{i-1,avg} > L_{i,avg}) \wedge (L_{i,avg} < L_{i+1,avg})$, $i = 2, \cdots, n - 1$. That is, a reversal time is when the average stress level achieves a peak or valley in the stress time series.*

*Our prediction problem is shown in Fig. 1. Given the stress candlestick line time series $< K_1, \cdots, K_n >$, we aim to predict: the time span from the next reversal time I_q $(q > n)$, called **reversal speed**, speed $= q - n$, i.e., how long the current uptrend/downtrend of the adolescent stress level will go on; the stress level change from the next reversal time, called **reversal range**, range $= |L_{q,avg} - L_{n,avg}|$, i.e., how much is the changing range of stress level between the current time and the next stress peak/valley time.*   □

4 Prediction Method

A stress candlestick K_i [12] on a time interval I_i can be determined through four values: $L_{i,open}$, $L_{i,close}$, $L_{i,high}$, $L_{i,low}$, as shown in Fig. 2. These values form a box with two lines. The box is called the real body which is the area between the open and the close stress level. If the close stress level is higher than the open stress level, the candlestick chart body is filled with red. Otherwise, it is filled with green. The two lines include the upper shadow line, constructed with the

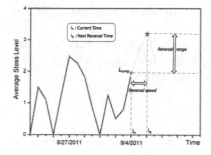

Fig. 1. Prediction problem

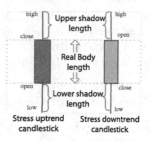

Fig. 2. Features for describing a candlestick line (Color figure online)

range between the high stress level and the higher value among the open and close level, and the lower shadow line, constructed with the range between the low stress level and the lower value among the open and close level.

4.1 Modeling Candlestick Lines

In Fig. 2, We extract four features to describe the shape and structure of a candlestick line: body color(bc), body length(bl), upper shadow length(usl) and lower shadow length(lsl). For body color, *black* represents that the open stress level is equal to the close stress.

Table 1. Features in modeling candlestick lines

	Feature	Formula
One candlestick	body color(bc)	$bc_i \in \{red, green, black\}$
	body length(bl)	$bl_i = |L_{i,close} - L_{i,open}|$
	upper shadow length(usl)	$usl_i = L_{i,high} - max(L_{i,open}, L_{i,close})$
	lower shadow length(lsl)	$lsl_i = min(L_{i,open}, L_{i,close}) - L_{i,low}$
Candlestick relationships	open style (os)	$os_i = L_{i,open} - L_{i-1,close}$
	close style (cs)	$cs_i = L_{i,close} - L_{i-1,close}$
	change rate (cr)	$cr_i = L_{i,avg} - L_{i-1,avg}$

As shown in Table 1, we also define three features to describe the candlestick lines relationship. Open style (os) is the difference between the open stress of the next day and the close stress of the previous day. This feature can indicate whether the last day's trend will continue. Close style (cs) is the difference of the close stress between two neighboring candlesticks. By observing the close style in a few consecutive days, we can judge the strength of the current trend. Change rate (cr) can be computed by the difference between the average stress of the next day and the previous day. It can measure how fast the average stress level changes.

A stress candlestick K_i at time interval $I_i(i = 1, \cdots, n)$ can then be represented with all the features: K_i =<*body color, body length, upper shadow length, lower shadow length, open style, close style, change rate*>.

4.2   Fuzzyfication of Candlestick Lines

Fuzzy set is a way to deal with vagueness uncertainty arising from human linguistic labels. On the universe of discourse $U = \{x_1, x_2, \cdots, x_n\}$, a *membership function* μ_A is assigned to measure the degree of each element x_i in U ($i = 1, \cdots, n$) satisfying the fuzzy set A, $\mu_A : U- > [0, 1]$. It can be represented as $A = \{\mu_A(x_1)/x_1, \mu_A(x_2)/x_2, \cdots, \mu_A(x_n)/x_n\}$.

We fuzzify all the features of candlestick lines through the membership functions, and generate fuzzy stress candlesticks. The body color feature takes values of linguistic labels *green, red, black*, thus we don't need to fuzzify it. On the universe of discourse $U = [0, 5]$, we define three fuzzy sets *small, middle, large* to represent the body length, upper shadow length, or lower shadow length. Terms describing the open or close style are usually "open low/high" or "going low/high". Thus, we use fuzzy linguistic variables *low, equal, high* to describe the open style, close style, and change rate of candlesticks lines. We take two methods to determine the membership functions based on the data distribution. We take *small, middle, large* for example to introduce the identification of membership functions as follows.

Trapezoid Membership Function. In defining the linguistic variable *small, middle*, or *large*, we think values within a certain interval can best represent the concept, and the values which are far from the interval are less likely to satisfy the concept. Thus we can use the classic trapezoid membership function to describe the fuzzy sets. By identifying the boundary values of the trapezoid, we can then obtain the membership function.

$$\mu_{small}(x) = \begin{cases} 1 & 0 \le x \le a_1 \\ \frac{a_2-x}{a_2-a_1} & a_1 < x \le a_2 \\ 0 & a_2 < x \le 5 \end{cases} \quad \mu_{middle}(x) = \begin{cases} 0 & 0 \le x \le a_1 \\ \frac{x-a_1}{a_2-a_1} & a_1 < x \le a_2 \\ 1 & a_2 < x \le a_3 \\ \frac{a_4-x}{a_4-a_3} & a_3 < x \le a_4 \\ 0 & a_4 < x \le 5 \end{cases}$$

$$\mu_{l\,arg\,e}(x) = \begin{cases} 0 & 0 \le x \le a_3 \\ \frac{x-a_3}{a_4-a_3} & a_3 < x \le a_4 \\ 1 & a_4 < x \le 5 \end{cases} \tag{1}$$

The problem is how to identify the four parameters of the membership function. The most direct way is to take the equidistance strategy. The universe of discourse can be partitioned into intervals with equal length by the parameters. In this way, the parameters (a_1, a_2, a_3, a_4) can take values (1.0, 2.0, 3.0, 4.0). However, this strategy doesn't consider the distribution of the body length or shadow length, and isn't suitable for biased data. The linguistic variables *small, middle, long* are relative concepts. For example, if the values of candlestick body length are rarely bigger than 4.0, then the boundary of the *long* set should be moved left.

We use the equal number strategy to identify the parameters by taking into account the data distribution. This strategy is to make the points falling into the five intervals separated by a_1, a_2, a_3, and a_4 have the same number. Let $X = x_1, x_2, \cdots, x_n$ represent the sample of the feature values in the experimental data set. Then (a_1, a_2, a_3, a_4) take values of the quantiles $Z_{0.8}$, $Z_{0.6}$, $Z_{0.4}$, $Z_{0.2}$. Here Z_α is the quantile of the sample, satisfying the percent of values bigger than Z_α is α, i.e., $percent(x > Z_\alpha) = \alpha$.

Membership Function Using Fuzzy C-Means Method. Fuzzy C-Means method is a fuzzy clustering algorithm that every point is considered to have a degree of belonging to different clusters rather than belonging completely to just one cluster [2]. Here we use this method to determine the membership degree μ_x. Let $C = \{c_1, c_2, c_3\}$ represent the center value of fuzzy set *small*, *middle*, *long* respectively. $\mu_{c_j}(x_i)$ is the membership degree that x_i belongs to the fuzzy set of the center value c_j, $j = 1, 2, 3$. $m \in [1, \infty)$ is a weighting parameter, and is commonly set to 2 in the absence of experimentation or domain knowledge. Then the fuzzy C-Means algorithm can obtain the values of $\mu_{c_j}(x_i)$ by minimizing the objective function: $\arg\min\limits_{C} \sum\limits_{i=1}^{n} \sum\limits_{j=1}^{3} \mu_{c_j}^m(x_i)|x_i - c_j|^2$, where

$$\mu_{c_j}^m(x_i) = \frac{1}{\sum\limits_{k=1}^{3} \left|\frac{x_i - c_j}{x_i - c_k}\right|^{\frac{2}{m-1}}}. \tag{2}$$

4.3   Prediction Model

A *stress pattern* P is a sequence of fuzzy stress candlesticks in a time period. Through a teenager's candlestick time series, we can obtain a lot of stress patterns with different number of candlesticks. Each pattern is followed with a reversal speed or range value for prediction. We divide all these patterns to different groups according to their lengths, and then get several pattern sets: $D_1, D_2, \cdots, D_w$. Here w is the number of candlesticks. Table 2 shows the stress candlestick patterns composed of one fuzzy candlestick.

On each pattern set D_i ($i = 1, \cdots, w$), we adopt the *Fuzzy ID3* algorithm [18], an effective decision tree method to extract knowledge in uncertain classification problems, to implement the fuzzy stress pattern classification for predicting the reversal speed and range. This method is an extension of classical decision tree, and represents the data set using the fuzzy set theory for tree growing and pruning. Similar to the classical ID3 algorithm, the fuzzy decision tree is built by choosing the attributes one by one according to their information gains. All the patterns can be classified to m classes $\{tr_1, \cdots, tr_m\}$ which are fuzzy sets defined on the reversal speed or reversal range.

In the fuzzy decision tree, each path from the root to a leaf node forms a fuzzy rule R. The leaf node of this rule can be classified to different classes with corresponding probabilities rather than only one class. Let $p(R, tr_k)$ represent the probability that the leaf node of R is classified to the class tr_k, $k = 1, \cdots, m$. An

Table 2. Fuzzy database of stress patterns

ID	bc_1	bl_1	usl_1	lsl_1	os_1	cs_1	cr_1	Reversal range
P_1	$\{1.0/r\}$	$\{1.0/lg\}$	$\{1.0/s\}$	$\{1.0/s\}$	$\{0.75/e,$ $0.25/h\}$	$\{0.5/e,$ $0.5/h\},$	$\{0.8/e,$ $0.2/h\}$	$\{0.3/samllIncrease,$ $0.7/largeIncrease\}$
P_2	$\{1.0/r\}$	$\{1.0/s\}$	$\{1.0/s\}$	$\{1.0/s\}$	$\{1.0/l\}$	$\{0.7/l,$ $0.3/e\}$	$\{0.6/l,$ $0.4/e\}$	$\{1.0/smallIncrease\}$
P_3	$\{1.0/r\}$	$\{0.8/lg,$ $0.2/m\}$	$\{0.9/lg,$ $0.1/m\}$	$\{1.0/s\}$	$\{1.0/l\}$	$\{1.0/l\}$	$\{0.7/l,$ $0.3/e\},$	$\{1.0/smallIncrease,$ $0.1/largeIncrease\}$

r:red, g:green, b:black, s:small, m:middle, lg:large, l:low, e:equal, h:high

example of a fuzzy rule R is in the form: "If the first day's body color is red, the second day's body color is red, the second day's body length is $large$, and the second day's upper shadow length is $small$, then the reversal range is $largeIncrease$ with probability 0.5 and is $middleIncrease$ with probability 0.5". It can be represented as $R = \{bc_1{:}red, bc_2{:}red, bl_2{:}large, usl_2{:}small\}$, $p(R, largeIncrease) = 0.8$, $p(R, middleIncrease) = 0.2$, $p(R, smallIncrease) = 0$. All the rules in the fuzzy decision tree comprise the rule set $\mathcal{R}$.

In the forecasting process, a test pattern P may match more than one branch with corresponding membership degree, and reach several leaf nodes in the fuzzy decision tree. Let $r \in R$ represent the value at one branch, $e.g.$, $bl_2{:}large$. If the pattern P reaches a leaf node according to the path of fuzzy rule R, then the probability that pattern P satisfies rule R and can be classified to the class tr_k is $p(P, R, tr_k) = p(R, tr_k) * \prod\limits_{r \in R} \mu_r(P)$.

In the entire fuzzy tree, the probability that pattern P is classified to the class tr_k can be computed as $p(P, tr_k) = \dfrac{\sum\limits_{R \in \mathcal{R}} p(P, R, tr_k)}{\sum\limits_{k=1}^{m} \sum\limits_{R \in \mathcal{R}} p(P, R, tr_k)}$, $\sum\limits_{k=1}^{m} p(P, tr_k) = 1$.

Reversal Speed Prediction. The fuzzification of the reversal speed is implemented in this way. Through observing all the patterns in the data set, we can obtain the maximal reversal speed value $speed_{max}$. Let u_1 be the minimal even number that is no less than $speed_{max}$. On the universe of discourse $U = [0, u_1]$, we partition this domain into s intervals with the same length 2: $w_1 = [0, 2], \cdots,$ $w_s = [u_1 - 2, u_1]$. Then s different fuzzy sets $tr_1, \cdots, tr_s$ can be defined as

$$tr_1 = 1/w_1 + 0.5/w_2 + 0/w_3 + 0/w_4 + \cdots + 0/w_{s-1} + 0/w_s$$
$$tr_2 = 0.5/w_1 + 1/w_2 + 0.5/w_3 + 0/w_4 + \cdots + 0/w_{s-1} + 0/w_s$$
$$tr_3 = 0/w_1 + 0.5/w_2 + 1/w_3 + 0.5/w_4 + \cdots + 0/w_{s-1} + 0/w_s$$
$$\cdots$$
$$tr_s = 0/w_1 + 0/w_2 + 0/w_3 + 0/w_4 + \cdots + 0.5/w_{s-1} + 1/w_s.$$

After we obtain the prediction results from the fuzzy decision tree, we defuzzify the fuzzy labels to real values. Let mid_k represent the midpoint of the interval w_k. Then the predicted reversal speed value is $speed = \sum\limits_{k=1}^{s} p(P, tr_k) * mid_k$.

Reversal Range Prediction. Let $range_{min}$ and $range_{max}$ be the minimal and maximal reversal range values in the experimental data. $u_1 = \lfloor range_{min} \rfloor$ is the largest integer no more than $range_{min}$. $u_2 = \lceil range_{max} \rceil$ is the smallest integer no less than $range_{max}$. We partition the domain of reversal range into s intervals with the same length 1 on the universe of discourse $U = [u_1, u_2]$, $w_1 = [u_1, u_1 + 1], \cdots, w_s = [u_2 - 1, u_2]$. The fuzzy sets and the defuzzification process are implemented in a similar way as the reversal speed prediction.

5   Performance Study

Experiment Setup. Our experimental data is crawled from the Chinese Sina Micro-blog platform. We identify the teen users through the user profile which contains the detailed birth dates. To obtain enough tweets for analyzing a teenager's behavior and modeling stress candlestick lines, we filter out users whose daily tweeting frequency (number of tweets/number of days) are lower than a threshold 1.0. Then we crawl all tweets of a teenager from his/her account creation time to May, 2015. Finally we fetch 50,000 tweets of 91 users whose ages are from 13 to 21 as our experimental data. Their average tweeting numbers are 632, varying from 342 to 1181, and their average daily tweeting frequency is 2.9, varying from 2.1 to 5.7. The stress detection tool [19] is applied on the tweets for detecting the stress level of a single tweet, whose detection precision is proved to be 82.6 %. Then we obtain the stress level sequences of teenagers in chronological order through the tweeting timelines. We aggregate the stress levels in day granularity, and generate daily average stress level time series and the daily candlestick lines time series. Based on these time series data, we implement the prediction model to forecast a teen's reversal speed and range.

5.1   Basic Performance

We modify the candlestick lines based prediction model in [9] as the contrast non-fuzzy method. This method doesn't fuzzify the candlestick lines. It defines a distance function to measure the similarity between two candlestick patterns. The next stress level change can then be predicted by pattern matching. We modify the model in this way. After finding the set of similar patterns with the current pattern, we then take the average of the reversal speed and range of all the matching patterns as the prediction result.

Table 3. Performance of reversal speed and range prediction

	Reversal speed					Reversal range				
	MAPE	MAD	MSE	RMSE	U	MAPE	MAD	MSE	RMSE	U
Trapezoid	19.2 %	0.397	0.439	0.603	0.292	23.3 %	0.357	0.208	0.443	0.092
Fuzzy C-Means	16.4 %	0.278	0.315	0.53	0.282	17.8 %	0.332	0.172	0.415	0.084
Non-fuzzy method [9]	24.4 %	0.419	0.446	0.637	0.332	25.6 %	0.395	0.238	0.491	0.137

In the experiment, we use the first 80 % data for training the prediction model for each teenager, and the rest 20 % is used for testing. Then we summarize the prediction results of each teenager, and take the average as the final result. Table 3 shows the prediction performance of the reversal speed and range prediction. We evaluate the prediction performance through five measures, *i.e.*, the Mean Absolute Deviation (MAD), the Mean Squared Error (MSE), the Root Mean Squared Error (RMSE), the Mean Absolute Percentage Error (MAPE), and the Theil's U-statistics (U).

In our fuzzy candlestick based model, the reversal speed values of stress patterns range from 0 to 14 in the experimental data, so the universe of discourse is [0, 14] and seven fuzzy sets can be defined. In both reversal speed and reversal range prediction, we can see our model using the membership functions from fuzzy C-Means method can make better prediction results than the trapezoid membership function on all the five measures, and they both perform better than the non-fuzzy method. On the MAPE metric, the MAPE of reversal speed prediction using fuzzy C-Means method is 16.4 % and the MAPE of trapezoid method is 19.2 %, while the MAPE of the non-fuzzy model is 24.4 %. In reversal range prediction, the prediction results of the fuzzy C-Means method (MAPE = 17.8 %) are also better than the trapezoid method (MAPE = 23.3 %), and the non-fuzzy method performs worst with a MAPE value 25.6 %. The results prove that the prediction performance can be improved by using the fuzzy linguistic variables to represent the candlestick lines. This fuzzy representation is more intuitive to users, and help them to discover stress candlestick patterns.

5.2   Different Membership Functions

In the fuzzification of candlestick lines, we use two different membership functions on basis of the data distribution: the trapezoid membership function and the membership function using the fuzzy C-Means method. Figure 3(a) shows an example of the membership functions of the change rate values(cr) between two neighboring candlesticks obtained from the fuzzy C-Means method. Three fuzzy sets *low*, *equal*, and *high* are generated, and they take the maximum membership degree 1.0 when the change rate value is −0.75, 0, and 0.75 separately. We can find the membership degree of the fuzzy set *low* decreases gradually with the decrease of the change rate when the change rate is lower than −0.75. That is because the fuzzy C-Means method takes the membership degree according to the distance from the center point. However, we regard the value to be more accordance with the linguistic variable "low" with the decrease of the change rate. Thus we use the sigmoid function in the form $\mu(x) = 1/(1 + e^{-b(x-c)})$ to simulate the left curve *low* and the right curve *high*. b and c are parameters to be determined. The modified membership functions are shown in Fig. 3(b), and seem more reasonable. In our experiment, we also do the sigmoid simulation to handle the two fuzzy sets in the left and right in the fuzzification of the body length, upper shadow length, lower shadow length, open style, and close style.

From the prediction results in Table 3, we find the reversal speed and range prediction performances of fuzzy C-Means are better than the trapezoid method. This may be because the fuzzy C-Means method generates the membership function according to the density of the data distribution. Compared the fuzzy

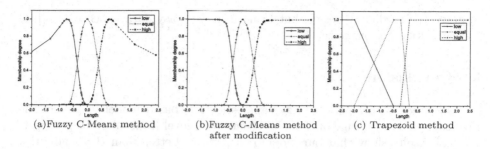

(a)Fuzzy C-Means method   (b)Fuzzy C-Means method   (c) Trapezoid method
after modification

Fig. 3. Membership degree functions

C-Means based membership function in Fig. 3(b) with the trapezoid membership function in Fig. 3(c) obtained from the same data set, we can see the trapezoid membership curves are sharp, while the membership functions of the fuzzy C-Means method are smoother. The membership function with vague boundary and gradual change may better match the habit of human cognition.

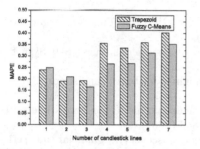

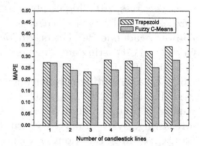

Fig. 4. MAPE of reversal speed with different number of candlestick lines

Fig. 5. MAPE of reversal range with different number of candlestick lines

5.3 Different Number of Candlestick Lines in the Stress Pattern

We generate stress candlestick patterns with different numbers of candlestick lines, and construct prediction models separately. The prediction results are shown in Figs. 4 and 5, and the number of candlestick lines vary from 1 to 7. We find the best prediction results of reversal speed (16.4 %) and reversal range (17.8 %) are achieved at the number of 3 for fuzzy C-Means method. The reversal speed prediction of trapezoid membership function based model has the smallest MAPE value (18.9 %) when the candlesticks number is 2. The prediction of reversal range using the trapezoid method achieves the least MAPE value 23.3 % at the number of 3. When the number of candlestick lines keeps increasing, the performance becomes worse. This proves that 2 or 3 candlesticks can provide enough information for the discovery of stress patterns. More candlesticks can't improve the prediction result, but bring in more noisy data which can reduce the prediction performance.

6   Conclusion

In this paper, we propose a fuzzy candlestick line based model to predict the reversal speed and range of the adolescent stress level from micro-blog. Experimental results show that our model can perform better than the candlestick theory based model without fuzzy processing.

Acknowledgement. The work is supported by National Natural Science Foundation of China (61373022, 61073004), and Chinese Major State Basic Research Development 973 Program (2011CB302203-2).

References

1. APA's 2013 Stress In America survey (2013). http://www.apa.org/news/press/releases/stress/2013/highlights.aspx
2. Bezdek, J.C.: Pattern Recognition With Fuzzy Objective Function Algorithms. Kluwer Academic Publishers, Norwell (1981)
3. Chen, S.: Forecasting enrollments based on fuzzy time series. Fuzzy Sets Syst. **81**, 311–319 (1996)
4. Chen, S.: Forecasting enrollments based on high-order fuzzy time series. Cybern. Syst. Int. J. **33**, 234–244 (2002)
5. Huang, K., Yu, T., Hsu, Y.: A multivariate heuristic model for fuzzy-time series forecasting. Syst. Manage. Cybern. **37**, 836–846 (2007)
6. Lan, Q., Zhang, D., Xiong, L.: Reversal pattern discovery in financial time series based on fuzzy candlestick lines. Complex. Syst. Eng. Manage. **2**, 182–190 (2011)
7. Lee, C.-H.L., Liu, A., Chen, W.-S.: Pattern discovery of fuzzy time series for financial prediction. IEEE Trans. Knowl. Data Eng. **18**(5), 613–625 (2006)
8. Li, Q., Xue, Y., Jia, J., Feng, L.: Helping teenagers relieve psychological pressures: a micro-blog based system. In: EDBT (2014)
9. Li, Y., Feng, Z., Feng, L.: Using candlestick charts to predict adolescent stress trend on micro-blog. In: ICTH (2015)
10. Li, Y., Huang, J., Wang, H., Feng, L.: Predicting teenager's future stress level from micro-blog. In: Proceedings of CBMS (2015)
11. Lin, H., Jia, J., Guo, Q., Xue, Y., Li, Q., Huang, J., Cai, L., Feng, L.: User-level psychological stress detection from social media using deep neural network. In: Proceedings of MM (2014)
12. Nison, S.: Japanese Candlestick Charting Techniques. Prentice Hall Press, Upper Saddle River (2001)
13. Park, M., McDonald, D., Cha, M.: Perception differences between the depressed and non-depressed users in twitter. In: Proceedings of ICWSM, pp. 476–485 (2013)
14. People's Daily Online (2014). http://hm.people.com.cn/n/2014/0831/c230533-25574055.html
15. Song, Q., Chissom, B.S.: Forecasting enrollments with fuzzy time series - Part I. Fuzzy Sets Syst. **54**, 1–9 (1993)

16. Song, Q., Chissom, B.S.: Forecasting enrollments with fuzzy time series - Part II. Fuzzy Sets Syst. **62**, 1–8 (1994)
17. Teens, Social Media & Technology Overview 2015 (2015). http://www.pewinternet. org/2015/04/09/teens-social-media-technology-2015/
18. Umano, M., Okamoto, H., Hatono, I., Tamura, H., Kawachi, F., Umedzu, S., Kinoshita, J.: Fuzzy decision trees by fuzzy id3 algorithm and its application to diagnosis systems. In: Proceedings of the Third IEEE Conference on Fuzzy Systems, vol. 3, pp. 2113–2118, June 1994
19. Xue, Y., Li, Q., Jin, L., Feng, L., Clifton, D.A., Clifford, G.D.: Detecting adolescent psychological pressures from micro-blog. In: Zhang, Y., Yao, G., He, J., Wang, L., Smalheiser, N.R., Yin, X. (eds.) HIS 2014. LNCS, vol. 8423, pp. 83–94. Springer, Heidelberg (2014)

Linking Obesity and Tweets

Mohd Anwar[✉] and Zhuoning Yuan

Secure and Usable Social Media and Networks Lab,
Department of Computer Science,
North Carolina A&T State University, Greensboro, NC, USA
manwar@ncat.edu, zyuan@aggies.ncat.edu

Abstract. Obesity has been a public health problem in the United States. The online social media platforms such as Twitter, Facebook, Google+ give users quick and easy way to engage in conversation about issues, problems, and concerns of their daily lives. In this exploratory research, our goal is to determine if the obesity conversation among Twitter users from fattest places is different than that among people from thinnest places. Our hypothesis is that the users in thinnest places would engage more, both in quantity and quality, in Twitter conversation about preventing obesity and promoting health than that of the users in fattest places. We conducted a comparative study of obesity conversations on Twitter by location of top ten fattest and thinnest cities as well as top ten fattest and thinnest states in the United States. Our results show that users in fattest cities and states participate significantly less in conversation covering the topics on and around obesity than that of thinnest cities and states.

Keywords: Obesity · Twitter · Tweet analysis · Online social networks · Sentiment analysis

1 Introduction

More than one-third (34.9 %) of U.S. adults are obese [22]. Obesity is related to serious health conditions such as heart disease, stroke, type 2 diabetes, as well as various cancers. The estimated annual medical cost of obesity in the U.S. was $147 billion in 2008 [22]. Therefore, obesity has become a serious public health problem that researchers from different disciplines have been trying to tackle.

Online social media has become an integral part of our daily social lives. Millions of conversations are taking place in OSN, and thereby generating huge amount of social content. Researchers have been successful in analyzing social content to discover new knowledge in many areas including user attribute and behavior analysis, location-based interaction analysis, recommender system development, and recently public health (e.g., flu outbreak [5]).

In addition to physical environment, social environment also contributes to obesity. Christakis and Fowler analyzed data from the Framingham Heart Study and reported that increases in an individual's weight correlates with weight gain in friends and family [25]. Online social media records a significant part of an individual's social life. Currently, Facebook has over 1.4 billion active users [23]. The more than 289 million active Twitter users post an average of 58 million tweets every day [24]. As a result,

© Springer International Publishing Switzerland 2016
X. Zheng et al. (Eds.): ICSH 2015, LNCS 9545, pp. 254–266, 2016.
DOI: 10.1007/978-3-319-29175-8_24

Twitter can offer a rich dataset to glean new insight on the social dimension of obesity. This new knowledge will contribute to the development of effective measures for obesity prevention and health promotion.

In this research study, we gather and analyze data from Twitter in order to determine whether the conversation about obesity are both quantitatively and qualitatively different among users of fattest and thinnest places in the United States. Fattest and thinnest places are determined by percentage of residents who are overweight. More specifically, we gather tweets from top 10 fattest and thinnest cities[1] as well as top 10 fattest and thinnest states[2]. For example, according to Gallup research, Huntington, WV is the fattest city in the U.S. that has almost 40 % overweight residents.

Building on the collected twitter dataset and our analysis algorithm, the contributions of this work is the comparative study of obesity conversation in fattest and thinnest places in the USA. The rest of the paper is organized as follows. Section 2 presents related work. Section 3 describes our approach to this research study. In Sect. 4, we present the results and the paper is concluded in Sect. 5.

2 Related Work

In this work we study Twitter as a platform for conversation about obesity. Over thirty-one days, we collected a corpus of obesity-related tweets together with relevant metadata, such as geographical locations, favorites, re-tweets, time of posting, etc. Our work is built upon and inspired by the existing literature.

Myslín et al. [1] use machine learning classification of tobacco-related tweets to detect tobacco-relevant posts and user sentiment towards tobacco products.

Paul and Dredze explored health-related tweets and topics on Twitter through the development of new computational models. They used supervised learning to filter tweets and find health-related messages.

Schwartz et al. [3] mined information on life satisfaction from Twitter and evaluated their approach using phone survey data. They use LDA classifier to find word topics, which correlate with demographics and socio-economic status. De Choudhury et al. [4] studied public tweets from new mothers as a method of identifying signals of postpartum depression. They examined linguistic and emotional correlates for postnatal changes of new mothers. Researchers study lifestyle factors such as physical activities from tweets [11].

Social media is in use for prediction and tracking of disease outbreaks [15]. Social media data can be analyzed for public health surveillance such as influenza surveillance using Twitter [5]. Sadilek et al. shows that user co-location and social ties information from social media can be used to learn very specific and fine-grained models of the spread of contagious disease [6].

Research of Gayo-Avello [7] shows that Social media like Twitter may provide a glimpse on electoral outcomes. An analysis of the tweets' political sentiment

---

[1] http://www.usatoday.com/story/money/business/2014/04/06/americas-thinnestcity/7306199/.

[2] http://stateofobesity.org/adult-obesity/.

demonstrates close correspondence to the parties' and politicians' political positions [10]. This research demonstrates that the content of Twitter messages reflects the offline environment.

Mitchell et al. [8] investigate the correlations between Twitter geo-tagged data (expressing in real-time sentiment of individuals) and emotional, geographic, demographic, and health characteristics and generate happiness maps of the United States from sentiment analysis. Wakade et al. [12] perform sentiment analysis from tweets related to iPhone and Microsoft using Naïve Bayes and decision tree classifier.

. Lee et al. [9] develop text-based and network-based classification models of trending topics of Twitter to understand which topic belongs to what category. De Silva and Riloff [14] address the problem of detecting whether a tweet comes from an organization or personal account.

Dredze et al. developed HealthTweets.org [13], a new platform for sharing the latest research results on Twitter data with researchers and public officials. The goal of this service is to transition results from research to practice.

Social pattern in obesity promotion and suppression was described from Facebook posts on watching television or going outdoors [16]. A literature survey of twelve studies found that interventions using social networking services produced a modest but significant 0.64 percent reduction in BMI from baseline for the 941 people who participated in the studies' interventions [17].

3   Approach

Twitter provides an accessible user data with broad demographic penetration across ethnicities, genders, age groups, income levels, education levels, etc.[3] As a result, Twitter dataset is a well-suited source to study obesity. Our study approach (presented in Fig. 1) involves building a corpus of obesity-related tweets and analyzing the corpus to detect quantitative and qualitative differences in the dataset across fattest and thinnest places.

3.1   Corpus Building Using Twitter API

Step 1: We created an app on Twitter developer website (https://apps.twitter.com/) and received *Consumer Key*, *Consumer Secret* and *Access Token* provided by Open Authentication (*OAuth*). It can be described as a passport to get access to retrieve and store these data from Twitter.

Step 2: Using Java in *NetBeans (IDE)* with a third party library, *Twitter4j* (http://twitter4j.org/en/index.html) (version: 4.04) [23], we implemented our query program. Our program retrieved obesity-related tweets for 31 days total, with 7 days' tweets (*a limit by search API for reaching only 7 days tweets*) at a time with obesity related hashtags. With *geolocation( )* filter, we fetched tweets from ten most fattest and thinnest cities and states.

---

[3] http://www.pewinternet.org/2014/01/08/social-media-update-2013/twitter-users/.

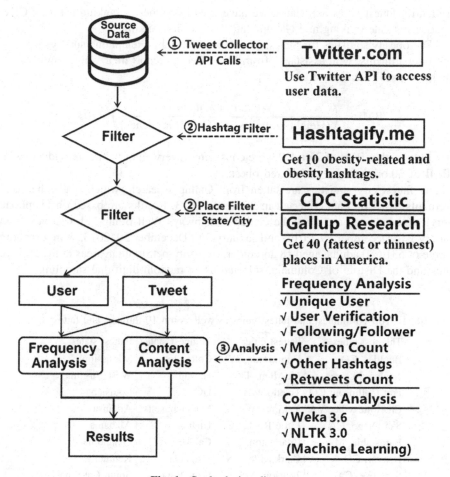

Fig. 1. Study design diagram.

Step 3: We used a library, *javacsv*, which can output data information as CSV format and be easily accessed by Excel. Thus, we get a dataset with "Time", "User", "Location", "Tweet", "Favorite Count", and "Retweet Number".

3.2   Obesity-Related Tweets Filtering

Place Filtering: The data collected from Twitter were filtered to find obesity-related tweets from top 10 fattest and thinnest cities and states (shown in Table 1). Excel functions are applied in this step. We set conditions as *20 fattest and thinnest cities (e.g., Boulder, CO is a thinnest city)* and *20 fattest and thinnest states (e.g., Mississippi is a fattest state)* using *advanced filter* and counting using *countif() function*. We dropped the tweets from users who never fill their location information and just fill a city without state information.

To identify fattest cities and states, we have used two Obesity ranking sources: CDC statistics for state ranking and Gallup statistics for city ranking.

CDC obesity statistics for States: The data are based on telephone surveys by state health departments, with assistance from CDC. People report their weight and height, which are used to calculate BMI [26].

$$BMI = \left(\frac{\text{Weight in pounds}}{(\text{Height in inches}) \times (\text{Height in inches})} \right) * 703$$

Adults with a BMI of 25 to 29.9 are considered overweight, while individuals with a BMI of 30 or more are considered obese.

The fattest city statistics are taken from Gallup research, which made the measurements based on data collected in 2012 and 2013. Results are based on telephone interviews conducted as part of the Gallup-Healthways Well-Being Index survey from January 2 to December 29, 2012, and January 2 to December 30, 2013, with a random sample of 531,630 adults, aged 18 and older, living in metropolitan areas in the 50 U.S. states and the District of Columbia, selected using random-digit-dial sampling.

Table 1. Top 10 thinnest and fattest cities as well as top 10 thinnest and fattest states.

Thinnest cities	Fattest cities	Thinnest states	Fattest states
Boulder, CO	Huntington, WV	Colorado	Mississippi
Naples, FL	McAllen, TX	Hawaii	West Virginia
Fort Collinson, CO	Toledo, OH	DC	Louisiana
Charlottesville, VA	Yakima, WA	Massachusetts	Arkansas
San Diego, CA	Little Rock, AR	Utah	Alabama
Barnstable, MA	Charleston, WV	California	Oklahoma
Denver, CO	Clarksville, TN	Montana	Kentucky
San Jose, CA	Jackson, MS	New York	South Carolina
Bridgeport, CT	Green Bay, WI	Vermont	Michigan
Bellingham, WA	Rockford, IL	New Jersey	Indiana

Topic Filtering: We have used 11 hashtags to filter obesity-related tweets. In order to determine which hashtags were most commonly used for obesity-related topics, the visual hashtag search engine Hashtagify[4] was used. Hashtagify collects tweets and examines hashtag usage patterns. To date, Hashtagify has analyzed 4,118,432,455 tweets collecting data about 49,078,312 hashtags. Hashtagify search engine identifies the following 10 most commonly used hashtags for obesity-related topics: #sugar, #fitness, #weightless, #health, #nutrition, #fat, #food, #diet, #overeating, and #diabetes.

---

4 www.hashtagify.me.

3.3   Data Analysis

Frequency Analysis. Twitter data is of two categories: *tweet* and *user*. We performed quantitative analysis of tweets and users of the tweets. Our program calculates counts for unique users, verified users, following/followers, mentions, and re-tweets. We also identified additional hashtags other than original 11 obesity-related hashtag filters.

Content Analysis. We conducted sentiment analysis on the content of tweets using Natural Language Tool Kit (NLTK [18]). Our goal is to categorize tweets into three categories: positive tweets (tweets promoting health), neutral (no definitive message related to obesity), and negative tweets (tweets promoting obesity). We also applied C4.5 algorithm for classification on our tweets from users of fattest cities using java implementation (J48) in Weka machine learning software toolkit [20].

4   Results

To understand the difference in obesity conversation among people of top 10 fattest and thinnest cities and states respectively, we performed several analysis tasks on our collected dataset from Twitter. We have collected 3,752,830 tweets on 11 obesity-related hashtags during the period of March 24 to April 27 of 2015. After filtering, we have total 356217 tweets that include 25927 tweets of 10 thinnest cities, 3372 tweets of 10 fattest cities, 280566 tweets of 10 thinnest states, and 46352 tweets of 10 fattest states.

We group these tasks into two categories: city-level analysis and state-level analysis. Table 2 shows total number of users who participated in obesity conversations from 10 fattest and thinnest cities and 10 most fattest and thinnest states. Table 3 shows tweet and re-tweet counts on and around obesity topic in fattest and thinnest places.

Table 2. Total number of users from 20 cities and 20 states.

Fattest cities	Thinnest cities	Fattest states	Thinnest states
382	3252	9047	41666

Table 3. Total number of tweets and re-tweets from 20 cities and 20 states.

Type/place	Fattest cities (10)	Thinnest cities (10)	Fattest states (10)	Thinnest states (10)
Total tweet count	2926	21138	25927	214877
Total re-tweet count	446	4789	20425	65679

Mention count is the number of times a user is mentioned in a tweet. A mention in a tweet is recognizable by the @ sign followed by a username. Number of tweets indicates total number of tweets with different mention counts. Mention is a "social" feature and indicates personal communication between Twitter users. In Table 4, we present mention counts for tweets from fattest and thinnest cities as well as fattest and thinnest states respectively.

Table 4. City-wise and state-wise mention counts.

Mention times	Number of tweet			
	Fattest cities	Thinnest cities	Fattest states	Thinnest states
=0	2752	18918	19455	178489
=1	453	5711	21605	74290
=2	110	887	3993	18865
=3	31	265	905	3961
=4	7	103	303	3060
=5	7	20	59	1684
=6	8	9	18	131
=7	0	6	9	43
=8	3	5	4	33
>=9	1	3	1	10

We further analyzed the tweets to identify 10 additional (other than the hashtags we used to search for obesity related conversation) high frequency hashtags that users in fattest and thinnest places used in their obesity related conversations. Table 5 shows high-frequency hashtags used in obesity conversation (tweets) from fattest and thinnest cities and states. The most commonly occurring hashtags across categories are #run, #running, #healthy, #exercise, #workout, etc.

Table 5. Top 10 additional (other than 11 search hashtags) high frequency hashtags found in tweets from 20 cities and 20 states.

10 fattest cities	10 thinnest cities	10 fattest states	10 thinnest states
#fatloss	#entrepreneur	#foodie	#workout
#packers	#exercise	#free	#best
#solution	#workout	#foodporn	#exercise
#free	#healthy	#healthy	#world
#endalz	#success	#running	#show
#radio	#entrepreneurs	#run	#internet
#run	#beauty	#everymomentcounts	#toxicemotions
#running	#kimkardashian	#win	#healthy
#talk	#hot	#wellness	#lifestyle
#everymomentcounts	#walking	#c25k	#fit

In order to detect the presence of influential users in the conversation, we explored how many users Twitter has verified and how many users have followers more than one

Table 6. Type of unique users among 20 states and cities

	Fattest city	Thinnest city	Fattest state	Thinnest state
Verified	6	33	59	494
Not verified	369	3130	8597	35549
Followers > 1k	86	939	1970	10352

thousand. Table 6 shows that among the users who participated in obesity conversation, thinnest cities have significantly more verified users (33 vs. 6) who participated in obesity conversation compared to fattest cities and thinnest states have significantly more verified users (494 vs. 59) than fattest states. In thinnest cities and states, users who participated in obesity related conversation have significantly more followers than fattest cities and states.

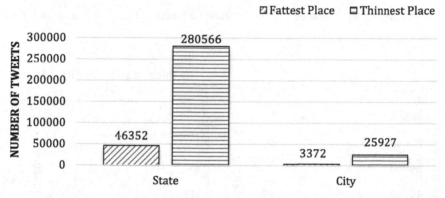

Fig. 2. A comparison of number of tweets in obesity conversation in fattest and thinnest states as well as fattest and thinnest cities.

Figure 2 shows that users from thinnest states have contributed significantly more tweets than the users in fattest states and the same trend is observed in fattest and thinnest cities. Figures 3 and 4 show that #health and #fitness and #food are the three most frequently occurring hashtags in the tweets from users of both thinnest and fattest cities and states respectively.

Content Analysis. We categorize tweets into three categories: neutral, positive (promoting health) and negative (promoting obesity). The following types of tweets are considered to be positive (promoting health):

- A tweet that encourages or announces exercise and/or physical activity
- A tweet that informs people of health advances in medicine
- A tweet that updates people on new health recipes
- A tweet that provides tips and steps for weight-loss or a healthier life

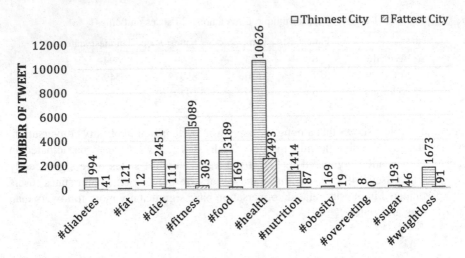

Fig. 3. A comparison of hashtag-wise tweet counts in fattest and thinnest cities (Color figure online).

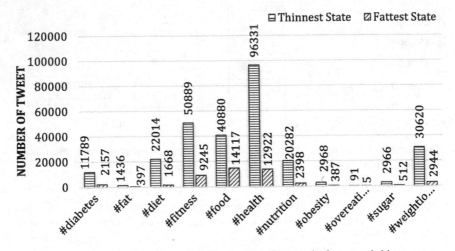

Fig. 4. A comparison of hashtag-wise distribution of tweets in fattest and thinnest states.

Examples of positive tweets that we captured:

- "11 Prime Nutrition rules fit people should follow"
- "Love this! Foods to avoid if you want to be healthy"
- "Make plans for tomorrow's workouts and meals now!"

Neutral tweets are as follows:

- A tweet that promotes both health and obesity or neither
- A tweet that proposes a recipe that cannot be determined healthy or unhealthy
- A tweet that has nothing to do with health or obesity

Examples of neutral tweets that we captured:

- "We can all dream!! #Sugar by @Maroon5 is a new favorite and bound to be a wedding must for..."
- "Yeah you show me good lovin, make it alright, need a little sweetness in my life #sugar"

Negative tweets (Promoting Obesity) are as follows:

- A tweet that encourages or announces inactivity
- A tweet that informs people of unhealthy recipes
- A tweet that is facetious concerning eating habits or health

Examples of negative tweets are as follows:

- "#DeathByChocolate #cookies and #cinnamon #orangezest and #sugar coated #donuts"
- "Anyone else in need of an afternoon sugar rush? #dumdums #lollipop #candy #sugar #flavor"
- "Cotton Candy for breakfast! #easter #sugar"

Sentiment Analysis using Natural Language Toolkit (NLTK). We trained a classifier on the collected tweets with the NLTK toolkit (Python 2.7.10). For using Naïve Bayes Classifier, we made a training set by manually selecting tweets. Two annotators analyzed manually and randomly picked 1472 total tweets including 520 positive posts, 432 negative posts and 520 neutral posts. When the software finished the "learning" step, we tested the rest of dataset and the program labeled these tweets with "positive", negative" and "neutral" tags.

In fattest cities, the majority (71 %) of the tweets of obesity-related conversation are neutral. In other words, the most conversation is not deeply rooted on obesity. However, 25 % of tweets contribute to promoting health. On the other hand, half of the tweets from thinnest cities are classified as neutral. This is an interesting finding that needs to be further investigated. Besides 36 % of tweets are related to promoting health.

In fattest states, about half (47 %) of the tweets are neutral. About one-fourth (26 %) of the tweets are about promoting health and other one-fourth (27 %) of the tweets are related to promoting obesity. On the other hand, the majority of the tweets (55 %) in obesity-related conversation in thinnest states are classified as neutral. This result is persistent with conversation type in thinnest cities. One third (34 %) of the tweets in thinnest states are supporting health promotion and about one-tenth (11 %) of the tweets are obesity promoting (Fig. 5 and Table 7).

Classification of Tweets and Obesity Rate. We further explored if it could be predicted whether a set of tweets are generated from a thinnest city or a fattest city. We applied J48 (Java implementation of C4.5 algorithm) algorithm on our tweet corpus using Weka toolkit [20].

The classification result is presented in Fig. 6. When the percentage of tweets containing #diet is greater than 3.66 %, the tweets' originating city is classified as thinnest place, if not, we need to check frequency of tweets with #fitness. If the percentage of tweets containing #fitness is greater than 40.26 %, further check on the

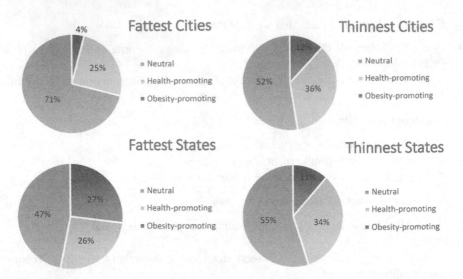

Fig. 5. Classification of obesity-related tweets in fattest and thinnest cities and states (Color figure online).

Table 7. Quality of obesity-related conversation measured through type of tweets (positive - health promoting, neutral, and negative - obesity promoting).

Sentiment	Fattest cities	Thinnest cities	Fattest states	Thinnest states
Neutral	2395	3073	12511	32383
Health-promoting	846	9239	12146	94320
Obesity-promoting	131	13615	21695	153863

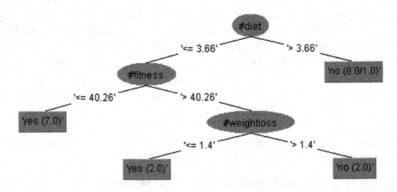

Fig. 6. Visualization tree for classification of thinnest and fattest city based on tweet hashtags.

frequency of #weightloss is required. And if tweets containing #weightloss is less than 1.4 %, and then the city from which tweets are collected is categorized as a fattest city. This prediction model achieved only 52.6 % of accuracy. Therefore, we will work on this classification task in future using a larger dataset and different algorithms.

5   Conclusion

We have conducted an exploratory research to determine whether the individuals in fattest cities engage in different type of obesity conversation than individuals in thinnest cities. This study is a precursor to the understanding of how social environment in general and Twitter in particular can inform us about social dimension of obesity condition. The key findings of our research are following:

- The individuals in thinnest places (both cities and states) engage significantly more in obesity conversation on Twitter than the individuals from fattest places.
- The obesity conversation in thinnest places are more socially and personally involved (more re-tweets, more mentions, more verified users, and users with more followers) than those of fattest places.
- Irrespective of thinnest or fattest places, a significant portion of conversation promotes obesity.
- The conversations among individuals in fattest places are not deeply rooted on obesity (a significant portion of tweets are neutral).
- We identified additional hashtags to capture obesity related conversation on Twitter.

We have developed algorithms and analytical tools to perform a larger study on obesity conversation on Twitter. Some of the findings warrant further study such as why significant percentage of the conversation are promoting obesity in both thinnest and fattest places. Or, why the obesity-related conversations are not very socially and personally rooted. Informed by this study, we plan to conduct a large-scale study on obesity conversation on Twitter.

References

1. Myslín, M., Zhu, S.H., Chapman, W., Conway, M.: Using Twitter to examine smoking behavior and perceptions of emerging tobacco products. J. Med. Internet Res. 15(8), e174 (2013)
2. Paul, M.J., Dredze, M.: You are what you tweet: analyzing Twitter for public health. Proc. ICWSM 2011, 265–272 (2011)
3. Schwartz, H.A., Eichstaedt, J.C., Kern, M.L., Dziurzynski, L., Lucas, R.E., Agrawal, M., Park, G.J., et al.: Characterizing geographic variation in well-being using tweets. In: Proceedings of the ICWSM 2013 (2013)
4. De Choudhury, M., Counts, S., Horvitz, E.: Predicting postpartum changes in emotion and behavior via social media. In: Proceedings of the SIGCHI Conference on Human Factors in Computing Systems, pp. 3267–3276. ACM (2013)
5. Lamb, A., Paul, M.J., Dredze, M.: Separating fact from fear: tracking flu infections on Twitter. In: HLT-NAACL, pp. 789–795 (2013)
6. Sadilek, A., Kautz, H.A., Silenzio, V.: Predicting disease transmission from geo-tagged micro-blog data. In: AAAI (2012)
7. Gayo-Avello, D.: A meta-analysis of state-of-the-art electoral prediction from Twitter data. Soc. Sci. Comput. Rev. 0894439313493979 (2013)

8. Mitchell, L., Frank, M.R., Harris, K.D., Dodds, P.S., Danforth, C.M.: The geography of happiness: connecting Twitter sentiment and expression, demographics, and objective characteristics of place. PLoS ONE **8**(5), e64417 (2013)

9. Lee, K., Palsetia, D., Narayanan, R., Patwary, M.M.A., Agrawal, A., Choudhary, A.: Twitter trending topic classification. In: 2011 IEEE 11th International Conference on Data Mining Workshops (ICDMW), pp. 251–258 (2011)

10. Tumasjan, A., Sprenger, T.O., Sandner, P.G., Welpe, I.M.: Predicting elections with Twitter: what 140 characters reveal about political sentiment. Proc. ICWSM **10**, 178–185 (2010)

11. Yoon, S., Elhadad, N., Bakken, S.: A practical approach for content mining of tweets. Am. J. Prev. Med. **45**(1), 122–129 (2013)

12. Wakade, S., Shekar, C., Liszka, K.J., Chan, C.C.: Text mining for sentiment analysis of Twitter data. In: International Conference on Information and Knowledge Engineering, pp. 109–114 (2012)

13. Dredze, M., Cheng, R., Paul, M.J., Broniatowski, D.A.: HealthTweets.org: a platform for public health surveillance using Twitter. In: AAAI Conference on Artificial Intelligence (2014)

14. De Silva, L., Riloff, E.: User type classification of tweets with implications for event recognition. In: Proceedings of the Joint Workshop on Social Dynamics and Personal Attributes in Social Media, vol. 98. ACL 2014 (2014)

15. Schmidt, C.W.: Trending now: using social media to predict and track disease outbreaks. Environ. Health Perspect. **120**(1), 30–33 (2012)

16. Chunara, R., Bouton, L., Ayers, J.W., Brownstein, J.S.: Assessing the online social environment for surveillance of obesity prevalence. PLoS ONE **8**(4), e61373 (2013)

17. Ashrafian, H., Toma, T., Harling, L., Kerr, K., Athanasiou, T., Darzi, A.: Social networking strategies that Aim to reduce obesity have achieved significant although modest results. Health Aff. **33**(9), 1641–1647 (2014)

18. Natural Language Toolkit. http://www.nltk.org/

19. Twitter API. https://dev.twitter.com/overview/documentation

20. Weka 3: Data Mining Software in Java. http://www.cs.waikato.ac.nz/ml/weka/

21. Twitter4J: A Java library for the Twitter API. http://twitter4j.org/en/

22. Adult Obesity Facts. CDC. http://www.cdc.gov/obesity/data/adult.html

23. Statistica Inc. Facebook: monthly active users 2015. In Statista - The Statistics Portal for Market Data, Market Research and Market Studies, Retrieved July 21, 2015. http://www.statista.com/statistics/272014/global-social-networks-ranked-by-number-of-users/

24. Statistic Brain. (n.d.). Twitter Statistics. Retrieved July 21, 2015. http://www.statisticbrain.com/twitter-statistics/

25. Christakis, N.A., Fowler, J.H.: The spread of obesity in a large social network over 32 years. N. Engl. J. Med. **357**(4), 370–379 (2007)

26. Obesity Rates and Rankings Methodology. http://stateofobesity.org/methodology/

Social Dynamics of the Online Health Communities for Mental Health

Ronghua Xu and Qingpeng Zhang[✉]

Department of System Engineering and Engineering Management,
City University of Hong Kong, Tat Chee Avenue, Kowloon, Hong Kong
ronghuaxu2-c@my.cityu.edu.hk, qingpeng.zhang@cityu.edu.hk

Abstract. Online Health Communities (OHCs) have become more and more prevalent with the advance of web 2.0 and social media. These platforms provide free, open and wide-sourced places for people to publicly discuss health-related problems, especially some mental health problems, such as depression. This paper aims to characterize the unique structural and dynamic patterns of users' interactions in depression related OHCs. Through the topological analyses of social networks, we identify the unique highly sticky structure of depression related OHCs as compared with other social communities. Besides, users in these communities spend relatively longer time on closely peer-to-peer messaging. Moreover, the evolutionary trends show that depression related OHCs present distinctive growth patterns in terms of user addition and user activeness, which could be further applied in differentiating the community types and the development stages.

Keywords: Online health communities · Social network analysis · Message exchange · Social dynamics

1 Introduction

Online health communities (OHCs) provide a novel means for patients and their families to learn an illness and connect with others in similar circumstances [1]. These communities have become more and more prevalent for knowledge exchange, information sharing and healthcare practising [2,3], especially for some sensitive issues, such as mental health problems. With the advantageous characteristics of effectiveness, always-available and unrestricted access to common people [1,4], OHCs can be extremely beneficial for patients to get both emotional and social support and improve their mental conditions [5–7], which may not be possible in the real world. Although the knowledge from these communities cannot be evaluated, it has been suggested that the formation of social connections in OHCs may serve as a coping mechanism to deal with high-stress situations and build resilience [8].

The social networks formed by peer-to-peer messaging in OHCs can not only reveal the social connections of users, but also shed light on the community

X. Zheng et al. (Eds.): ICSH 2015, LNCS 9545, pp. 267–277, 2016.
DOI: 10.1007/978-3-319-29175-8_25

structures [1]. In [3], the authors showed that the level of peer-to-peer messaging is a strong indicator of social interactions and social tie strength. With respect to OHCs, if two users exchange information frequently, it may imply that these users have similar interests or the same health problems [9]. Besides, the structural information is also effective in detecting and differentiating the polarisation of users' opinions [12].

Furthermore, the dynamics of peer-to-peer messaging in OHCs also uncover the dynamics of users' online behaviours and the evolution of social networks. From the perspective of individual users, the actions such as the message posting and receiving, community visiting frequency and duration, provide valuable clues to characterize the activeness and the role of the user [9,13]. From the other perspective of the overall community, the dynamic messaging reveals the evolution of user interactions and the development of the community [16]. Both are important factors for stakeholders to provide more reasonable and easy-get support and help in OHCs [14].

In this paper, we study the network properties, users' interaction behaviours and network evolutions in OHCs. Taken the disease of depression as an example, the main datasets include two closely related OHCs, named *Depression* and *Major Depressive Disorder (MDD)*. Both are operating on a popular Chinese social media platform, *Douban*, which allows and encourages its users to launch communities with various topics. The reason why we choose these two communities is that they both have a clear objective to provide support and help for depressed users.

We mainly focus on the following three questions,

- What are the network properties of peer-to-peer messaging in OHCs? And whether there are unique properties as compared with other social networks?
- What are the characteristics of user participation and messaging frequency in OHCs?
- What are their interaction patterns with respect to network evolution? Are there any differences between different OHCs in terms of the dynamic patterns?

2   Data Preparation

2.1   Datasets

The data set is collected from *Douban*, a comprehensive social media platform with various daily life topics such as books, music, and travel. Most of the contents are generated by its users. *Douban* allows users to form peer-peer communities, also called interest groups, where other users can post messages and publicly discuss around some specific topics. Among the thousands of communities, a large portion is about mental health, and the mainframe in mental health is the depression related OHCs.

There are two specific communities highlighted in this work, the Depression[1] and Major Depressive Disorder (MDD)[2]. The reason for choosing these two communities is that both have a clear purpose of providing support and help for the depressed patients. For comparison and verification of the interaction patterns, we also collect other related OHCs, including Youth Loneliness Depression (YLD)[3], Autism (AUT)[4], Anxiety Disorder (AND)[5], and also another different type of community of young Scientists (use Scientists for short)[6].

Within the user-created communities, any user can initiate a thread and each thread is denoted by a specific *threadID*. Others can join the thread by posting replies to the creator, or to some other users in the thread. For every piece of message, the pre-defined items include the owner of the message, the target receiver, the post time, and the thread it belongs to. The post-reply connection implies the users interactions and possible relationships between them, and thus is the focus of our work. For privacy concerns, all the users are denoted by a unique *userID*.

2.2   Network Construction

User interactions are embodied by the post-reply connections, which are further captured by the analysis of networks patterns. To construct networks, we treat each user in OHCs as a node, and every node is identical. When a piece of message is exchanged from one user to another, there is a directed edge from the former to the latter. As user may communicate many times, multiple edges exist between some nodes. The detailed procedure of network construction is as follows,

– If a user, A, initiates a new thread, A becomes one node in the network. To denote the opening message that A posts, a sell-loop edge from A is added. Note that the self-loop is only used to denote the opening of the thread but will be removed in network analysis.
– If another user, B leaves a message in the thread that A has created, a directed edge from B to A is constructed.
– If a user, C, also joins and leaves a message directly replying to B, then a directed edge from C to B is constructed. If C does not target to any users, then by default, it responds to A, the initiator, and a directed edge form C to A is drawn.
– If no other users join the thread that A initiates, there will not be any more edges to A with respect to this thread.

---

[1] http://www.douban.com/group/fly_vs_free/.
[2] http://www.douban.com/group/151898/.
[3] http://www.douban.com/group/16530/.
[4] http://www.douban.com/group/zibi/.
[5] http://www.douban.com/group/worrying/.
[6] http://www.douban.com/group/Scientists/.

3   Empirical Results

3.1   Network Properties

In this section, the largest network from the starting date of OHCs until the crawling date is constructed. The results are shown in Table 1. N denotes the number of nodes in the network, E is the number of edges removing all the self-loops. $Comp$ stands for the number of weakly connected components, N' is the number of nodes in the largest connected component, D is the density, $Diam$ is the diameter, which is the largest path length of all paired nodes that can be connected. L is the average shortest path length. C is the clustering coefficient, and it measures the probability that any two neighbours of a certain node are also connected. R is the reciprocity ratio, and it is the percentage of paired nodes with mutual connections. e is the power-law exponent if the degree distribution has a power-law feature. max denotes the maximum in-degree and out-degree. Finally, $Assor$ represents the degree assortativity, which measures to what degree the nodes with larger degree tend to connect to those of smaller degree (negative), or to those of larger degree (positive). Some of these properties will be extended into dynamic ones in subsequent sections of network evolution. Figure 1 presents the structure of the social network formed by the user interactions in MDD, where the nodes are users and edges denote their communications. The size of the node stands for the intensity of user connections.

As MDD is founded later than Depression, there are only 5,050 nodes in the MDD network, which accounts for half of nodes in the latter. However, the density is almost twice higher than *Depression*, which indicates *MDD* users may

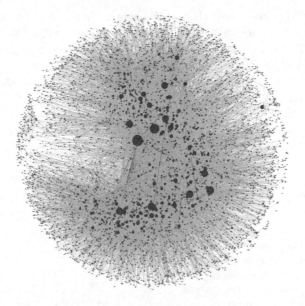

Fig. 1. The communication network in MDD community

Table 1. Comparison of network properties, where Myspace is from [10] and MedHelp from [11]

Propertiy	Depression	MDD	Myspace	MedHelp	YLD	AUT	AND	Scientist
N	11,659	5,050	36,459	30,915	3,267	2,318	774	1,691
E	100,884	36,657	80,675	113, 273	8,012	5,954	2,133	4,421
$Comp$	276	162	1	2	157	70	68	70
N'	11,369	4,881	36,459	30,870	3,034	2,240	689	1,611
D (E-5)	74.2	143.8	6.07	23.7	75.1	110.9	365.5	154.7
$Diam$	13	10	11	-	20	14	14	13
L	4.30	4.11	5.14	3.81	7.16	5.58	5.51	5.23
C (E-2)	4.26	4.47	0.031	3.1	2.11	2.01	7.70	2.95
R (E-2)	33.1	34.0	1.45	-	4.30	3.531	22.2	4.84
$e(in/out)$	1.99/2.10	2.13/2.20	2.65/2.0	2.12	2.18/3.35	2.06/3.2	2.9/3.2	2.17/2.83
max	2,391/1,553	451/942	558/6,077	-	411/82	374/84	64/51	189/198
$Assor$	0.34	0.029	−0.032	−0.075	−0.15	−0.10	−0.11	−0.002

have much closer interactions. This observation can also be verified by the last three networks, *AUT*, *AND*, and *Scientist*. But the densities of the other two OHCs, Depression and YLD, are quite similar.

Even with different length of existence period, the reciprocities in MDD and Depression are almost at the same level. Both are extremely high, and about thirty times larger than Myspace and seven or eight times than other networks except AND. The much higher reciprocity implies that users in these communities tend to be mutually connected so as to form a sticky network structure. To eliminate the effect of the network density, another normalized reciprocal metric is defined in [17] as $(R-D)/(1-D)$. Because D is three orders of magnitude lower than R, the results of both reciprocity metrics are consistent. The stickiness in these communities also applies even when users have sparse connections.

As for assortativity, it should be noted that *Depression* presents a very strong assortative property, which means the tendency is very prominent that nodes of higher degrees connect to the nodes also of larger degrees.

3.2   Messaging Frequency and User Participation

In this section, we will first show the peer-to-peer messaging along with the overall growth of OHCs and then analyze the detailed behaviours in terms of the individual user participation in the community and their averaged messaging.

Along the overall growth of OHCs, the number of daily messages is presented in Fig. 2. As there are fewer users in *MDD*, its daily messages are less than *Depression* and the maximum number is around 150 and 350 respectively. But both communities are growing with the steadily increasing tendencies and several periodical peak days. As the daily-generated messages are too much detailed, we aggregate the daily into monthly scale and the overall trends are shown in Fig. 3. Note that in this figure, all the OHCs and the other *Scientist* community mentioned in the previous section are included. To stand out the trends and

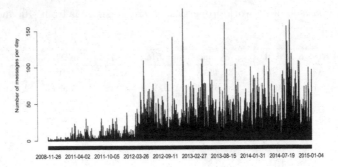

(a) MDD

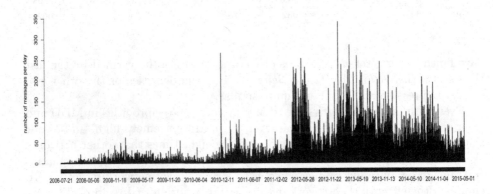

(b) Depression

Fig. 2. The number of daily messages in total (a) 2,234 days in MDD and (b) 3,217 days in Depression

make descriptions clear, we layer the monthly messages into **Level I** (below 1,000), **Level II** (1,000 to 2,000) and **Level III** (2,000 to 4,000) denoted by the two horizontal lines in Fig. 3.

In terms of monthly messages, *MDD* and *Depression* show concordant increasing patterns, but the increasing rates are different. MDD raises up to **Level II** in around the 40th month, whereas Depression achieves the same level 12 months later. Starting from the 70th month, Depression suddenly explodes and steps into **Level III**. As similar patterns are observed between these two communities, it can be predicted that the messages in MDD will also break up to 4,000 or even a higher limit in some subsequent months. Comparatively, the other four communities, *YLD*, *AUT*, *AND* and *Scientist*, are always at **Level I** along the whole procedures of development.

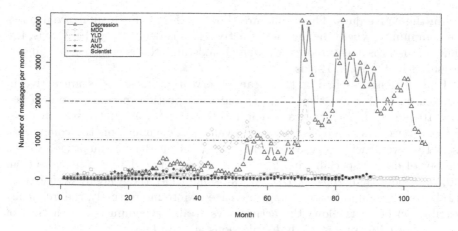

Fig. 3. The number of monthly messages

For individual users, we define two closely related metrics, *active days*, the number of days that a user visits the community, and *averaged messaging*, that is, the average quantity of messages users post during the same active days. On the one hand, these two metrics evaluate the attractiveness of the community to the user. On the other hand, they also show the dependency of the user on the OHCs and the degree to which the user would like to provide or ask for social support from the community.

All the six communities mentioned above are included. We calculate the count of users with specific active days, and the average messages posted by the users

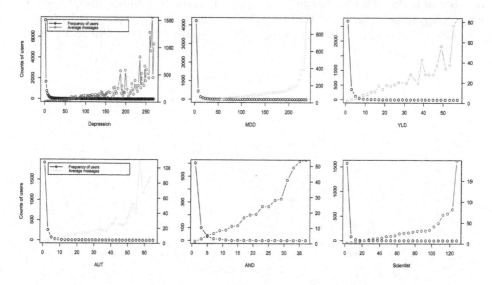

Fig. 4. The count of users and averaged messaging during the active days

within the active days. The results are shown in Fig. 4. Each subfigure denotes one community, where the number of active days is denoted by the *X*-axis, the count of users is measured by the *left Y*-axis and the averaged messaging is measured by the *right Y*-axis.

From the figures in Fig. 4, we can observe that most users are active in the community for less than 10 days, and their posting messages are also less than 10 pieces. It may indicate that most users are only interested in some of the discussions in OHCs, but not loyal and dependent on the community itself. However, there are also some users who consult the community for a large number of days. Especially, in *Depression*, users' active days can be more than 250, and more than 200 in *MDD*. At the same time, these highly active users also have a large number of average messages. More interestingly, the frequency distribution of users along the active days is almost symmetric with that of average posted messages. Both distributions are non-linear.

3.3   Network Evolution

In this section, we build dynamic networks and observe the growth patterns of different OHCs. We sample the communities every month and adopt the 'memorising past' strategy as compared to the 'missing past' in [16]. That is, as long as a user leave some message during the period from the starting date of the community to the sampled date, it is included in the network. Based on this strategy, there are in total 106 networks sampled in *Depression*, 74 in *MDD*, 103 in *YLD*, 107 in *AUT*, 90 in *AND* and 82 in *Scientist*. For the evolutionary network properties, we explore the number of nodes and the number of edges.

In [16,18], it is shown that the number of edges grows super linearly with the number of nodes. This trend can be extended into piecewise linear in OHCs, see Fig. 5. Apparently, there are three successively increasing growth phases (separated by the two vertical lines) in terms of the number of nodes. **Phase I** ranges

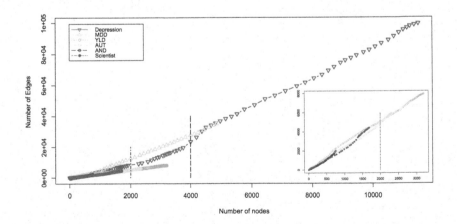

Fig. 5. The number of edges change with the number of nodes

from 0 to 2,000, **Phase II** from 2,000 to 4,000 and **Phase III** from 4,000 to more than 10,000. In Phase I, the growth rates are slower for all communities, increase in Phase II, and then they become extremely higher in Phase III, which means the community is expanding much faster than before. According to this division, we can identify that *AND* (the blue line) and *Scientist* (the purple line) are experiencing **Phase I**, *AUT* and *YLD* are stepping into **Phase II**. However, *MDD* and *Depression* have already been in **Phase III**.

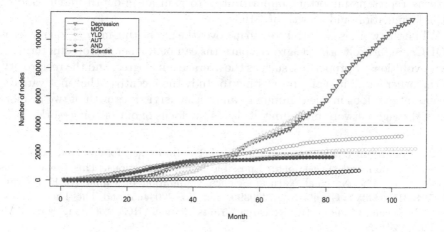

Fig. 6. The number of nodes change with time

The increase of nodes along time is shown in Fig. 6. Generally, we can see that *Depression* and *MDD* have concordant growth patterns. This observation is also consistent with the increasing patterns of monthly messages. Therefore, it can be concluded that *Depression* and *MDD* are highly coordinated although the reason is not clear at this moment. Besides, all communities except AND, start to approach Phase II in around 50th month. But thereafter users in MDD and Depression explode quickly for the next 20 months and step into Phase III whereas other communities still grow slowly. Starting from the 80th month, Depression community expands even more quickly.

The graph densification and the increasing trend of nodes can explain some peaks in monthly messages in Fig. 3. As for MDD, two peaks are achieved in around the 40th and 70th month, and these two time slots are exactly when the increasing rate of MDD users turns to rise up. That is, the quickly addition of users causes the sharp addition of messages. This pattern can also be validated in Depression, where both the monthly messages peak and the increasing rate of users rises in around 70th and 80th month. However, the first peak is mainly caused by the addition of nodes as the increase rate of edges with nodes is slow during that period whereas the second peak is caused by both the addition of nodes and the addition of edges as both the increase rate of nodes and the increase rate of edges are high.

4   Conclusion

This paper analyzed the structure and dynamics of the social networks formed by the user interactions in depression related OHCs. We have observed the unique sticky community structure of depression related OHCs as compared to other OHCs and social networks. The findings shed light on the understanding of several hidden factors that lead to the success and sustainability of OHCs in terms of user participation and mutual interaction. In particular, the unique evolution patterns represent important opportunities to gain an in-depth understanding of the formulation and growth of OHCs.

While this work is an initial step to uncover the interesting interaction patterns in OHCs, in future work, the growth patterns can be further explored in terms of other evolutionary properties, such as the average out-degree, and the reciprocity. On the other hand, it is also interesting to study the incentives that motivate the mutual interactions in one community and the synergistic growth of two or more OHCs through network modelling, which is the focus of our ongoing work.

Acknowledgments. We would like to thank Dr. Ron Chen for his kind advices of dataset selection and suggestions of possible research questions. This research was supported by The National Natural Science Foundation of China (NSFC) Grant No. 71402157, CityU Grants No. 7200399. and No. 7004465, and The Theme-Based Research Scheme Grant of the Research Grants Council (RGC) of Hong Kong SAR No. T32-102/14N.

References

1. Neal, L., Oakley, K., Lindgaard, G., Kaufman, D., Leimeister, J.M., Selker, T.: Online health communities. In: CHI 2007 Extended Abstracts on Human Factors in Computing Systems, pp. 2129–2132. ACM, April 2007
2. Bonniface, L., Green, L.: Finding a new kind of knowledge on the HeartNET website. Health Inf. Libr. J. **24**(s1), 67–76 (2007)
3. Jadad, A.R., Enkin, M.W., Glouberman, S., Groff, P., Stern, A.: Are virtual communities good for our health?: they seem to be good at managing chaotic information—and may have other virtues too. BMJ Br. Med. J. **332**(7547), 925 (2006)
4. Eysenbach, G., Powell, J., Englesakis, M., Rizo, C., Stern, A.: Health related virtual communities and electronic support groups: systematic review of the effects of online peer to peer interactions. BMJ Br. Med. J. **328**(7449), 1166 (2004)
5. Hybye, M.T., Dalton, S.O., Deltour, I., Bidstrup, P.E., Frederiksen, K., Johansen, C.: Effect of internet peer-support groups on psychosocial adjustment to cancer: a randomised study. Br. J. Cancer **102**(9), 1348–1354 (2010)
6. Gill, P.S., Whisnant, B.: A qualitative assessment of an online support community for ovarian cancer patients. Patient Relat. Outcome Measures **3**, 51 (2012)
7. Griffiths, K.M., Calear, A.L., Banfield, M.: Systematic review on internet support groups (ISGs) and depression (1): do ISGs reduce depressive symptoms? J. Med. Internet Res. **11**(3), e40 (2009)
8. Phan, T.Q., Airoldi, E.M.: A natural experiment of social network formation and dynamics. Proc. Nat. Acad.Sci. **112**(21), 6595–6600 (2015)

9. Wagner, C., Rowe, M., Strohmaier, M., Alani, H.: Ignorance isn't bliss: an empirical analysis of attention patterns in online communities. In: 2012 International Conference on Privacy, Security, Risk and Trust (PASSAT) and 2012 International Confernece on Social Computing (SocialCom), pp. 101–110. IEEE, September 2012

10. Suvakov, M., Mitrovic, M., Gligorijevic, V., Tadic, B.: How the online social networks are used: dialogues-based structure of MySpace. J. Roy. Soc. Interface. 10(79), 20120819 (2013)

11. Vydiswaran, V.V., Liu, Y., Mei, Q., Zheng, K., Hanauer, D.: User-created groups in health forums: what makes them special. In: Proceedings of the Conference Weblogs and Social Media (ICWSM). Association Advancement Artificial Intelligence, pp. 515–524, May 2014

12. Agrawal, R., Rajagopalan, S., Srikant, R., Xu, Y.: Mining newsgroups using networks arising from social behavior. In: Proceedings of the 12th International Conference on World Wide Web, pp. 529–535. ACM, May 2003

13. Alani, H., Rowe, M., Angeletou, S.: Modelling and analysis of user behaviour in online communities. In: Aroyo, L., Welty, C., Alani, H., Taylor, J., Bernstein, A., Kagal, L., Noy, N., Blomqvist, E. (eds.) ISWC 2011, Part I. LNCS, vol. 7031, pp. 35–50. Springer, Heidelberg (2011)

14. Morrison, D., McLoughlin, I., Hogan, A., Hayes, C.: Evolutionary clustering and analysis of user behaviour in online forums. In: ICWSM, May 2012

15. Chuang, K.Y., Yang, C.C.: Interaction patterns of nurturant support exchanged in online health social networking. J. Med. Internet Res. 14(3), e54 (2012)

16. Leskovec, J., Kleinberg, J., Faloutsos, C.: Graph evolution: densification and shrinking diameters. ACM Trans. Knowl. Discov. Data 1(1), 2 (2007)

17. Garlaschelli, D., Loffredo, M.I.: Patterns of link reciprocity in directed networks. Phys. Rev. Lett. 93(26), 268701 (2004)

18. Leskovec, J., Chakrabarti, D., Kleinberg, J., Faloutsos, C., Ghahramani, Z.: Kronecker graphs: an approach to modeling networks. J. Mach. Learn. Res. 11, 985–1042 (2010)

Impact of Flavor on Electronic Cigarette Marketing in Social Media

Yunji Liang[1,2(✉)], Xiaolong Zheng[3], Daniel Dajun Zeng[2,3], and Xingshe Zhou[1]

[1] School of Computer Science, Northwestern Polytechnical University, Xi'an, China
[2] Department of Management Information Systems, University of Arizona, Tucson, AZ, USA
yunjiliang@email.arizona.edu
[3] State Key Laboratory of Management and Control for Complex Systems,
Institute of Automation, Chinese Academy of Sciences, Beijing, China

Abstract. The electronic cigarette (e-cigarette) marketing is unregulated on social media currently. Flavor is one of the potent marketing strategies for e-cigarette manufactures and vendors. In this paper, we investigate the flavor-related e-cigarette marketing and online users' response to flavor-related e-cigarette marketing in Facebook. We find that the fruit flavor is most frequently promoted on social media e-cigarette marketing with a share of 33.19 %, followed by nut (17.72 %), candy & sweet (9.28 %), alcohol (7.43 %) and menthol (6.75 %). With regard to the users' response to e-cigarette marketing, 85 % of comments on flavor-related content (FC) happened within 84 h, while it is 243 h for 85 % comments on content unrelated with flavor (named as miscellaneous content, MC). Furthermore, the ratio of positive content to negative content in FC (R_{FC}) is 1.4857; while R_{MC} is 0.8801. According to this work, we conclude that flavor plays an important role for online e-cigarette marketing with the boosting of user interaction and positive emotion.

Keywords: Electronic cigarette · Flavor · Facebook · Electronic liquid

1 Introduction

Electronic cigarettes - battery-powered devices that convert liquid nicotine into a vapor inhaled by the smoker, or "vaper" - were invented in China and came to the U.S. in 2007. Currently, there are an estimated 20 million American vapers. As the most important feature of e-cigarettes, the flavor contained in the liquid solution (also known as e-liquid or e-juice) is promoted widely. Meanwhile, e-cigarette manufacturers provide consumers with not only classic tobacco and menthol flavors but also a variety of youth appealing flavors including fruit, dessert, spice, candy, beverage, and bakery. A recent online survey finds that fruit flavors are the most popular with a 31 % market share, followed by tobacco flavors (22 %) and dessert flavors (19 %) [1]. It is obvious that flavors of e-liquids become one of the potent marketing strategies for e-cigarettes.

Due to the similar impact that flavors have on tobacco, it is concerned that the variety of e-cigarette flavors might attract users, especially youths to start using e-cigarettes. Current e-cigarette use among high school students increased from 4.5 percent in 2013

© Springer International Publishing Switzerland 2016
X. Zheng et al. (Eds.): ICSH 2015, LNCS 9545, pp. 278–283, 2016.
DOI: 10.1007/978-3-319-29175-8_26

to 13.4 percent in 2014, rising from approximately 660,000 to 2 million students [2]. There are a large variety of e-cigarette flavors available in the market. On average, each e-cigarette consumer uses three flavors [3]. However, there is little research about the impact of flavors for online users. In this paper, we investigate users' responses to flavor-related content in online e-cigarette marketing to reveal the impact of flavor on online users.

The remainder of this paper is organized as follows. The data collection is presented in Sect. 2. In Sect. 3, we present how to extract flavor-related content from user-generated content. We elaborate our preliminary findings including flavor distribution in online e-liquid marketing and users' response to e-liquid marketing in Sect. 4. Section 5 concludes this paper.

2   Collection of E-cigarette Related Content on Social Media

To collect e-liquid flavor content, we reuse the data collection program implemented in our previous work [4, 5]. This data collection program can retrieve user-generated content from Facebook fan pages. Facebook fan page is a public profile that enables users to share their business and products with Facebook users. The data collection on Facebook consists of two steps: offline data preparation and online data collection.

Table 1. E-cigarette related keywords for Facebook searches

Keywords	electronic cigarette, disposable cigarette, e-cig, e-cigarette, rechargeable cigarette, rechargeable kits, flavor cartridge, vaporizer, vaporized, vapor, vaping, mod, apv, refill cartridges, vaping pen, refills, cigalikes, mechs, vape pen, electronic pipe, cartomizer, clearomizer, atomizer, hookah, electronic hookah, shisha, electronic shisha, e-hookah, e-shisha, electronic cigar, e-cigar, electronic juice, electronic liquid, e-juice, e-liquid, electronic joint, e-joint, electronic spliff, e-spliff, vape, vaping, istick, coil tank, coil, rda

For the offline data preparation, we need to find out e-cigarette related fan pages using the keywords. We have defined a set of e-cigarette related keywords according to keyword lists[1]. The partial keywords are shown in Table 1. Based on the keyword searching, we find a large number of fan pages related with the given keywords. However, due to the ambiguity of keywords, some retrieved fan pages are unrelated with e-cigarette. To rule out the fan pages unrelated with e-cigarette, we manually classify the retrieved fan pages into 2 types (0: unrelated with e-cigarette; 1: related with e-cigarette) by two coders according to the profiles of fan pages. A third coder coded the fan pages for which there was no agreement between the first two coders. If the third coder disagreed with each of the first two coders, that fan pages are excluded. Meanwhile, the coders also checked whether the fan pages are written in English or not. In this paper, we only focus on the e-cigarette related fan pages written in English.

---

[1] http://www.bestclearomizer.com/ultimate-vaping-glossary/.

In the online data collection, we collect the content (including posts and comment) and interaction records in e-cigarette related fan pages using the Facebook APIs. Through the APIs, we can collect the public historical data on the fan pages. The data collection lasted from to March 8 2015 to April 12 2015. Totally, we got 4778 e-cigarette related fan pages with 472,435 posts and 5,606,020 comments.

3   Identify Online E-cigarette Marketing from Social Media

Online marketing refers to use a set of powerful tools and methodologies to promote products and services through the internet. Generally, the information is embedded in the user-generated content and disseminated through the user activities (such as like, comment, and sharing) to increase the visibility of the products. To identify the content related with online e-cigarette marketing, we assume the content should cover three topics: e-cigarette topics, flavor topics, and business activities. The workflow to identify the online e-cigarette marketing is presented in Fig. 1.

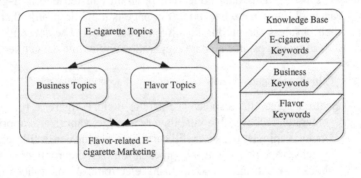

Fig. 1. Workflow to identify the flavor related e-cigarette marketing

First, we use the e-cigarette keywords to decide whether the textual inputs (posts) are related with e-cigarette. The e-cigarette keywords are partially presented in Table 1. Second, we check whether the content is related with business activities or flavor based on the outputs of first step respectively. To find business-related content, we integrate several keyword lists related with business activities[2, 3]. While for the flavor keywords, we assemble the flavor lists from different flavor manufacturers[4] to maximize the coverage of flavor-related keywords. Finally, we calculate the overlapping of the outputs of second step. The overlapping is the content which not only promotes e-cigarette products, but also is related with flavor. In total, we get 12,391 posts with 85,989 comments. This is the dataset for the following analysis.

---

[2] http://nichehacks.com/buyer-keywords-list/.

[3] http://miscellanea.hubpages.com/hub/How-to-Sell-your-Products-with-Buying-Keywords.

[4] http://www.missionflavors.com/flavorlist.aspx.

4   Users' Response to Online E-cigarette Marketing

4.1   Distribution of E-cigarette Flavor in Social Media

Due to the variety of e-cigarette flavors, we try to group similar flavors into one flavor category. However, the flavor category varies by e-juice manufacturers and retailers. Even worse, the product names themselves often give no guidance, can be misleading, or can even be counterintuitive. To address this question, we adopt the vapor digest flavor categorizing system (VDFCS)[5] to place individual flavors from many different manufacturers into the appropriate flavor category. The creation of VDFCS is based on the 'primary flavor' of an e-liquid. In VDFCS, 12 flavor categories including *alcohol*, *beverage, candy & sweets, coffee & tea, fruit and tobacco* are defined. In this paper, we use the 11 flavor categories except *miscellaneous*.

To reveal the flavor-related content, we need to create the mapping from flavor-related keywords to 11 flavor categories. In the mapping step, we want to setup matches between keywords and flavor categories. To ensure the reasonability of mapping, two coders manually create the mapping respectively. When there is no agreement between the two coders, they will discuss together to decide the reasonable mapping.

As shown in Fig. 2, the fruity e-liquid is most frequently promoted on social media with a share of 33.19 %, followed by nut (17.72 %), candy & sweet (9.28 %), alcohol (7.43 %) and menthol (6.75 %). This means that fruity e-liquid is frequently promoted by the e-liquid vendors and manufacturers in social media. According to the findings in [1], fruity e-liquid is the most popular with a 31 % market share. Our result explains why the fruity e-liquid has the largest market share. The nut e-liquid (17.72 %) is the second most frequently promoted e-liquid in social media. The flavors in nut e-liquids contain almond, pecan, cashew, pistachio, etc.

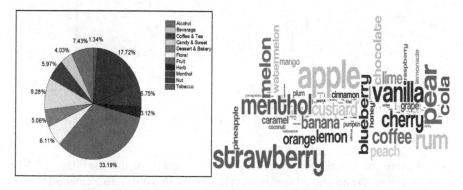

Fig. 2.   The distribution of flavor in online e-cigarette marketing

Certain e-liquids even contain alcohol such as vodka, margarita, and rum. Although the amount of alcohol used in the e-liquids is very small, the flammable alcohol could ignite the vapor resulting in a fire. Additionally, poisoning can easily occur when vaping

---

[5]   http://www.vaporlives.com/eliquid-flavor-categories/.

alcohol as the body has no way to reject the alcohol when inhaled. Despite of these consequences, the alcohol flavored e-liquids are still widely promoted on social media with a share of 7.43 %.

4.2   Users' Response to Online E-liquid Marketing

To measure the impact of advertised flavor in e-liquid marketing in social media, we compare the users' response including comment patterns and emotional patterns in flavor-related content (FC) and miscellaneous content (MC). Here, MC refers to the content unrelated with e-liquid flavor.

To reveal the impacts of online e-liquid marketing to online user activities, we compare the temporal patterns of comments on FC and MC. As shown in Fig. 3a, the response time of comments has a heavy tail. The heavy-tailed distribution of response time means that most comments happened instantly after the posts is related. For FC, 77.02 % of comments happened within 24 h after the releasing of posts; which it is 74.04 % for MC. On the other hand, the time range of response time for FC is shorter, which means the user interaction happened in a shorter time period. The cumulative distribution function (CDF) of response time is presented in Fig. 3b. According to Fig. 3b, 85 % of comments on FC happened within 84 h, while it is 243 h for 85 % comments in MC. It demonstrates the flavor-related content in online e-liquid marketing can attract more user interaction within a shorter time period and the flavor-related content may boost the user activities in social media.

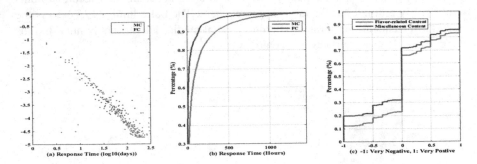

Fig. 3.   The distributions of response time in FC and MC

To measure the emotional patterns in the comments, we use the Stanford NLP package to extract the emotional words and classify those words into 5 categories: very negative, negative, neutral, positive, and very positive. In addition, the emoticons in the comments are classified into the 5 categories as well, according to the definitions of emoticons. As shown in Fig. 3c, for the flavor-related content, 12.29 % is very negative; while it is 20.00 % for MC. In terms of very positive emotion, it is 17.05 % for FC vs. 14.24 % for MC. In addition, we compare the ratios of positive content and negative content (R) in FC and MC. According to R, we find that the ratio for FC (R_{FC}) is 1.4857, while R_{MC} is 0.8801. This demonstrates that the comments for flavor-related content in e-cigarette marketing are more positive, and flavor-related cigarette marketing have positive effects for users' emotion.

5 Conclusions

In this paper, we focus on the impact of flavor for online users and investigate the users' response to flavor-related e-cigarette marketing in social media. We find the fruit flavor is most frequently promoted on social media with a share of 33.19 %, followed by nut (17.72 %), candy & sweet (9.28 %), alcohol (7.43 %) and menthol (6.75 %). With regard to the users' response, flavor-related content in online e-cigarette marketing can attract more user interaction within a shorter time period and the flavor-related content may boost the user activities in social media. Meanwhile, users' response to flavor-related content in online e-cigarette marketing is more positive.

Acknowledgements. This work was supported by the National Natural Science Foundation of China (Grant No. 71472175, 71103180), the National Institutes of Health (NIH) of USA (Grant No.1R01DA037378-02), and the Ministry of Health (Grant No. 2013ZX10004218).

References

1. Mclaren, N.: Big survey 2014: initial findings e-liquid. http://vaping.com/data/big-survey-2014-initial-findings-eliquid. Accessed on 2015
2. CDC. E-cigarette use triples among middle and high school students in just one year. http://www.cdc.gov/media/releases/2015/p0416-e-cigarette-use.html. Accessed on 2015
3. Farsalinos, K.E., Romagna, G., Tsiapras, D., et al.: Impact of flavour variability on electronic cigarette use experience: an internet survey. Int. J. Env. Res. Public Health **10**, 7272–7282 (2013)
4. Liang, Y., Zheng, X., Zeng, D., et al.: Characterizing social interaction in tobacco-oriented social networks: an empirical analysis. Sci. Rep. **5**, 10060 (2015)
5. Liang, Y., Zhou, X., Zeng, D., et al. An integrated approach of sensing tobacco-oriented activities in online participatory media. IEEE Syst. J. (2014)

Health-Related Spammer Detection on Chinese Social Media

Xinhuan Chen[1(✉)], Yong Zhang[1], Jennifer Xu[2], Chunxiao Xing[1], and Hsinchun Chen[1,3]

[1] Department of Computer Science and Technology,
Research Institute of Information Technology, Tsinghua University, Beijing, China
xh-chen13@mails.tsinghua.edu.cn
[2] Department of Computer Information Systems, Bentley University, Waltham, USA
jxu@bentley.edu
[3] MIS Department, University of Arizona, Tucson, USA
hchen@eller.arizona.edu

Abstract. Weibo (Chinese microblog) has become a popular social media platform for users to share health-related information. However, illegitimate users or spammers often generate and spread false or misleading health information so as to advertise and attract more attention. To address this issue, we propose a health-related spammer detection approach on Chinese social media. Our approach is a deep belief network (DBN) based model incorporating a comprehensive feature set, including burstiness-based features, profile-based features, and content-based features, to identify spammers who spread misleading health-related information. Especially, we create a medical and health domain lexicon to better extract content-based features. The experimental results show the approach achieves an F1 score of 86 % in detecting spammer and significantly outperforms the benchmark methods using baseline features.

Keywords: Spammer detection · Health · Chinese · Weibo · Deep belief network

1 Introduction

In recent years, microblogs (e.g., Twitter and Weibo) have become a popular social media platform, where people post short messages to "tweet" about a wide variety of topics ranging from politics, sports, music, culture, health, to everyday life or even rumors. It is reported that the monthly number of active users of Weibo, the microblogging platforms in China, has reached 167 million as of September 30, 2014.

Health is an important topic closely related to people's lives. Because it is convenient and easy to generate tweets, many people turn to Weibo to discuss medical and health-related topics. Meanwhile, many medical and healthcare professionals use Weibo as a communication channel to share with the public health-related information and educational materials and answer medical questions posted by concerned users.

However, spammers could also take advantage of the microblogging services to generate and post a large number of false messages for advertisement purposes. Some of the spammers are virtual accounts controlled by malicious computer programs; others may be so-called Internet Water Army [2], who are a group of users hired and paid by

© Springer International Publishing Switzerland 2016
X. Zheng et al. (Eds.): ICSH 2015, LNCS 9545, pp. 284–295, 2016.
DOI: 10.1007/978-3-319-29175-8_27

certain individuals or organizations to spread misleading information. Spammers may behave like ordinary users. As a result, detecting spammers and separating them from real, non-spammer accounts are difficult.

In the past a few years, some research has been done for spammer detection. Features that are based on text content of messages [1, 9, 17] or user profiles [15] have been used to identify spammers. Some researchers use the features of burstiness of product reviews to detect spammers in e-commerce applications [3, 16]. Social media also have the characteristics of burstiness. Tweets appearing in a sudden may mean that spammers are working together to generate a large number of tweets to attract the attention of regular users. However, burstiness has rarely been considered in applications that detect spammers on social media.

Spammer detection on English social media, such as Twitter, has been studied extensively [1, 17]. However, little research has been done to detect spammers posting health-related topics in Chinese on Weibo. In this paper, we propose a health-related spammer detection approach on Chinese social media. The contribution is three-fold. First, to the best of our knowledge, our study is the first to address the problem of spammer detection on Chinese microblogs for the health domain. Second, we propose to employ the Deep Belief Network (DBN) [7], a type of deep learning model, together with the a comprehensive set of features including burstiness-based features, user's profile-based features, and tweets' text content-based features, to enhance the detection performance. Third, unlike many previous English spammer detection studies that can leverage existing medical knowledge bases like the UMLS (Unified Medical Language System), our research provides a medical lexicon that we have collected and constructed because there has been no existing, standard Chinese medical lexicon available. Our experiments using real data collected on Weibo show that our health-related spammer detection approach significantly outperforms the benchmark methods using baseline features.

The remainder of the paper is organized as follows. We present a review of literature on spammer detection in Sect. 2, and then describe our research design in Sect. 3. Next, we report on our experiments and discuss the results. We conclude the paper in Sect. 5.

2 Related Work

Heydari et al. [6] conducted a comprehensive survey and reviewed methods for detecting spam product reviews, individual spammers, and group spammers. We review some related literature about spammer detection technologies, which can be categorized into two types: meta-data based and content-based.

Meta-Data Based Spammer Detection. A microblog user account usually has associated meta-data (e.g., user's identity, age, the number of friends, the timestamps of tweets, and the users' computer IP addresses, etc.). Many researchers [3, 5, 15, 16, 18] analyzed these data to find users with malicious behaviors. For example, a user may be a spammer if a user has a large number of followers or fans but few subscriptions, which are other accounts that the user follows [18]. Because in order to spread spamming contents to as many people as possible, spammers often strive to attract many followers but do not tend to follow others.

Content-Based Spammer Detection. Text content generated by users is very important for understanding the meaning of tweets and detecting spammers. Linguistic features, such as n-grams [8], topic distribution [10] and stylistic [11], can be extracted from text content to identify malicious behaviors. Lin et al. [9] used content similarity for detecting spams in product reviews. However, content-based features alone are not enough to accurately detect all types of fake messages. A professional and experienced spammer may be able to fabricate contents so deliberately that even a real person cannot distinguish them from truthful reviews or tweets. Liu et al. [10] proposed a hybrid model for spammer detection on Weibo by combining user behaviorial features, social attributes, and text content characteristics.

In the health domain, there has been little research on spammer detection. Only a few studies can be found to examine the information trustworthiness of medical claims or statements. Vydiswaran et al. [14] studied the trustworthiness of medical claims based on community based knowledge and ranked the claims. Mukherjee et al. [11] analyzed the credibility of user-provided medical statements and extracted the side-effects of medical drugs as supplement of medical knowledge. Gao et al. [4] also explored Chinese user's perceived credibility of health and safety information on Weibo using questionnaires. In this research, we propose a DBN-based model combining three types of features for Chinese spammer detection on Weibo in the health domain. The following section describes in detail our research design.

3   Research Design

In this section, we introduce our research design for health-related spammer detection. We introduce two properties of spammer tweets, based on which we propose three types of features: time burstiness, user's profile attributes, and tweets' text content. The three types of features are used in the DBN-based model to distinguish spammers from regular Weibo users.

3.1   Properties of Spammer Accounts

The temporal patterns of normal users' tweeting activities, i.e., the number of tweets generated by regular users in any period time, are usually random with very little burstiness. Here, the burstiness refers to the situation where the number of tweets generated by users in a period of time increases sharply. Prior research has shown that the burstiness of tweets can be caused either by a sudden public event (e.g. a massive earthquake), about which people tweet extensively during a short period of time, or by spammer attacks which result in a sharp increase in the number of fake or misleading tweets [3]. Based on this observation, we introduce the first property of spammer accounts:

Property 1. *Spammers are likely to generate tweets in the period of the beginning (valley) of a burst to the middle (peak) of a burst.*

Three basic statistics are readily available in each Weibo account: the number of *tweets*, the number of *followers* (or *fans*), and the number of *subscriptions* (other users whom the current user follows). Regular users tend to maintain mutual relationships with other users. Thus, a user's number of followers and number of subscriptions usually are comparable. Spammers, especially Internet Water Army, often have a large number of followers but few subscriptions [18]. Thus, we derive the second property of spammer accounts based on the social attributes:

Property 2. *Spammers are likely to have a large number of followers and few subscriptions.*

3.2 Features

In this research, we select three types of features, namely time burstiness, user's profile attributes, and tweets' text content, to represent each user.

Burstiness. We use KDE (Kernel Density Estimation) [12] for burstiness detection. KDE can estimate the probability density function of a random variable and will be used to generate a smooth and continuous curve for our Weibo dataset. It is a commonly-used [3] technique for burstiness detection.

Let $X = \{x_1, x_2, \ldots, x_n\}$ be a sample with n values drawn from an unknown density function $f(x)$ of a random variable x. We need to estimate the shape of the function $f(x)$, whose estimated kernel density is

$$\hat{f}_h(x) = \frac{1}{nh} \sum_{i=1}^{n} K(\frac{x - x_i}{h}),$$ (1)

where K is the kernel function that integrates to one and has mean zero; h is the smoothing parameter called the bandwidth. h can be set experimentally to make the curve of the function $f(x)$ not too jagged or too smooth.

On Weibo, a user generates some health-related tweets, each of which has a time-stamp. As a result, the tweets of users in a dataset have a set of timestamps $\{t_1, t_2, \ldots, t_m\}$ corresponding to m tweets in the temporal order. The span of all tweets is $span = t_m - t_1$. Subtracting t_1 from the timestamps we get $T = \{t_1 - t_1, t_2 - t_1, \ldots, t_m - t_1\}$.

We use the Gaussian kernel function for K:

$$K(x) = \frac{1}{\sqrt{2\pi}} e^{-\frac{x^2}{2}},$$ (2)

and set $X = T$ as the sample over the range $[0, span]$. As a result, formula (1) becomes

$$\hat{f}_h(t) = \frac{1}{nh\sqrt{2\pi}} \sum_{i=1}^{m} (e^{-\frac{(t-t_i)^2}{2h^2}}).$$ (3)

By taking the derivative of the density function $\hat{f}_h(t)$ and setting it to zero, we obtain a set of time points for peaks $\{t_{p_1}, t_{p_2}, \ldots\}$ and a set of time points for valleys $\{t_{v_1}, t_{v_2}, \ldots\}$.

To detect the burstiness, we need to select burst peaks. Although all peaks represent sharp increases in the number of tweets in a period of time, they vary in magnitude. We remove those peaks whose density values are below the half of the maximum density value. The remaining peaks and corresponding valleys are considered to be *bursts*:

$$bursts = \left\{ \left[t_{v_1}, t_{p_1} \right], \left[t_{v_2}, t_{p_2} \right], \ldots \right\}, t_{v_i} < t_{p_i} \quad , i = 1, 2, \ldots \tag{4}$$

According to **Property** 1, we calculate the number of tweets generated in all *bursts* for each user as b_{u_j}. Thus burstiness-based features of two dimensions are represented as

$$B_{u_j} = \left\{ \frac{b_{u_j}}{max\left(b_u\right)}, \frac{b_{u_j}}{w_j} \right\}, \tag{5}$$

where w_j is the number of tweets of user u_j. In the experiment section, we will demonstrate the effectiveness of the burstiness feature.

User Profile Attributes. We consider three types of profile attributes for each Weibo user, namely the number of *tweets, followers,* and *subscriptions.* Based on **Property** 2, a spammer is very likely to have a large number of followers, most of whom are also spammers rather than regular users. On the other hand, spammers do not have many subscriptions and often post a large number of tweets. Thus we define a measure based on the three profile attributes:

$$profile_{u_j} = \frac{\frac{followers_{u_j}}{\max(followers)} * \frac{tweets_{u_j}}{\max(tweets)}}{\frac{subscriptions_{u_j}}{\max(subscriptions)}}. \tag{6}$$

To ensure the integrity of user's profile-based features, we consider the features of four dimensions for each user as follow:

$$A_{u_j} = \left\{ profile_{u_j}, \frac{followers_{u_j}}{\max\left(followers\right)}, \frac{tweets_{u_j}}{\max\left(tweets\right)}, \frac{subscriptions_{u_j}}{\max(subscriptions)} \right\} \tag{7}$$

Text Content. Word segmentation for health-related Chinese text is different from that for documents in other domains. Health-related text content usually contains many professional vocabulary (e.g. 迟发性低血糖 [late-onset hypoglycemia]). Without the help of a health and medical lexicon, the word segmentation will result in the loss of important information. For example, the term "迟发性低血糖" will be parsed and separated into "迟发性" (late-onset) and "低血糖" (hypoglycemia). As a result, the performance of spammer detection will be affected. Thus, a high quality health and medical lexicon is critical for parsing texts into meaningful segments of words with their original meanings preserved.

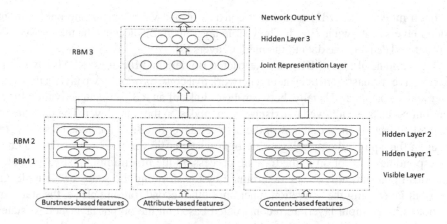

Fig. 1. The DBN-based model for combining features

We collected and synthesized a set of medical vocabulary including disease names (31,450 terms), disease diagnoses (3,475 terms), foods (26,808 terms), body organs (6,086 terms), and medicine names (38,144 terms) from a set of professional sources, including Sogou, and Xywy.

We use jcseg [19], a open source project, to perform word segmentation for text contents of tweets. Then, we apply the TFIDF method [13], which is a statistical method that finds weights of the most frequently used terms in a document, to extract text content based features from tweets. Thus, the content-based features can be represented as a feature vector of k dimensions:

$$C_{u_j} = \{tfidf_1, tfidf_2, \ldots, tfidf_k\}, \tag{8}$$

where k is the number of terms used in TFIDF and is often associated with the number of distinct words in the dataset.

The three types of features are used as input to the DBN-based classifier for spammer detection.

3.3 DBN-Based Model

The most straightforward way to use the three types of features is to simply combining them, resulting in a feature space of $2 + 4 + k$ dimensions. For example, the burstiness-based features is related to the number of tweets, which is also used for profile-based features. Simply combining the three types of features would not produce the optimal classification performance.

In order to incorporate the three types features effectively, we employ a Deep Belief Network (DBN) based model to combine the features. Figure 1 presents the DBN-based model, which consists of four modules: the burstiness-based feature training module (on the bottom left), the profile-based feature training module (on the bottom center), the content-based feature training module (on the bottom right), and the joint representation output module (on the top).

Each module is a DBN model that consists of one visible layer and one or more hidden layers as shown in Fig. 1. The visible layer of a DBN accepts the feature vectors of input and delivers the data to the hidden layers [7].

The building blocks of DBN are Restricted Boltzmann Machines (RBMs), which is a generative stochastic artificial neural network that consists of only two layers: the input layer and output layer. Usually, between-layer links of an RBM use an activation function, but no links are allowed to exist between nodes on the same layer. The parameters of an RBM include the weights w of the between-layer links and the node biases b. The nodes in the input and output layers are binary stochastic variables with values 0 or 1, corresponding to off or on in the training process. In the first training phase, the states of nodes in the output layer are determined by transforming the states of the nodes in the input layer using the activation function. In the second training phase, the states of the nodes in the input layer are reconstructed based on the output layer nodes' states generated in the first training phase. The training process can be expressed as

$$p\left(O_i|I\right) = sigmoid\left(-b_i - \sum_j I_j w_{ij}\right), \tag{9}$$

$$p\left(I_j|O\right) = sigmoid(-b_j - \sum_i O_i w_{ij}), \tag{10}$$

where O_i and I_j are the states for the i_th node in the output layer and the j_th node in the input layer, respectively. The sigmoid activation function is defined as: $sigmoid(x) = \frac{1}{(1 + e^{-x})}.$

The parameters are updated after each iteration. The weights w_{ij} are updated based on

$$\Delta w_{ij} = \varepsilon \cdot (< I_j O_i >_{first} - < I_j O_i >_{second}), \tag{11}$$

where ε is the training rate from 0 to 1; $< I_j O_i >_{first}$ is the pairwise product of the state vectors for the nodes in the first phase; and $< I_j O_i >_{second}$ is the pairwise product of the state vectors in the second phase. The biases b are updated similarly. This process stops until it reaches the predefined maximum number of iterations.

After layer-wise pre-training for a DBN in the above processes, all parameters of the DBN can be fine-tuned using the back-propagation algorithm with a supervised method. The process stops when it reaches the maximum number of iterations.

When the DBNs of the three modules on the bottom finish the training processes, a joint representation layer with the outputs of the three modules appended is regarded as a visible layer for a new DBN's input. In the joint representation output module, we add an output layer to output two probability values representing spammer or non-spammer by applying a logistic regression classifier.

All parameters obtained from the model training process are saved and used to test the performance of the model in the experiments.

4   Experiments

The experiments were indented to evaluate the performance of our spammer detection method, which incorporates a medical and health domain lexicon, a DBN-based model combining three types of features: burstiness-based, user profile-based, and content-based, and a logistic regression classifier. We aim to answering two research questions:

- Does the domain lexicon that we created help improve the performance of the spammer detection based on tweet contents?
- Does the DBN-based method using the combined feature set perform better than the benchmark methods using the baseline features?

4.1   Dataset

We used an automatic crawler to collect Sina Weibo data using health-related keywords (e.g., diabetes). The data include the profiles of Weibo users, their tweet text and associated timestamps between October 2013 and May 2015. Spammers in the dataset were labeled using the Sina Weibo Community Management service, which depends on manual efforts to identify violations of users' right and obligations.

Data about 338,533 distinct users were collected, in which 7,494 users were labeled as spammers. In order to create a balanced sample with roughly the equal number of regular users and spammers, we randomly selected 7,500 regular users from the total users and labeled them as non-spammers. Thus, the final sample consisted of 14,994 users.

To verify **Property** 1 regarding the burstiness characteristics, we depicted the probability density for regular users and spammers in Fig. 2. The horizontal axis is the time span of all tweets in days; the vertical axis is the probability density value; and the red dots represent the timestamps of tweets. The burstiness distribution in Fig. 2(b) contains a number of spikes over time. The sharp contrast between the probability density distributions of regular users and spammers demonstrates the validity of **Property** 1, and shows that burstiness is helpful for spammer detection on Weibo.

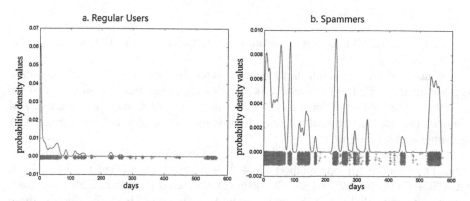

Fig. 2.   The burstiness distributions of regular users' tweets and spammers' tweets

4.2 Evaluation Metrics and the Baseline Features

We adopted *precision*, *recall*, and *F1 score* to assess the performance of the our spammer detection method. These metrics have been widely used in data mining and machine learning studies.

We conducted a comprehensive study comparing the performance of our DBN-based method using the combined feature set and a logistic regression model using the following baseline feature sets:

- A: profile-based features only;
- B: burstiness-based features only;
- C: content-based features only;
- C no-lexicon: content-based features without the medical lexicon;
- A + C: profile-based and content-based features combined;
- A + B: profile-based and burstiness-based features combined;
- B + C: burstiness-based and content-based features combined;
- A + B + C: simple combination of the three types of features.

4.3 Results

Table 1 lists the number of dimensions for the input and output layers in the DBN-based model, which includes the three training modules based on the burstiness-based features (Module 1), profile-based features (Module 2), content-based features (Module 3), and the joint representation output module (Module 4). In addition, there is only one hidden layer in the four modules. The learning rate during the pre-training and fine-training is 0.1 and 0.01, respectively. The maximum number if interactions is 500.

Table 1. The default parameters in the DBN-based model

	Module 1	Module 2	Module 3	Module 4
Input layer	2	4	333*	339
Output layer	2	4	333	2

* Determined using TFIDF.

We conducted 10-fold cross validation for each feature set. The performance is reported in Table 2.

To answer the first research question, we conducted a one-tail paired t-test to compare C no-lexicon and C. The F-score of C is significantly higher than that of C no-lexicon ($p < 0.01$) (see the first highlighted box). This indicates that when using content-based features, the medical and health domain lexicon can help improve the performance of spammer detection significantly.

A one-tail paired *t*-test was also conducted to examine the second research question. The F-score for our method (A + B + C with DBN) and the benchmark (A + B + C) is 86.41 % and 85.5 %, respectively (see the second highlighted box). The result shows that the DBN-based model for effectively incorporating the three

Table 2. Performance comparison with 10-fold cross validation

	Precision%	Recall%	F1 Score%
A	70.34	51.44	58.78
C no-lexicon	71.39	71.43	**71.41**
C	72.68	72.68	**72.68** *
B	86.80	84.31	85.57
A+C	72.53	72.48	72.78
A+B	86.66	83.14	84.86
B+C	86.06	84.04	85.04
A+B+C	86.36	84.67	**85.50**
A+B+C with DBN	87.32	85.49	**86.41 ***

*$p < 0.01$; ***$p < 0.0001$

types of features is significantly better than simplifying combining them together for spammer detection.

Table 2 also shows that the DBN-based model outperforms all other seven methods (logistic regression model with different feature sets) for health-related spammer detection. Because of the space limit, we cannot present the results of paired t-tests for comparing our method with the other seven methods.

5   Conclusion

In this study, we propose a health-related spammer detection approach on Chinese social media (Weibo). Our approach uses a DBN-based model to incorporate a comprehensive feature set, including burstiness-based features, user's profile-based features, and content-based features, to identify spammers. Especially, we created a medical and health domain lexicon to better extract content-based features. The experimental results show that our approach outperforms the benchmark methods (a logistical regression model with different baseline feature sets), and that the domain lexicon helps improve content-based spammer detection.

Acknowledgments. This work was supported by the National High-tech R&D Program of China (Grant No. SS2015AA020102), National Basic Research Program of China (Grant No. 2011CB302302), the 1000-Talent program, Tsinghua University Initiative Scientific Research Program.

References

1. Amleshwaram, A.A., Reddy, N., Yadav, S., Gu, G., Yang, C.: CATS: characterizing automation of twitter spammers. In: Fifth International Conference on Communication Systems and Networks (COMSNETS), pp. 1–10. IEEE (2013)
2. Chen, C., Wu, K., Srinivasan, V., Zhang, X.: Battling the internet water army: detection of hidden paid posters. In: Proceedings of the 2013 IEEE/ACM International Conference on Advances in Social Networks Analysis and Mining, pp. 116–120. ACM (2013)
3. Fei, G., Mukherjee, A., Liu, B., Hsu, M., Castellanos, M., Ghosh, R.: Exploiting burstiness in reviews for review spammer detection. In: ICWSM. Citeseer (2013)
4. Gao, Q., Tian, Y., Tu, M.: Exploring factors influencing chinese user's perceived credibility of health and safety information on weibo. Comput. Hum. Behav. **45**, 21–31 (2015)
5. Ge, L., Gao, J., Li, X., Zhang, A.: Multi-source deep learning for information trustworthiness estimation. In: Proceedings of the 19th ACM SIGKDD International Conference on Knowledge Discovery and Data Mining, pp. 766–774. ACM (2013)
6. Heydari, A., ali Tavakoli, M., Salim, N., Heydari, Z.: Detection of review spam: a survey. Expert Syst. Appl. **42**(7), 3634–3642 (2015)
7. Hinton, G., Osindero, S., Teh, Y.W.: A fast learning algorithm for deep belief nets. Neural Comput. **18**(7), 1527–1554 (2006)
8. Jindal, N., Liu, B.: Opinion spam and analysis. In: Proceedings of the 2008 International Conference on Web Search and Data Mining, pp. 219–230. ACM (2008)
9. Lin, Y., Zhu, T., Wang, X., Zhang, J., Zhou, A.: Towards online review spam detection. In: Proceedings of the Companion Publication of the 23rd International Conference on World Wide Web Companion, pp. 341–342. International World Wide Web Conferences Steering Committee (2014)
10. Liu, Y., Wu, B., Wang, B., Li, G.: SDHM: a hybrid model for spammer detection on Weibo. In: IEEE/ACM International Conference on Advances in Social Networks Analysis and Mining (ASONAM), 2014, pp. 942–947. IEEE (2014)
11. Mukherjee, S., Weikum, G., Danescu-Niculescu-Mizil, C.: People on drugs: credibility of user statements in health communities. In: Proceedings of the 20th ACM SIGKDD International Conference on Knowledge Discovery and Data Mining, pp. 65–74. ACM (2014)
12. Rosenblatt, M., et al.: Remarks on some nonparametric estimates of a density function. Ann. Math. Stat. **27**(3), 832–837 (1956)
13. Salton, G., McGill, M.J.: Introduction to Modern Information Retrieval. ACM Press, New York (1986)
14. Vydiswaran, V., Zhai, C., Roth, D.: Gauging the internet doctor: ranking medical claims based on community knowledge. In: Proceedings of the 2011 Workshop on Data Mining for Medicine and Healthcare, pp. 42–51. ACM (2011)
15. Wang, G., Xie, S., Liu, B., Yu, P.S.: Review graph based online store review spammer detection. In: IEEE 11th International Conference on Data Mining (ICDM), pp. 1242–1247. IEEE (2011)
16. Xie, S., Wang, G., Lin, S., Yu, P.S.: Review spam detection via temporal pattern discovery. In: Proceedings of the 18th ACM SIGKDD International Conference on Knowledge Discovery and Data Mining, pp. 823–831. ACM (2012)
17. Yang, C., Harkreader, R., Gu, G.: Empirical evaluation and new design for fighting evolving twitter spammers. IEEE Trans. Inf. Forensics Secur. **8**(8), 1280–1293 (2013)

18. Zhang, Y.: Detect spammers in online social networks (2015)
19. A open source project for Chinese word segmentation. http://code.google.com/p/jcseg/

Healthcare Intelligent Systems and Clinical Practice

DiabeticLink: An Internationally Collaborative Cyber-Enabled Patient Empowerment Platform

Grace Samtani[1(✉)], Lubaina Maimoon[2], Joshua Chuang[2], Casper Nybroe[1], Xiao Liu[1], Uffe Wiil[3], Shu-Hsing Li[4], and Hsinchun Chen[1]

[1] Artificial Intelligence Lab, University of Arizona, Tucson, AZ, USA
{gsamtani,xiaoliu}@email.arizona.edu,
casper@nybroe.com, hchen@eller.arizona.edu
[2] Caduceus Intelligence Corporation, Tucson, USA
lubainamaimoon@email.arizona.edu, joshua.chuang@gmail.com
[3] University of Southern Denmark, Odense, Denmark
ukwiil@mmmi.sd.dk
[4] Health Information Research, National Taiwan University, Taipei, Taiwan
shli@management.ntu.edu.tw

Abstract. Diabetes mellitus is a leading cause of death in both developed and emerging countries, and a chronic disease that requires a substantial amount of financially difficult and time-consuming healthcare provisions. However, patients' quality of life can be significantly improved with appropriate education and tools for self-management. In order to improve health outcomes among populations largely prone to or already suffering from diabetes, the University of Arizona Artificial Intelligence Lab developed DiabeticLink, a free diabetes self-management patient portal. This system is utilizable on mobile devices and personal computers. It incorporates novel methods for health status monitoring and trend projections, assessment and prediction of risks for major health events, recommendations of educational materials, and social functionalities. It was evaluated in 2014 prior to launching through an IRB-approved usability study. This internationally collaborative system has been launched in Taiwan and the United States (2013 and 2014, respectively), while a Danish version is currently being developed.

Keywords: Diabetes · Patient empowerment · System evaluation · Health social media · Dashboard · Self-management · Collaborative

1 Introduction

The International Diabetes Foundation reported a total of 387 million cases of diagnosed diabetics in the world in 2014 [1]. This number is expected to increase to 592 million in 2035. In the US alone, more than 9.3 % (29.1 million people) of the population is affected by diabetes and this number is expected to grow further, affecting 1 in every 3 people in the US by 2050 [2]. The total estimated costs associated with treatment and management of diabetes in the United States in 2012 was $245 billion [2].

© Springer International Publishing Switzerland 2016
X. Zheng et al. (Eds.): ICSH 2015, LNCS 9545, pp. 299–310, 2016.
DOI: 10.1007/978-3-319-29175-8_28

The current healthcare system in the United States is designed to cater to acute and symptom-driven diseases/conditions [3], and often fails at providing the appropriate level of care required for chronic diseases such as diabetes. However, diabetes is still a manageable chronic disease [4]. With a collaborative environment where patients are empowered by healthcare providers and educators to manage their condition, treatments, and diet, their quality of life can be significantly improved. Recognizing this need for patient education and empowerment, several organizations such as the American Diabetes Association, the International Federation for Diabetes, World Health Organization and others have begun to develop websites and mobile applications that can provide patients and caregivers with diabetes self-management education. Furthermore, many healthcare and fitness companies also promote daily activity tracking to monitor fitness on the go. However, each website or mobile application currently on the market lacks comprehensibility. They all cater to one aspect of disease management, but not to the other. This often leads to hopping from website-to-website in search of relevant information and patient support.

To better address user needs, we developed DiabeticLink, an all-encompassing patient empowerment portal that uses information technology to provide access to easy-to-use tools for better self-management of diabetes for diabetics as well as their family members and health care providers. DiabeticLink is a free online health portal that can help reduce the need to rely heavily on other health care systems.

2   Literature Review and Related Systems

In order to examine the current tools and technological advances made in the field of diabetes management, we searched the diabetes online portal markets and diabetes related mobile applications. There are more than 20 different types of online portals and more than 50 reliable mobile applications that cater to one or more aspects of diabetes management. We will review these products in the following categories: diabetes-related websites and social communities, diabetes health tracking and visualization tools, health data integration from medical devices and risk engines for health prediction.

2.1   Online Diabetes Websites and Social Communities

With the widespread reach of the Internet and social media, people resort to the web for most disease-related information. To cater to this need, there are several informative websites online that provide an extensive array of reputable data. Examples of such web portals include the American Diabetes Association, DiabeticConnect, and Dlife. These websites feature a host of credible, high quality health reference materials such as diabetes related articles, online guides, videos and scholarly articles, nutrition and dietary plans, diabetes friendly recipes and new tools, and treatments for disease management. A common feature on most sites is the social community section that allows users to connect to others like them via forums and blogs. For instance, some of the most popular diabetes forums include PatientsLikeMe, DiabetesForum, DiabetesDaily, and tuDiabetes.

2.2 Health Tracking and Visualization Tools

Due to the complexity associated with the development of tracking tools and applications, these products often tend to offer services limited to tracking diabetic measurements such as blood glucose, Hemoglobin A1c, carbohydrate intake, and physical activity. Most products in this category are either focused on weight management (e.g. SparkPeople.com, or MyFitnessPal.com) or mobile diabetes management with tracking parameters limited to weight, food and activity levels only. The most popular diabetes tracking applications are Glucose Buddy, BG Monitor Diabetes, Diabetes Logbook and OnTrack Diabetes. Some advanced applications also exist that allow download of data from different medical devices such as glucometers in order to easily follow trends and monitor patterns. Glooko is an application (FDA approved) that can directly connect with a doctor's devices to measure and log blood sugar levels.

2.3 Risk Engine for Health Prediction

Personalized preventive care for diabetics can lead to patient empowerment. Patients aware of their risks are motivated to better manage their health to improve overall outcomes. To achieve the goals of risk prediction, several studies were undertaken to investigate different predictive modeling techniques using patient health indicators from longitudinal patient data [5]. The UKPDS risk engine, used widely, can predict the risk of heart disease and stroke in a patient suffering from Type 2 diabetes. However, this model only predicts risk for two events and is limited to Type 2 Diabetics [5]. Possibilities of predicting different types of risk will be greatly influenced by the amount of patient information that becomes available through EHR integration.

2.4 DiabeticLink's Research Motivation

A major motivation behind the development of the DiabeticLink system was the technical limitations of existing diabetes self-management tools. First, most do not consider mobile devices as a platform for the health monitoring applications. Furthermore, existing tools do not translate self-monitoring data to patient-interpretable implications and meanings. In addition, the tools ignore an individual's health status and unique needs, and are therefore deficient in providing personalized alerts, tailored educational materials, and actionable recommendations [6].

DiabeticLink is an all-inclusive, free, and intelligent self-management web portal that provides access to credible educational resources, advanced tracking capabilities, a unique risk management module, and a sense of community through its social blogs and discussion forums. Family members, physicians, and nurses of diabetics also have a place on DiabeticLink, as it provides comprehensive information on all aspects of diabetes management.

3   Target Populations

3.1   User Population 1: Patients

There are three main patient populations who could benefit from the DiabeticLink system: Type 1 diabetics, Type 2 diabetics, and pre-diabetics. The first patient population, Type 1 diabetics, consists of diabetics who are insulin-dependent, whereas Type 2 diabetes is manageable through lifestyle changes, as the pancreas is still able to secrete limited amounts of insulin [7]. The third patient population, pre-diabetics, consists of proactive people who are in danger of developing Type 2 Diabetes and want to take better control of their health. Both long-time diabetics and those recently diagnosed can turn to DiabeticLink as a resource for figuring out how to track their blood glucose, food intake, and log their insulin dosages daily, as well as a tool to access diabetes educational resources and assess their future health risk factors.

3.2   User Population 2: Caregivers

Caregivers include family members or friends of a diabetic patient-those who are providing care to the diabetic when he or she cannot care for him/herself. They provide a support system for the diabetic, which may include mental, emotional, physical, and/or financial support. Caregivers would be most interested in using DiabeticLink to learn about new treatments and possible cures for the disease.

3.3   User Population 3: Healthcare Providers

Healthcare providers include doctors, nurses, nurse practitioners, and researchers. They are able to provide clinical and medical care or treatments to diabetic patients of all populations. They would be most interested in using DiabeticLink to recommend the latest research information on treatments and technology to their patients and caregivers and to help their patients self-manage their blood sugars, insulin dosages, and other health data.

4   DiabeticLink System Functionalities

DiabeticLink has been launched in two countries, namely, the US (September 2014) and Taiwan (August 2013). DiabeticLink's system functionalities were developed to cater to each market individually based on country specific needs, policies, and regulations. Hence, even though the basic value provided by the system remains the same, certain functionalities are unique to the two systems.

4.1   DiabeticLink US

Features and Benefits. DiabeticLink's strength lies in its tools that aid in diabetes self-management. Where DiabeticLink's competitors may offer a subset of features, this system provides a multi-feature, one-stop site to patients for a complete diabetes management solution. There are four main types of features that are provided, as detailed below.

Health Resources. The Health Resources module is designed as an educational resource, where the user finds up-to-date health information, such as the latest diabetes-related information (in the form of articles, videos, blogs, tweets, and research) sourced from credible diabetes sites (American Diabetes Association, NIH, etc.) created via daily information aggregation and mash-up of third-party user-generated content. This part of the website is dedicated to bringing together all relevant information on one platform. This module is interactive and has a variety of options for how users want to receive their educational information. It also provides a sub-module known as "Healthy Eating," which offers the latest diabetes-friendly recipes and a guide for eating out locally, powered by *nutritionix* and *factional* (Fig. 1).

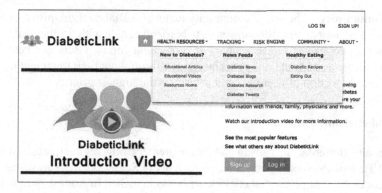

Fig. 1. Health resources module on DiabeticLink US; provides the latest information on diabetes and diabetes management

Health Tracking. The tracking segment of DiabeticLink provides a dynamic platform to track 8 different health parameters including insulin, glucose, cholesterol, HbA1c, weight, food intake, activity and blood pressure. These health logs are automatically displayed in color coded graphs and can be exported/downloaded in .csv or excel formats. This allows for easy monitoring of all health parameters on one website, while ending the hassle of manual consolidation of tracking data (Fig. 2a).

Risk Engine. DiabeticLink has developed a unique risk engine based on an experiment that used about 2,000 diabetic patients [8]. DiabeticLink provides two scientific approaches to profile patient risk. Both tools are based on results published in scientific journals. One predicts the 5-year risk of stroke and coronary heart disease (CHD) based on the U.K. Prospective Diabetes Study [9]. The other predicts the risk of diabetes-induced hospitalization based on the research in the Artificial Intelligence (AI) Lab at the University of Arizona (Fig. 2b).

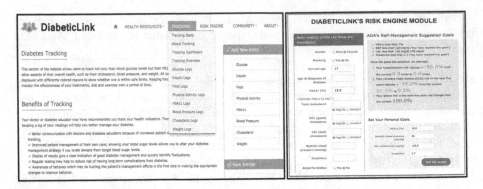

Fig. 2. (a) (left) Tracking module (DiabeticLink US) allows tracking of 8 different health parameters and (b) (right) Risk engine module (DiabeticLink US) predicts risk of stroke, CHD and hospitalization and allows users to set health goals based on recommendations

Social Community. The social community feature on DiabeticLink provides forums, blogs and a list of members, allowing users to befriend people with similar health-related issues and challenges and seek support in convenient forms. Users can benefit from readily available and critical online social support throughout their treatment journey in this section. Protection of user data and privacy is the highest priority.

4.2 DiabeticLink Taiwan

Features and Benefits. In Taiwan and for the greater China region (partnered with the National Taiwan University and Chinese Academy of Sciences), the Taiwanese version of DiabeticLink (at http://tw.diabeticlink.org/) was launched in August 2013 with more than 25,000 unique visitors and a Facebook fan following of more than 500 people.

Health Resources. DiabeticLink-Taiwan currently provides hundreds of news articles, healthcare and medication related articles, research reports, and healthy recipes much like its US counterpart. It also offers a Knowledge Quick Search (provided by the Taiwanese National Health Insurance Database) that provides answers to some of the most frequently asked questions from diabetes patients and caretakers.

Social Connections. This feature of the website is similar to the social community functionality on the DiabeticLink US website and provides a safe and anonymous platform to share treatment management questions, experiences, successes, challenges and search for similar patients across multiple discussion forums.

Health Tracking. This module allows tracking of nine different health parameters and provides advanced visualization tools for easy data comprehension, similar to the DiabeticLink US tracking module.

Drug Safety Module. The Taiwanese version of DiabeticLink also includes a total of 139 drug names that are commonly prescribed to diabetic patients and their comorbidity from US Federal Drug Administration (FDA) Adverse Event Reporting System (FAERS) database in the Taiwanese Drug Safety module. Taiwanese users can review the adverse drug effect reports in the FAERS system to have a better understanding of the drugs prescribed to them. Several physicians and educators in National Taiwan University Hospital (NTUH) were consulted to determine the accuracy of the Chinese translation of this drug related information.

5   DiabeticLink US System Evaluation

The US user study was conducted prior to the DiabeticLink US system launch in September 2014 in order to obtain feedback on system design, functionalities, ease of use and other factors. The main objectives of this user study were to test the website in real world settings with potential users and to obtain direct feedback to determine areas of improvement for the system prior to its launch. At this point, the system was not available to the public for viewing and was offered in its beta version to subjects. The Institutional Review Board (IRB) at the University of Arizona approved the study design and material.

5.1   Evaluation Metrics

Ten major factors were considered during the user study, modeled after Jakob Nielsen's Usability Heuristics [10]. The factors are as shown in Table 1:

Table 1. Usability heuristics [10] employed in 2014 DiabeticLink US user study design

Heuristic	Relates to
"Visibility of system status"	System ability to provide feedback to users
"Match between system and the real world"	User's ability to understand the system and the testing in layman's language, with appropriate logic and order
"User control and freedom"	Ease of website's navigation
"Consistency and standards"	User's evaluation of the convention of the platform of the website
"Error prevention"	User's determination of which parts of the website are most error-prone
"Recognition rather than recall"	System reliance on user memory or easily visible and self-explanatory organization of website
"Flexibility and efficiency of use"	Effectiveness for both novice and experienced users
"Aesthetic and minimalist design"	Relevance of included information and visuals
"Help users recognize, diagnose, and recover from errors"	Easily understandable error messages
"Help and documentation"	Ease of instruction and ability to search the website

5.2   User Study Design

The user study was conducted through expert review, hallway testing, and remote usability testing. Expert review involved those who designed the DiabeticLink system testing it internally. Then, the populations (highlighted below in "User Study Populations") were chosen and IRB approval was secured. The next step involved selecting participants for testing and determining whether they would participate in hallway or remote usability testing. Those who were hallway tested came to the University of Arizona to be observed and recorded while they tested the system. Those who participated in remote usability testing were given specific written instructions on how to access the system (while their computer screen was recorded), as well as all of the pre and post-test materials to complete.

The user study materials consisted of a pre-test survey, an interactive test, and a post-test survey. The pre-test survey was aimed at gauging the user's expectations of the system and to gather information on existing competition on the market. In the interactive system testing, users sat at a computer and were recorded (voice and mouse movements only) as they used the DiabeticLink website. The post-test survey evaluated user feedback on the DiabeticLink system from each specific population.

User Study Subjects Groups. There were three subject groups in this user study, with 3–5 participants in each. The first subject group consisted of diabetic patients (Type 1 and Type 2). The second group consisted of caregivers of diabetic patients (spouses, children, or other relatives). Lastly, the third group consisted of healthcare providers (physicians, nurses, nurse educators). There was one secondary population in this user study, which was composed of 13 college students with no previous relation to diabetes. In total, there were 24 subjects.

Participant Demographics. The age range for this study varied from 20 to 75 years of age, with fourteen participants aged 20–25, three aged 26–45, and seven aged 45–75. Figure 3 (below) shows the number of participants in each age group:

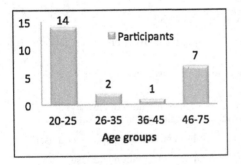
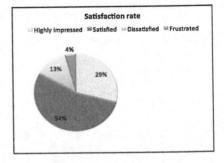
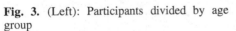

Fig. 3. (Left): Participants divided by age group

Fig. 4. (Right): Overall satisfaction rate of four populations in 2014 user study

5.3 Results

The 2014 User Study on the DiabeticLink US system showed that most users were, overall, at least satisfied (54 %), if not highly impressed (29 %), as shown in Fig. 4 (above). A minority was dissatisfied and/or frustrated (17 %) with the system (Fig. 4). The user study subjects reported that an online portal that allows tracking and easy report generation while providing important information on nutrition, all on the same platform, is exceedingly helpful and is a tool that they would use and recommend.

The satisfaction rates for the individual modules and overall website design are shown in Table 2 (below).

Table 2. User satisfaction with DiabeticLink modules and website design

Module	Percentage of satisfied users	Percentage of dissatisfied users	Percentage of neutral users
Tracking	75 %	25 %	0 %
Health resources	52 %	46 %	2 %
Risk engine	41 %	33 %	26 %
Community section	29 %	42 %	29 %
Website design	88 %	12 %	0 %

The most popular module on both a quantitative and qualitative basis amongst the test subjects was the Tracking module. As shown in Table 2 (above), the user satisfaction rate was much higher than the dissatisfaction rate (75 % versus 25 %). Users were pleased with the wide variety of options for health tracking and the easy-to-use log and chart formats, with reviews from such as "I like how it's all here; super easy to use, how it SHOULD be" and "this is the primary reason I might use this".

The Health Resources module was the next most affinitive with users, with a 52 % overall satisfaction rate. Reasons for user dissatisfaction included little proof of reliability of the sources of information and the reduced clarity of the diabetes videos sourced from YouTube, which was remedied after the user study.

The Risk Engine received a mixed review, which is shown above in Table 2 with the 41 % satisfaction rate, 33 % dissatisfaction rate, and 26 % rate of neutrality. The users who were satisfied with this module provided feedback such as "Nice, very tempting, even if I'm not a Diabetic, I would like to come back and use it again and again every time I get my blood tested," and, "It's good that you include your references. If I had diabetes I would want to make sure it's an evidence-based system," whereas those who expressed dissatisfaction found the risk engine "scary" and did not want to test it on themselves.

The Community section also received a mixed review. Quantitative data recorded from post-test surveys showed that 29 % of the users were satisfied with this section of the website, while 42 % were neutral and 29 % were dissatisfied. Those who were happy with this tool made comments such as "blogs are great so users can know they are not alone and can find answers from people in similar situations," while there was no direct qualitative negative feedback.

Next, the website design and layout was evaluated by users. As shown in Table 2 (above), there was an 88 % overall satisfaction rate with the layout, ease of accessibility, and aesthetics of the DiabeticLink US system. One nursing student stated that the website was "easy to navigate" with "attractive colors and layouts."

As shown in this study, the Tracking and Health Resources features were found to be the most popular with the test group of users (ages 20–75). They received comments such as "I love that you can track each of these things. Diabetes management includes all of these things" (Nursing student) and "the news section is great-always wanted to be able to see it all in one location" (Type 1 diabetic).

After the DiabeticLink US user study was completed, user feedback was taken into account and system improvements were made prior to the launch in September 2014, such as providing personalized guides on how to use each module, adding a calorie counter to the food tracking module, and improving search speed for the restaurant search in the Health Resources module. In addition, the tracking visualization was improved and superimposed graphs were made available in the Tracking module, and the system was made compatible with all iOS devices and most Android devices.

6   System Adoption and Usage Statistics

6.1   Digital Marketing Strategy

The DiabeticLink US website post-launch was promoted using several online marketing tools, including Search Engine Optimization (SEO), Google adwords, Facebook ads, guest blogging, YouTube videos and daily/weekly posts on popular social media websites such as Facebook and Twitter.

6.2   Social Media Statistics

Since the DiabeticLink US launch in September 2014 up until August 2015, the website has been promoted on two main social forums: Facebook and Twitter. The goal of this promotion was to increase the number of unique visitors on the DiabeticLink US website. Table 3 (below) displays statistics on the popularity of the DiabeticLink US social media accounts over time (quarter over quarter) since the launch of the website.

There has been an increasing trend in the popularity of DiabeticLink US on Facebook and Twitter since 2014, as shown in Table 3 (below). In approximately one year, the DiabeticLink US Facebook page has reached nearly 860 likes, while the Twitter fanbase has reached nearly 2,650 followers.

Table 3. Statistics for DiabeticLink social media accounts from September 2014 to August 2015

Time period (quarter)	Facebook likes	Twitter followers
Q3 2014	0	0
Q4 2014	197	943
Q1 2015	618	2,208
Q2 2015	836	2,606
Q3 2015	858	2,634
Total to date	858	2,634

6.3 Views and Members

The quarter over quarter growth in the usage of the DiabeticLink US website, broken down by total page-views, number of sessions, the number of unique visitors and number of registered members, is shown in Table 4 (below). The number of page-views and unique visitors to the website increased from quarter 1 to quarter 2 (in 2014), but decreased in the first quarter of 2015. The sudden growth in the first two quarters can be attributed to the use of paid advertising using Google adwords and Facebook ads. These paid advertisements were stopped in the end of quarter 2 (2014) and the reduced presence online led to a reduction in the number of unique visitations in the following quarters. Due to increased presence on social media sites like Facebook and Twitter, the site gained more audience in the second quarter of 2015. Even though the number of unique visitors declined, the number of registered users increased over the quarters. The increase is not significant in quarter 3 (2015) mainly because the figures shown in Table 4 have data that was collected before the end of quarter 4 (in August 2015).

Table 4. Number of page views, sessions, unique visitors, and registered members on DiabeticLink from September 2014 to August 2015

Time period (quarter)	Total page views	Sessions (visitors)	Users (unique visitors)	Registered members
Q3 2014	24,823	1,179	596	63
Q4 2014	28,142	6,102	4,487	203
Q1 2015	9,384	1,581	907	220
Q2 2015	6,565	2,401	2,125	221
Q3 2015	2,384	1,227	1,176	224
Total to date	71,298	12,490	9,291	224

7 Future Development Plans

In the near future, the DiabeticLink development team plans to incorporate direct data transmission from diabetic devices such as glucometers, insulin pumps, and insulin pods, which will make the tracking of diabetic health information easier. Our team will also add innovative features to appeal to a variety of populations, such as a youth forum for newly diagnosed young adults and a suggestion board for all members of the website. We hope that these developments will encourage the progress of the community aspect of DiabeticLink, as well as increase the number of page views and unique members. A third DiabeticLink system is currently being developed for Patient@Home, a healthcare initiative in Denmark. This Danish version of the website will cater to the requirements of the Danish healthcare system in adherence to their policies and regulations.

Acknowledgements. This work is supported by the University of Arizona Artificial Intelligence Lab, the Caduceus Intelligence Corporation (funded by the National Science Foundation IIP-1417181), the National Taiwan University (NTUH), and Patient@Home Denmark. We wish to acknowledge our collaborators in the US, Taiwan, and Denmark for their research support.

References

1. North America Internet Usage Statistics, Population and Telecommunications Reports. Internet World Stats: Usage and Population Statistics. http://www.internetworldstats.com/stats14.htm. Accessed 20 August 2015
2. National Diabetes Statistics Report. Center for Disease Control and Prevention (2014). Accessed 20 August 2015
3. Funnell, M.M., Anderson, R.M.: Empowerment and self-management of diabetes. Clin. Diab. J. Am. Diab. Assoc. http://clinical.diabetesjournals.org/content/22/3/123.long. Accessed 29 August 2015
4. Diagnosis and Classification of Diabetes Mellitus. Diabetes Care 27 (2004). American Diabetes Association. Accessed 10 August 2014
5. Coleman, R.L., Stevens, R.J., Holman, R.R.: The Oxford risk engine: a cardiovascular risk calculator for individuals with or without type 2 diabetes. Diabetes **56**(1), A170 (2007). Accessed 10 June 2015
6. Chuang, J., Hsiao, O., Wu, P.-L.,Chen, J., Liu, X., De La Cruz, H., Li, S.-H., Chen, H.: DiabeticLink: an integrated and intelligent cyber-enabled health social platform for diabetic patients. In: Zheng, X., Zeng, D., Chen, H., Zhang, Y., Xing, C., Neill, D.B. (eds.) ICSH 2014. LNCS, vol. 8549, pp. 63–74. Springer, Heidelberg (2014)
7. Type 1 Diabetes. Mayo Clinic (2015). http://www.mayoclinic.org/diseases-conditions/type-1-diabetes/basics/definition/con20019573
8. Calculate Your Hospitalization Risk for Diabetes. DiabeticLink. CIC (2015). http://www.diabeticlink.org/risk_engine
9. A1C Test: MedlinePlus Medical Encyclopedia. U.S. National Library of Medicine. U.S. National Library of Medicine (2015). http://www.nlm.nih.gov/medlineplus/ency/article/003640.htm
10. Nielson, J.: 10 Heuristics for User Interface Design. Nielsen Norman Group, 1 January 1995. http://www.nngroup.com/articles/ten-usability-heuristics/

MedC: A Literature Analysis System for Chinese Medicine Research

Xin Li[1(✉)], Yu Tong[1], and Wen Wang[1,2]

[1] Department of Information Systems,
City University of Hong Kong, Kowloon, Hong Kong
{Xin.Li,yutong}@cityu.edu.hk, wwang222-c@my.cityu.edu.hk
[2] School of Management, Xi'an Jiaotong University, Xi'an, Shannxi, China

Abstract. Chinese medicine research documents a significant amount of knowledge. However, compared to Western medicine, there are limited studies that take advantage of and summarize findings based on the Chinese medicine literature. This paper builds a literature analysis system based on information extraction and visualization technologies, which allow users to select and analyze a subset of Chinese medicine literature. The system provides complex search functionalities and makes a set of analyses (summary statistics on medicine/disease/acupuncture points, medicine co-occurrence analysis, and acupuncture point analysis) available to support Chinese medicine scholars and alleviate their workload. The system may facilitate Chinese medicine research and theorization.

Keywords: Chinese medicine · Text mining · Visualization · Literature analysis

1 Introduction

Chinese medicine is a treasure of Chinese culture. It reflects Chinese people's long-term wisdom in treating diseases and pursuing a healthy life. In its long history, Chinese medicine developed many effective disease treatments, which is documented in medicine monographs. Since the 1950s, Chinese medicine researchers have been systematically publishing cases, studies, and findings in journals.

This paper argues that it is necessary to examine the existing Chinese medicine publications, since they contain a large amount of empirical evidence from practice and hold the potential to derive theoretical explanations for Chinese medicine. Literature analysis is widely used in Western medicine to summarize previous findings, develop theories, and direct future research. However, literature analysis on Chinese medicine is rare, and difficult to many Chinese medicine scholars. To ease their research using the literature analysis approach, it is necessary to develop a system that provides automated literature analysis and visualization.

In this research, we propose a literature analysis system for Chinese medicine that is developed based on information extraction and knowledge mapping techniques [1, 2]. In this system, we collect Chinese medicine publications (especially journal papers), and extract disease, medicine, treatment, and acupuncture point information from the

© Springer International Publishing Switzerland 2016
X. Zheng et al. (Eds.): ICSH 2015, LNCS 9545, pp. 311–320, 2016.
DOI: 10.1007/978-3-319-29175-8_29

text of papers using text mining methods. We develop functionalities for descriptive statistics, medicine co-occurrence network, and body-based acupuncture point co-occurrence visualization. With this system, scholars can search and select some papers in their areas of interest and generate visualizations to help them digest the selected publications and have an overview of the empirical evidence published in that area.

We built a prototype system (http://medc.is.cityu.edu.hk/). We collect the abstracts and meta-data of about 1 million Chinese medicine papers published since the 1950s in the prototype. The system works in a cloud-computing fashion in which scholars can make multiple analyses and save the results. The system is open to the public.

2   Literature Review

2.1   Literature Analysis in Western Medicine

Medical literature records human experience in fighting diseases. The development of information technologies makes it possible to automatically extract and summarize information from medical literature. Information extraction and knowledge mapping reduce the work required to read and comprehend medical literature. By integrating findings from multiple medical literature, statistical methods and visualization tools can help further reduce errors in information extraction and identify the most important scientific discoveries. Text mining and knowledge mapping have been widely used to analyze and understand Western medical literature [1].

By the end of the last century, the National Library of Medicine (NLM) had supported a number of studies on searching and mining of medical literature [3]. NLM built the PubMed (formerly called MEDLINE) system, which is now the world's largest literature database on life sciences and biomedical information. Many knowledge extraction and mapping tools were developed based on this system to extract genetic relations [2], gene information [4], and other types of information [5]. The data extracted from MEDLINE literature are also being used to carry out further biomedical research [6–8].

2.2   Literature Analysis in Chinese Medicine

In recent years, Chinese scholars have gradually adopted text mining and knowledge mapping techniques to analyze Chinese medical literature [9]. For example, Zhou et al. proposed to mine both Chinese medicine and MEDLINE literature for gene functional networks [10]. Zheng et al. studied the shared biological networks between rheumatoid arthritis and coronary heart disease by simultaneously using Chinese medicine literature and MEDLINE literature [11]. In Taiwan, Fang et al. extracted Chinese medicine information (in English) from MEDLINE literature and developed a database that includes the links between Chinese medicine, genes, and disease [12]. Xue et al. developed a database for herb molecular mechanism analysis based on information extracted from literature [13]. In the past years, there is a group of related scholars who published about 40 papers analyzing various diseases in Chinese medicine literature [14, 15]. Nevertheless, for most Chinese physicians, it is a challenge to learn text mining and knowledge mapping skills and use them to digest literature.

From the knowledge mapping perspective, prescription analysis is related to literature analysis. In 2011, the Institute of Automation at the Chinese Academy of Sciences and the Chinese Academy of Traditional Medicine developed a prescription analysis software, TCMISS (http://www.tcmnd.com/detail.aspx?id=441). Although it uses basic visualization methods and does not have time-mining functions, it still significantly improved the ability of Chinese scholars to analyze prescriptions. This software supported over 30 papers to analyze prescriptions of some famous doctors [16].

Despite the above efforts, in general, existing efforts to analyze Chinese medicine literature are relatively simple. These studies usually report words frequency, word correlation analysis (network visualization) for a selected area or disease [14, 17, 18]. There are no generic Chinese medicine literature analysis systems for scholars.

This paper takes text mining and knowledge mapping approaches to fill the gap. We develop a Chinese medicine literature analysis system to support scholars who have no information processing experience conducting literature analysis.

3   System Architecture

Following the design science paradigm, we develop a Chinese medicine literature analysis system (named MedC) and evaluate its effectiveness in helping Chinese medicine scholars. Figure 1 presents the general framework for this study, including testbed development, system development, and user studies. Before system development, in the testbed development part we collect Chinese medicine literature from CNKI (the largest literature database in China), which will be mined and analyzed. We also collect medical knowledge bases on medicine, diseases, and syndromes to facilitate the text mining task. After system development, for the user study we will interview domain experts and conduct studies with students to validate the proposed approach. This paper focuses on reporting the system development component, which is shown in detail in Fig. 2.

Information Extraction Module Design and Development. After collecting the Chinese medicine literature, we built an automatic information extractor based on existing research in Chinese NLP. We convert the collected papers to text format and build a heuristic filter to filter out irrelevant information, such as header on each page, and keep only paper content. We conduct Chinese word segmentation and POS tagging by using the ICTCLAS package (http://ictclas.nlpir.org) developed by NLPIR. We incorporate Chinese medicine-specific dictionaries, which are built upon the collected medical knowledge bases, to extract terms such as disease names, symptoms, etc. We conduct rule-based term aggregation and disambiguation to address typos and synonyms in literature, so that each term has a unified identifier in our system. (This step is supported by a thesaurus of medicine and disease names collected and compiled by us.) We then extract co-occurrence relations between terms within and across sentences and paper sections. We pre-process our collection and conduct information extraction for later visualization.

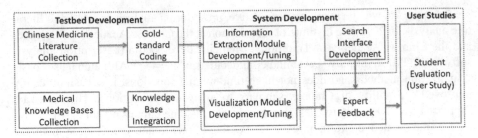

Fig. 1. The framework for the study on MedC system

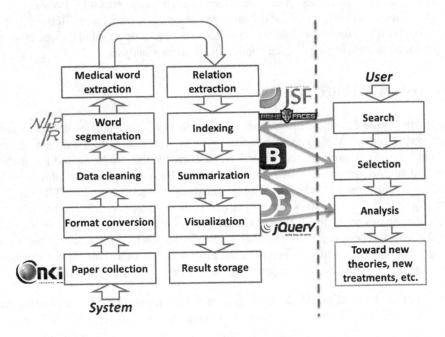

Fig. 2. System development

Search Interface Development. Different from previous researchers' work, we do not specify any scope of literature. We leave the selection of literature to be analyzed to researchers, i.e., potential users of our system. To facilitate users finding the literature they are interested in for visualization and analysis, we develop a Web interface that contains complicated literature search and selection functionalities. The interface is built on Html, Ajax, Java, and JSP techniques. It is based on the JavaServer Faces (JSF) framework[1] using primefaces[2] with the help of bootstrap[3]. The webpage logic was

---

[1] https://en.wikipedia.org/wiki/JavaServer_Faces.
[2] http://primefaces.org/.
[3] http://getbootstrap.com/.

written with the help of JQuery[4]. The system also has basic account management and report management functionalities to ease the use of visualization modules.

Visualization Module Design and Development. The visualization module is a key component of the project. We customize an open source package, D3[5], to build the interface. The visualizations are designed considering Chinese medicine researchers' requirements. Specifically, we provide summary statistics of diseases, medicines, and acupuncture points, in which we highlight the inter-correlations among the three types of entities. We provide medicine co-occurrence graph visualization together with their medicine properties (药性, Chinese medicine classifies medicines to four types: cold, hot, warm, and cool; note that such classifications may not match their chemical properties) and GuiJing (归经, a unique construct in Chinese medicine to annotate which part-of-human-body the medicine belongs to; note that the part-of-human-body in Chinese medicine does not always match anatomy). We provide an acupuncture point visualizer based on the human body. While we are still developing other visualization modules, the three visualizers provide us unique perspectives on understanding the selected literature.

4 System Implementation/Functionality

4.1 Testbed

We developed a spider and crawled all the abstracts and meta-data of CNKI publications (the full-text of papers requires purchase). By November 2014, we collected the abstracts of 1,098,014 articles, including 1,081,864 journal papers, 2,995 doctoral dissertations, and 12,118 master theses. Our customized text segmentation system contains a lexicon with 979,079 unique words integrated from multiple sources. By applying the text segmentation tool to the 1 M papers, we extract 494 unique disease names occurring 672,226 times, 877 unique medicines occurring 669,604 times, and 331 unique acupuncture points occurring 151,925 times.

Chinese medicine literature abstracts usually do not contain enough information on treatments, prescriptions, and symptoms of the subjects, which are necessary for this research. In the future, we will purchase full-texts of papers to improve the system. For a case study, we retrieved asthma research papers with the help of some Chinese medicine scholars. Such literature is used to illustrate the functionalities of the system. The system also allows users to upload full-texts of papers for analysis.

4.2 System Functionality

Literature Search and Selection. The MedC system provides several searching functions for Chinese medicine scholars. Users can start with simple search functionalities,

---

[4] https://jquery.com/.
[5] http://d3js.org/.

such as title, keyword, and abstract. The system also provides advanced search functionalities. Users can use author, acupuncture point, medicine, disease, and year to search
the results. After the initial query, the related publications are listed as shown in Fig. 3,
on which users can further shortlist publications by applying filtering criteria, including
time, journal names, and words in title/abstracts. On the shortlisted search results, users
can browse and select papers into an analysis candidate list. The left half of Fig. 4 shows
the analysis candidates. Here users can search and select publications, so they have the
flexibility to analyze any subset of the 1 M publications in our system. We assume, after
this step, the users can identify a small set of related documents that are worthwhile and
relevant for further analysis.

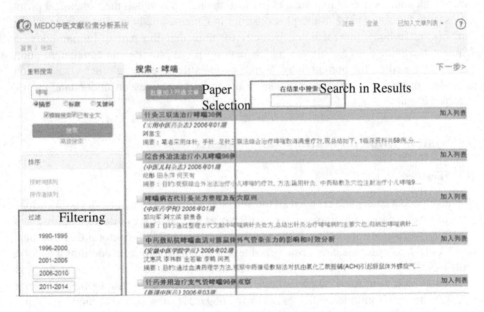

Fig. 3. Literature search and selection

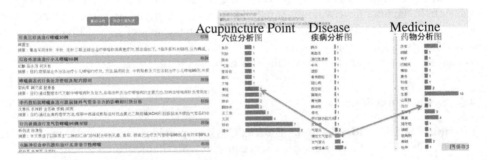

Fig. 4. Analysis candidates and summary statistics

Summary Statistics. The system provides three ways to visualize Chinese medicine literature. The summary statistics function reports the occurrence frequency of acupuncture points, diseases, and medicine in the selected literature. Since our collected dataset is abstracts, the co-occurrence relations are at the abstract level. The right part of Fig. 4 illustrates this functionality; by selecting any term on the bar charts, the co-occurrence of two other types of terms in the charts will be highlighted. As a result, the highlighted bars show the co-occurred elements surrounding a specific disease and medicine in the selected literature. This analysis can aid researchers to have some initial idea of the disease and treatment relations in existing literature.

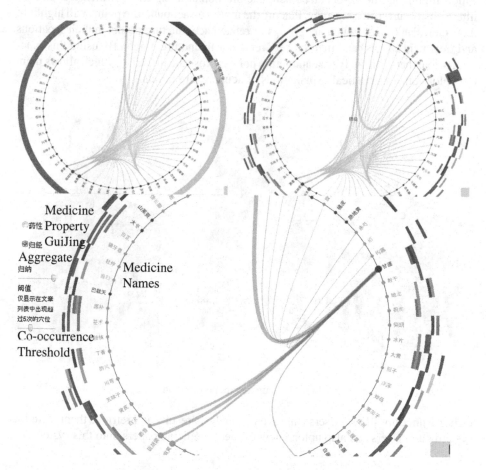

Fig. 5. Medicine co-occurrence graph

Medicine Co-occurrence Graph. Figure 5 shows the medicine co-occurrence graph, which shows the medicines that are often used together. Here, we visualize the co-occurrence network in a ring-layout. We organize medicines according to their properties as shown in the upper left part of Fig. 5. The system can also show the GuiJing of medicines using colors outside of the rings, as shown in the upper right part of Fig. 5.

The interface can filter out links with a small co-occurrence frequency and group similar types of links closer, which makes them more distinct on the interface, as shown in the lower part of Fig. 5. Moving the mouse over a medicine will show its GuiJing and highlight its related medicines. This function allows researchers to identify the interesting relations among medicines, such as the effective collocation or prohibition of using medicines, and conduct follow-up analysis.

Acupuncture Point Graph. Figure 6 illustrates the acupuncture point graph, which places acupuncture points according to their position on the human body. The visualization highlights the co-occurred acupuncture points using links, which can also be filtered by occurrence frequency. Placing the mouse on acupuncture points will highlight their meridian (经络, which are groups of related acupuncture points in their locations and treatment effects) and their closely related acupuncture points. By using this function, researchers can analyze acupuncture points across the meridian, which allows them to explore other theoretical explanations of acupuncture points.

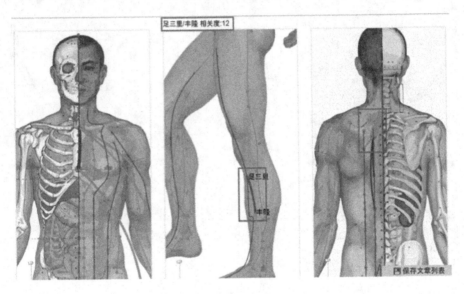

Fig. 6. Acupuncture point graph

Other Functionalities. Users can save the analysis results and retrieve them from the system later. Users can also upload new Chinese medicine papers onto this system.

5   Discussion and Future Work

This paper develops a tool (MedC) to help Chinese medicine scholars retrieve literature, extract key information, and analyze their relations. The system contains more than 1 million Chinese medicine publications and works in a cloud-computing fashion. Users can access it using a browser. MedC can be used to support scholars to comprehend the key information from literature and direct their explorations in Chinese medicine research. This paper discusses the development and functionalities of the system.

In order to validate the effectiveness of our proposed approach, we need to conduct follow up user studies to evaluate system functionalities. Such evaluation, which is missing in this paper, is critical for a design science paper, especially for the development of design theories. We plan to recruit Chinese physicians and conduct an interview regarding the usefulness and ease-of-use of the information extraction, visualization, and knowledge integration components. We will also conduct another round of evaluation among senior students majoring in Chinese medicine. These senior students have experience in participating in clinic decisions and hence can be considered as junior-level practitioners in Chinese medicine. The purpose of the evaluation is to evaluate how much the platform has changed the efficiency and effectiveness of physicians' work. We will adopt a randomized, between-groups design to conduct the evaluation.

In future research, we will continue improving the system, including information extraction effectiveness and visualization functionalities. Nevertheless, it is one of the earliest efforts to reduce manual efforts in Chinese medicine literature analysis. It allows scholars without IT background to employ state-of-the-art text mining and visualization methods to analyze empirical evidence related to their interest.

Acknowledgements. The research is partially supported by National Natural Science Foundation of China grant 71572169, GuangDong Natural Science Foundation grant 2015A030313876, and CityU SRG 7004287.

References

1. Chen, H., Fuller, S., Friedman, C., Hersh, W.: Medical Informatics: Knowledge Management and Data Mining in Biomedicine. Springer, Heidelberg (2005)
2. Leroy, G., Chen, H.C.: Genescene: an ontology-enhanced integration of linguistic and co-occurrence based relations in biomedical texts. J. Am. Soc. Inf. Sci. Technol. **56**, 457–468 (2005)
3. Houston, A.L., Chen, H.C., Hubbard, S.M., Schatz, B.R., Ng, T.D., Sewell, R.R., Tolle, K.M.: Medical data mining on the internet: research on a cancer information system. Artif. Intell. Rev. **13**, 437–466 (1999)
4. Wei, C.H., Harris, B.R., Kao, H.Y., Lu, Z.Y.: tmVar: a text mining approach for extracting sequence variants in biomedical literature. Bioinformatics **29**, 1433–1439 (2013)
5. Savova, G.K., Masanz, J.J., Ogren, P.V., Zheng, J.P., Sohn, S., Kipper-Schuler, K.C., Chute, C.G.: Mayo clinical text analysis and knowledge extraction system (cTAKES): architecture, component evaluation and applications. J. Am. Med. Inform. Assoc. **17**, 507–513 (2010)
6. Wong, A., Shatkay, H.: Protein function prediction using text-based features extracted from the biomedical literature: the CAFA challenge. BMC Bioinform. **14**, S14 (2013)
7. Li, J.X., Zhang, Z., Li, X., Chen, H.: Kernel-based learning for biomedical relation extraction. J. Am. Soc. Inf. Sci. Technol. **59**, 756–769 (2008)
8. Li, X., Chen, H.C., Li, J.X., Zhang, Z.: Gene function prediction with gene interaction networks: a context graph kernel approach. IEEE Trans. Inf. Technol. Biomed. **14**, 119–128 (2010)

9. Zhou, X.Z., Peng, Y.H., Liu, B.Y.: Text mining for traditional Chinese medical knowledge discovery: a survey. J. Biomed. Inform. **43**, 650–660 (2010)
10. Zhou, X.Z., Liu, B.Y., Wu, Z.H., Feng, Y.: Integrative mining of traditional Chinese medicine literature and medline for functional gene networks. Artif. Intell. Med. **41**, 87–104 (2007)
11. Zheng, G., Jiang, M., He, X.J., Zhao, J., Guo, H.T., Chen, G., Zha, Q.L., Lu, A.P.: Discrete derivative: a data slicing algorithm for exploration of sharing biological networks between rheumatoid arthritis and coronary heart disease. Biodata Min. **4**, 18 (2011)
12. Fang, Y.C., Huang, H.C., Chen, H.H., Juan, H.F.: TCMGeneDIT: a database for associated traditional Chinese medicine, gene and disease information using text mining. BMC Complement. Altern. Med. **8**, 58 (2008)
13. Xue, R.C., Fang, Z., Zhang, M.X., Yi, Z.H., Wen, C.P., Shi, T.L.: TCMID: traditional Chinese medicine integrative database for herb molecular mechanism analysis. Nucleic Acids Res. **41**, D1089–D1095 (2013)
14. Zhang, Z.H., Guo, H.T., Zheng, G., Feng, F.H., Li, S.W.: Exploration drug characteristics of Sjogren's syndrome using text mining. Tradit. Chin. Med. Res. **26**, 72–74 (2013)
15. Zha, Q.-l., Yu, J.-Y., Yu, F., Zheng, G., Guo, H.-T., Lv, A.-P., Yu, Z., Jiang, M.: Biological characteristic of five flavours categorized Chinese herbs used for cough treatment based on metabolism related mesh text mining. Chin. J. Basic Med. Tradit. Chin. Med., 616–618 (2010)
16. Liu, T., Liu, J.C.Z.T., X.F., Liu, X.S., Zhang, W.D.: Based on TCM inher-itance assist system to analyze the mdication experience of Liu Yun-Shan for treating Diarrhea in children. Clin. J. Chin. Med. **5**, 10–13 (2013)
17. Tan, Y., Yang, J., Zhao, N., Zheng, G., Cai, F., Jiang, C.Y., Guo, H.T., Jiang, M., Lv, A.P.: Regularity of Chinese and western medicine application for chronic hepatitis b with text mining technique. Chin. J. Exp.Tradit. Med. Formulae **17**, 232–235 (2011)
18. Zhou, C.Y., Chen, H.J., Tao, J.H.: Graph: a domain ontology-driven semantic graph auto extraction system. Appl. Math. Inform. Sci. **5**, 9–16 (2011)

Design of a Mobile Application to Support Non-pharmacological Therapies for People with Alzheimer Disease

Angie K. Reyes[1], Jorge E. Camargo[1($\boxtimes$)], and Gloria M. Díaz[2]

[1] Laboratory for Advanced Computational Science and Engineering Research, Antonio Nariño University, Bogotá, Colombia
{angreyes,jorgecamargo}@uan.edu.co

[2] Grupo de Investigación en Automática, Electrónica y Ciencias Computacionales, Instituto Tecnológico Metropolitano, Medellín, Colombia
gloriadiaz@itm.edu.co

Abstract. As the number of elderly people increase in the world age-related diseases are arising public health problems. Particularly, dementia is one of the most challenging diseases that affect not only to patient but also relatives and specially caregivers. Non-pharmacological therapies have shown to be useful to improve life quality of patients and caregivers but its applications are actually restricted by the presence of a therapy specialist. In this paper we present the designing process of a mobile application for helping caregivers in non-pharmacological therapies to early and moderate Alzheimer disease patients.

Keywords: User-centered design · Alzheimer · Mobile app · Cloud computing

1 Introduction

Neurodegenerative diseases are characterized by a progressive loss of neurons in the central nervous system that generates cognitive impairment and causes several psychological and behavioral symptoms (SBS) such as aggressiveness, hallucinations, apathy, among others [16]. According to the World Alzheimer report, 46 million people worldwide live with dementia in 2015, which generates a total estimated cost of US$818 billion. This number will almost double every 20 years, so that in 2050 there will be 131.5 million people with dementia around the world [14].

Although the Alzheimer disease (AD) is not curable, it has been shown that therapeutic interventions can be effective in treating depression, improving cognitive function, caregiver mood and, consequently, quality of life of patients. Particularly, non-pharmacological therapies (NPT) have received special attention by its low cost and its possible effect on the treatment of the behavioral symptoms, although preliminary results are not conclusive [3,5]. Therefore, it is

© Springer International Publishing Switzerland 2016
X. Zheng et al. (Eds.): ICSH 2015, LNCS 9545, pp. 321–332, 2016.
DOI: 10.1007/978-3-319-29175-8_30

important to evaluate the effectiveness of various NPT with a wide range of participants and settings. However, this is not an easy task due to the complexity of intervening and following continuously each patient and his/her caregiver.

Recently, pervasive computing systems such as home based monitoring, ambient assisted living and daily activity reminders, have shown to be useful in the identification of individuals at risk of developing dementia and in the monitoring of treatment advances [7]. However, its use on the application of therapeutic interventions is still incipient. Some technologies aim to support people with dementia through communication, which has generated therapeutic effects on patients [17]. Armstrong et al. [1] analyze Alzheimer patient needs and propose a system based on smart phone technology that includes an activity of daily living reminder, a picture dialing telephone, short messaging service, a geo-fencing, and one-hour reminder application. Similarly, Zhang [19] developed and evaluated a mobile-based system in which users (AD patients) could receive messages and reminders to manage various daily activities. Reminiscence therapy aspects have been studied in [4,6], where it is possible to create a digital memory of patients in which images, videos and context information (feels, places, event notes, etc.) are stored and retrieved to help AD patients to recall past events or friends.

In this paper we propose a mobile system to support specialists and caregivers in the intervention of early and moderate cognitive impairment of patients thorough non-pharmacological therapies. This system is composed of three main components: (1) A mobile component that implements a set of non-pharmacological therapies using a friendly graphic user interface; (2) A web component aimed at specialists and caregivers to guide therapeutic processes and to register patient events; and (3) A cloud component to store information of therapeutic exercises and patient performance.

2   Non-pharmacological Therapies

According to the World Alzheimer report [13], one of the main barriers to access care services when Alzheimer is diagnosed is "the false belief that nothing can be done for people with dementia and their families". Therefore, promoting the application of different types of treatments is as important as early detection of the disease. The term non-pharmacological therapies refers to all interventions that aim at improving the quality of life of patients without the use of drugs or chemical treatments [12]. In the case of the Alzheimer disease, NPTs emerge as a useful and potentially cost-effective approach that delays psychological and behavioral symptoms.

NPTs can be divided into four main categories: movement, sensory, cognitive-based and psycho-social. In the following paragraphs these categories are described.

Movement therapy corresponds to physical activities aimed at preventing functional impairment, which has demonstrated benefits to reduce symptoms of depression and sleep-wake, and even improving cognitive capacities [8].

Sensory therapy is based on stimulation of the patient's senses to enhance the feeling of well-being. Some examples of this kind of therapy are aromatherapy, music therapy, light therapy and snooze (multisensory) therapy.

Cognitive-based interventions are founded on the hypothesis of brain neuro-plasticity, which suggests that even when a person has been affected by neurode-generation, he/she is able to learn new knowledge and develop new skills [12]. Cognitive training aims at improving cognitive functions such as verbal mem-ory, verbal fluency, attention, comprehension, language and executive functions, by performing a set of tasks or exercises with frequency, duration and difficulty depending on the patient's abilities. Cognitive rehabilitation is defined as the use of "any intervention strategy intended to enable patients, and their families, to live with, manage, bypass, reduce or come to terms with deficits precipitated by injury to the brain" [5]. Cognitive stimulation involves subjects in discussions and activities that require enhancing cognitive and social functions. Reality orienta-tion therapy is a kind of cognitive stimulation that aims to reduce the time/place disorientation present in most Alzheimer disease patients.

Finally, psycho-social therapies are focused on improving feeling of well-being, social and communication skills, and on stimulating patient's residual memory. Reminiscence therapy is one of the most used non-pharmacological interven-tions for enhancing social and familiar abilities. In this therapy a wide variety of elements (images, text, videos, fragrances, etc.) are systematically presented to patients in order to evoke memories associated with his/her own life [12]. Vali-dation therapy is the most specialist-dependent therapy, in which the patient is motivated to remember the skills required to carry out proper communication. It is a highly criticized therapeutic scheme and its effectiveness has not been demonstrated [5].

The system presented in this paper implements a set of these non-pharmacological therapies, which can be performed individually and does not require the presence of a specialist or caregiver. The proposed system architec-ture enables the future inclusion of other therapies.

3   User-Centered Design

One of the most relevant aspects in the development of mobile applications to assist elderly people with cognitive impairment is user satisfaction. In the last years there have been different techniques that apply quality factors to achieve user satisfaction. One of the most relevant approaches for achieving this goal is the *User-Centered Design* (UCD). The UCD is a development methodology based on the interaction between user and application during all the develop-ment process [11]. The UCD helps to ensure the success in a customer-based application involving the user in each phase [18] of the development process.

In this paper we adapt the UCD methodology for the development of a mobile application focused on elderly people. Alzheimer patients have other difficulties related to the age that should be considered in the design of a system. The requirement definition process is very important and for this reason we involved Alzheimer professionals in the system development process.

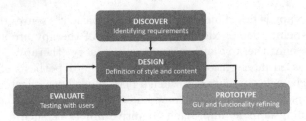

Fig. 1. User-centered design process used to build the proposed system.

As shown in Fig. 1, the development process is composed of two main phases: *discover* and *design*. At the same time, the *design process* is an iterative process composed of *prototyping and evaluation* phases. The first main stage consisted of meetings with therapy professionals of different institutions. In each session, we recorded observations, ideas, recommendations, which was very important to define functional requirements of the system.

Based on a literature review and the recommendations performed by professionals, a first prototype was built with some functionality. With this prototype and the support of an Alzheimer Institute, we carried out a first evaluation of the application, which was conducted by two therapy professionals. From this phase we obtained the observations described below, which were considered for improving the user interface of the system prototype:

- The therapists manifest that the application should not be developed just for the patients, and must include the caregivers at home.
- The application should be *intuitive* and *easy to use*, and this should be considered for the GUI design.
- The text submitted in the application should be larger, due to some patients presenting vision problems.
- Illustrations should be included to facilitate the meaning of the components.
- The use of colors should be *striking*, and avoid the use of light colors because of the difficulty of reading such text.
- The images used in the application should be real because animated images can affect the patients' sensibility.

On the other hand, based on the proposed methodology, it is important to carry out constant evaluations to measure the impact and application performance. However, carrying out some tests generate high costs and involve a lot of time [2]. For this, one of the most applied techniques is the *Guerrilla usability testing* that includes the *thinking aloud* method. This is a test in which the participant that uses the system is asked to think out loud continually, expressing his/her opinion with respect to the user interface [10]. According to this approach, we performed a new evaluation with *caregivers*. This process is described in detail in next Section.

4   System Description

The proposed system is composed of two main elements: a mobile component, that is developed for implementing non-pharmacological therapies to the patients such as reminiscence, reality orientation and cognitive training; and a server component that allows health professionals to have access to statistical information on the use of the application and make configurations about how to proceed with the therapies. Both components are supported on a *cloud computing* platform that allows data synchronization and storage of patient information.

4.1   Server Components

Back-End Component. A back-end component is a critical part of a *cloud computing*-based system because it allows to manage key elements of the system [15]. The back-end was developed using web technologies hosted in the *Amazon Web Services* (AWS) infrastructure. *Amazon Elastic Compute Cloud* (Amazon EC2) was used to run a web server in which a user can access to back-end and front-end components through a web browser.

Off-Line Functionality. *Amazon Cognito* was used to support off-line functionality in the mobile component. This service facilitates the storage and synchronization of data when an Internet connection is not available on the smartphone. To this aim, we used the *Amazon Simple Storage Service* (Amazon S3). The main reason for choosing this platform is the high availability that Amazon offers and the possibility to scale to support a large number of users. In addition, it provides a set of cloud characteristics such as backup support, security, data analytics, among others.

Front-End Component. The front-end component allows therapists and caregivers to track non-pharmacological therapies. It is worth to note that caregivers and therapists can manage information of more than one patient. This component offers the following functionalities:

- To manage aspects dealing with the patient memories. Accordingly, the user has the option of uploading patient data, which is stored with the identity of each user, a *tag* and the date.
- To select and upload photos from the mobile photo gallery. Users can select a *tag* for each photo. Additionally, users can create photo albums that allow patients relate and understand past events. Similarly, users can do the same with audio and video records.
- To add information about dates, events, tasks or more about the patient life events. For instance, add an event for taking medicine at an established hour.
- To view a contact list previously added or add a new contact, an image, and a tag based on the relationship with other people.
- The caregiver or health professional can see the patient's answers and compare them to the correct answer. Additionally, he/she can visualize the results in a graphical way.

4.2   Mobile Component

The objective of this component is to provide caregivers a tool to control patient daily activities and, at the same time, to allow patients to perform cognitive exercises with the assistance of caregivers. This component is focused on elderly people with memory problems, and early or moderate stage AD patients. The next subsections describes each module of the component.

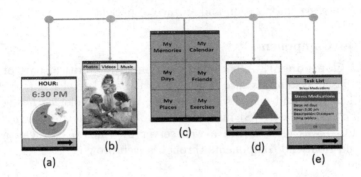

Fig. 2. Modules of the mobile application component organized by non-pharmacological therapies.

Reminiscence Therapy Module. As shown in Fig. 2(c), the application contains 6 modules, two of them are based on reminiscence therapy (*my memory* and *my places*), which aim to illustrate images, videos and audios significant to patients. For instance, autobiographical photographs, home videos and family/friends love messages.

Reality Orientation Therapy Module. One of the symptoms of Alzheimer patients is disorientation. For this reason, we designed a module based on *temporary location* (see Fig. 2). This module shows the time zone where the user can visualizes time, actual day and an image that supports the information and changes depending on the current time zone.

Psycho-Social Therapy Module. Based on the psycho-social therapy, we created the *My Friends* module. This module offers a customized diary, which registers the names of persons. By pressing on each person patients or caregivers can associate to the selected one an image and a tag. In this case, a tag indicates the relationship between the patient and the person registered in the diary.

Cognitive Rehabilitation Therapy Module. The *my exercises* module is designed to support specific cognitive stimulation. Through daily training functions users can stimulate their cognitive abilities. In Fig. 2(d), an example of this module is illustrated: The elderly person loses some of their skills, therefore, it is necessary to motivate her/him through simple but useful cognitive exercises. It is worth noting that the system should not show negative messages to users. Instead, a positive score is displayed in the web component. If patients select a question incorrectly, the system allow to try up to a limit of 3 attempts. The success of this module is based on the simplicity of questions and answers.

5   System Evaluation

The followed UCD methodology described in Sect. 3 allowed us to obtain a more stable application prototype for validation purposes. We recruited five Alzheimer caregivers to validate the proposed system as recommended in [9]. We conducted an evaluation test using a combination of two techniques: one based on the *thinking aloud technique* and the other one based on a *questionnaire*.

5.1   Tasks

For the first evaluation test we established three simple tasks by increasing the difficulty order as follows:

1. Access the application main menu, go to the *my diary* module, and read some notes included in the *my notes* module.
2. Return to the main menu and play a video in the *my memories* module.
3. Access personal information of one of the contacts, read aloud its phone number and name.

For each task we gather information about whether or not the task was completed, execution time and steps taken to complete the activity. Afterwards, the user could freely to explore the application while we recorded their opinions about this process.

5.2   Questionnaire

In the second stage, each caregiver answered a series of questions related to terminology and graphic aspects of the user interface such as colors, fonts, image content and location. We also ask for how useful the application is in general terms. Each question scored a value between 1 to 5. There were the questions used in the questionnaire:

1. Is the terminology used in the *my memory* module appropriate to its functionality?
2. Is the terminology used in the *my diary* module appropriate to its functionality?
3. Is the terminology used in the *my calendar* module appropriate to its functionality?
4. Is the terminology used in the *my people* module appropriate to its functionality?

5. Is the terminology used in the *my place* module appropriate to its functionality?
6. Is the terminology used in the *my exercises* module appropriate to its functionality?
7. Are colors and font size suitable?
8. How useful is the application in your opinion?

Besides, it was asked if the participant thinks that the use of the application is feasible to support the daily development of the patient.

5.3   Participants

The evaluation was conducted by five caregivers. In Table 1 the information gathered of the participants is presented. Each participant was a caregiver of an a specific Alzheimer patient. Some patients were in early stage and others in moderated stage. Patient age range between 60 and 82 years old. The average age of participants was 41 years old. The lowest age was 29 years old and the elder was 50 years old. Most of the participants were women, just one participant was man. Professions of the participants were two housewives, a lawyer, an electrical engineer and an entrepreneur.

Table 1. Participants and patients information

Participant				Patient		
Participant	Age	Gender	Profession	Stage	Age	Gender
Participant 1	39	Female	Lawyer	2	82	Male
Participant 2	44	Female	Housewife	2	73	Female
Participant 3	50	Female	Housewife	2	71	Female
Participant 4	43	Female	Entrepreneur	1	81	Female
Participant 5	29	Male	Engineer	1	60	Male

Participants were asked about his/her fluency in the use of touch screens in mobile devices. In level from 1 to 5 (being five the highest), two participants said to have level 3, two participants level 4, and one participant level 5.

6   Results

In this Section we present the obtained results using the Thinking Aloud technique and questionnaire techniques.

6.1   Qualitative Results

Figure 3 shows the sequence of steps that every participant followed for each of the established tasks. The black lines represent the ideal flow. Note that Participant 3 was the only one that does not complete correctly the task 1. Task 3 presented difficulties caused by unclear instructions, which were not enough descriptive. This caused that participants had to explore the application to achieve the aim.

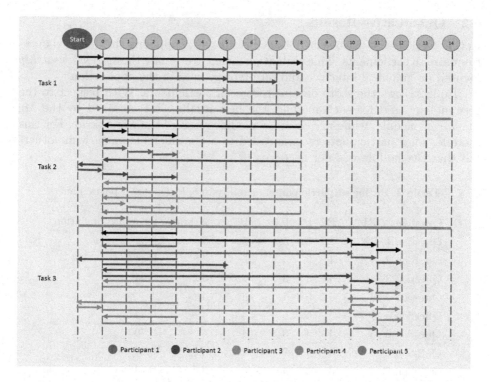

Fig. 3. Navigation path of each participant in each task of the valuation process. The number inside the circle represents the system functionality: (1) *My memories*; (2) *Photos* (3) *Videos* (4) *Recordings* (5) *My date* (6) *Tasks* (7) *Notes* (8) *Meets* (9) *My calendar* (10) *My contacts* (11) *Contact list* (12) *Personal information* (13) *My places* (14) *My exercises*.

Some problems were identified by participants as follows: (1) There were not direct access to the menu in the *my exercises* module; (2) The application does not had a return option; (3) In the *my calendar* module participants did not find difference between the presented three tools. These problems were addressed in the final application prototype.

Other participant suggestions were also considered and are summarized as follows: (1) Customization of colors in the application; (2) Change the name of *My calendar* by *My days or My hours*; (3) Establish just one function in the *My agenda* module; (4) Add an order to instructions (as "press here to reproduce" instead of "reproduce"); (5) Include questions to the questionnaire about history and significant prominent figures of the country; and finally, (6) Bring the possibility to establish the *My calendar* module as screen saver.

In this part of the evaluation we highlight the fact that to include different roles (relatives, keepers and therapists) in the system calls the attention of participants.

6.2   Quantitative Results

In this section we describe the obtained results after applying the designed questionnaire to participants. This evaluation aimed to evaluate the *system's usability* focused on graphical interface and terminology used in the application.

Table 2 shows the score obtained from all participants. With respect to the terminology used for each module, the best results were obtained by the *My memories* module, while *my calendar* module received the worst score. For this module, some participants recommended to use a different name, while others felt that the module was not necessary.

Table 2. Rating of participants: usability test. P denotes a participant.

Question	P1	P2	P3	P4	P5	Average	Standard deviation
Question 1	5	5	5	5	5	5	0
Question 2	5	4	5	5	5	4.8	0.44
Question 3	3	4	3	3	3	3.2	0.44
Question 4	3	5	5	4	3	4	1
Question 5	5	5	5	5	4	4.8	0.44
Question 6	5	4	4	3	4	4	0.70
Question 6	5	5	5	5	4	4.8	0.44
Question 7	4	3	3	4	3	3.4	0.54
Question 8	4	5	5	5	4	4.6	0.54
Average	**4.875**	**5**	**5**	**4.875**	**4.375**	**4.825**	**0.5739**

The initial average score for the design in relation with font size, colors and images was 3.4. Application usefulness (question 8) was scored 4.6. All participants indicate the feasibility of the application for supporting therapeutic activities in Alzheimer disease patients.

7   Conclusions and Future Work

Although the use of mobile applications in the field of health has not been studied systematically, many patients and health professionals use them as a mechanism to support activities such as therapy and diseases tracking. This paper described a system that will serve as support for diseases therapy that cause cognitive impairment. A mobile application was developed following a user-centered design approach. Special attention was paid to caregivers, since these applications are not usually developed to patients but his/her caregiver. Using this methodology we had a more accurate definition of requirements as to the needs of AD patients and their caregivers. The assessment techniques known as *thinking aloud* allowed us to obtain more information about the design, the features that should be considered and the great challenges that we face to counter the use of technology in elderly people. Usability testing helped us to identify different characteristics in the system design and functionality. Participants had difficulty with some of the tasks, mostly on the location and signage absence, although in some of these cases it was due to the inability to use the tablet device. We need to perform more systematic evaluations in order to improve application usability. Some suggestions such as to include voice recognition should be carefully evaluated, due that most of the caregivers could be also elderly people. As future work we will evaluate the system usability in caregivers and patients. We also want to include more therapy options such as music and other cognitive therapies.

Acknowledgments. This work was funded by Universidad Antonio Nariño through the project 20131088 "Desarrollo de herramientas diagnósticas basadas en anńalisis de neuroimágenes para la identificación de pacientes con enfermedades neuropsiquiátricas". This work was partially funded by BIGDATA SOLUTIONS SAS. Our thanks to the therapists and caregivers of the "CENTRO DIA PARA EL DESARROLLO DE LA MEMORIA Y LA COGNICION" for their support and invaluable feedback.

References

1. Armstrong, N., Nugent, C., Moore, G., Finlay, D.: Using smartphones to address the needs of persons with alzheimers disease. Ann. Telecommun. **65**(9–10), 485–495 (2010)
2. Boivie, I., Åborg, C., Persson, J., Löfberg, M.: Why usability gets lost or usability in in-house software development. Interact. Comput. **15**(4), 623–639 (2003)
3. Ballard, C., Khan, Z., Clack, H., Corbett, A.: Nonpharmacological treatment of alzheimer disease. Can. J. Psychiatry **56**(10), 589 (2011)
4. Dobbins, C., Merabti, M., Fergus, P., Llewellyn-Jones, D.: Creating human digital memories with the aid of pervasive mobile devices. Pervasive Mob. Comput. **12**, 160–178 (2014)
5. Gardette, V., Coley, N., Andrieu, S.: Non-pharmacologic therapies: a different approach to ad. Can. Rev. Alz. Dis. Other Dem. **13**(3), 13–22 (2010)
6. Good, A., Wilson, C., Ancient, C., Sambhanthan, A.: A proposal to support well being in people with borderline personality disorder: applying reminiscent theory in a mobile app. (2013). arXiv preprint. arxiv:1302.5200
7. Tung, M., Snyder, H., Hoey, J., Mihailidis, A., Carrillo, M., Favela, J.: Everyday patient-care technologies for alzheimer's disease. IEEE Pervasive Comput. **12**(4), 80–83 (2013)

8. Netz, Y., Axelrad, S., Argov, E.: Group physical activity for demented older adults-feasibility and effectiveness. Clin. Rehabil. **21**(11), 977–986 (2007)
9. Nielsen, J.: Estimating the number of subjects needed for a thinking aloud test. Int. J. Hum. Comput. Stud. **41**(3), 385–397 (1994)
10. Nielsen, J.: Guerrilla hci: using discount usability engineering to penetrate the intimidation barrier. Cost-justifying usability, pp. 245–272 (1994)
11. Nielsen, J.: Usability Engineering. Elsevier, Amsterdam (1994)
12. Olazarán, J., Reisberg, B., Clare, L., Cruz, I., Peña-Casanova, J., Del Ser, T., Woods, B., Beck, C., Auer, S., Lai, C., et al.: Nonpharmacological therapies in alzheimers disease: a systematic review of efficacy. Dement. Geriatr. Cogn. Disord. **30**(2), 161–178 (2010)
13. Prince, M., Bryce, R., Ferri, C.: World Alzheimer Report 2011: The Benefits of Early Diagnosis and Intervention. Alzheimer's Disease International, London (2011)
14. Prince, M., Wilmo, A., Guerchet, M., Ali, G.-C., Wu, Y.-T., Prina, M.: World Alzheimer Report 2015: The Global Impact of Dementia. Alzheimer's Disease International, London (2015)
15. Reese, G.: Cloud Application Architectures: Building Applications and Infrastructure in the Cloud. O'Reilly Media Inc., Sebastopol (2009)
16. Reyes-Figueroa, J.C., Rosich-Estragó, M., Bordas-Buera, E., Gaviria-Gómez, A.M., Vilella-Cuadrada, E., Labad-Alquézar, A.: Síntomas psicológicos y conductuales como factores de progresión a demencia tipo alzheimer en el deterioro cognitivo leve. Rev. Neurol. **50**(11), 653–660 (2010)
17. Rodriguez-Rodriguez, A., Martel-Monagas, L.: Enhancing the communication flow between alzheimer patients, caregivers, and neuropsychologists. In: Arabnia, H.R. (ed.) Advances in Experimental Medicine and Biology, pp. 601–607. Springer, New York (2010)
18. Shneiderman, B.: Designing the User Interface: Strategies for Effective Human-Computer Interaction, vol. 3. Addison-Wesley, Reading (1992)
19. Zhang, D., Hariz, M., Mokhtari, M.: Assisting elders with mild dementia staying at home. In: Sixth Annual IEEE International Conference on Pervasive Computing and Communications, PerCom 2008, pp. 692–697. IEEE (2008)

A Speech-Based Mobile App for Restaurant Order Recognition and Low-Burden Diet Tracking

Xiaochen Huang and Emmanuel Agu[✉]

Computer Science Department, Worcester Polytechnic Institute,
Worcester, MA, USA
emmanuel@cs.wpi.edu

Abstract. Obesity is a public health problem in the US. Diet tracking helps control obesity but manual entry is tedious. Proposed solutions such as food recognition from photographs and scanning barcodes have limitations. We investigate the use of speech recognition for diet recording. We improved the accuracy of food order recognition at restaurants by (1) limiting words in the speech recognizer's corpus to only items on the menus of nearby restaurants (2) implementing an acoustic model to recognize the speaking style of the smartphone owner. Building on these mechanisms, we propose DietRecord, a smartphone application that automatically recognizes and records restaurant orders. Results of our user studies to evaluate DietRecord were encouraging.

1 Introduction

Obesity rates have more than doubled since the 1970s [1]. Obesity increases the risk of many health conditions including hypertension and diabetes. Diet tracking helps control obesity, and to manage ailments requiring controlled diets. Manually recording food is tedious, which reduces compliance. Several proposed solutions have limitations. Recognizing foods from photographs [2] cannot recognize certain foods. Scanning food QR codes [9] or barcodes [10] works but not all foods have barcodes. Improved user entry interfaces have also been proposed but are also manual [8].

Speech is one of the most natural methods of interaction. However, in practice, factors such as environmental noise and individual speaking styles make speech recognition not accurate enough for food entry. Our work focuses on recognizing spoken food orders at restaurants since 25 % of Americans consume fast food daily [3]. We improve speech recognition accuracy and speed using two concepts:

1. *Location-dependent speech recognizer vocabularies:* Just before a user orders food at a restaurant, we limit the words the speech recognizer can guess was spoken (recognition range) by pre-populating the speech recognizer's corpus with only menu items from nearby restaurants.
2. *Speaker Personalization:* Since the speech recognizer may pick up the orders of other customers and restaurant staff, we train the recognizer on the speaking style and accent of the smartphone owner.

© Springer International Publishing Switzerland 2016
X. Zheng et al. (Eds.): ICSH 2015, LNCS 9545, pp. 333–339, 2016.
DOI: 10.1007/978-3-319-29175-8_31

Leveraging these mechanisms, we propose *DietRecord*, a smartphone app that automatically recognizes and records foods ordered by its owner at restaurants. DietRecord users can browse order history and nutrition information using its interfaces.

2   Investigating Speech Recognition Accuracy

CMU Sphinx [4] and Google Voice Service [5] are currently the most widely used speech recognition systems. Using Google Voice, a user can initiate a Google search by speaking into their smartphones. CMU Sphinx is a non-commercial speech recognizer that has features useful for our work. Developers can modify the set of words that can be recognized by building a special corpus (vocabulary). They can also adapt the voice recognition system to individual accents and speaking styles by building an acoustic model. Since we wanted to leverage these customizations, we adopted Pocketsphinx [6], a mobile implementation of CMU Sphinx for our work.

To establish a baseline against which to compare our novel ideas, we initially evaluated unmodified PocketSphinx and Google Voice Speech Recognition demos and their error rates under various conditions. We define the error rate as the percentage of incorrect words in a test sentence. We investigated two factors that affect error rates: (1) the length of spoken sentences and (2) the background noise (in decibels) since restaurants may be noisy. Our test sentences consisted of typical food orders such as "I want a big mac" of different lengths. PocketRTA, a software-based spectrum analyzer was run to generate various noise levels.

Without our proposed enhancements, Pocketsphinx had low speech recognition accuracy, with an error rate of about 65.5 % (Fig. 1) and performs worse than Google Voice. While recognition accuracy is inversely proportional to noise levels, we found no relationship between speech recognizer accuracy and sentence length.

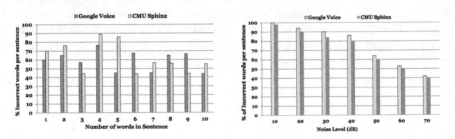

Fig. 1. Accuracy of PocketSphinx unmodified vs Google Voice Speech Recognition for different sentence lengths (left) and background noise (right)

3   Improving Speech Recognition Accuracy

We then explored location-dependent vobularies and speaker personalization to improve the accuracy of spoken order recognition.

(1) *Location-Dependent Vocabularies to limit Speech Recognizer Range:* The corpus of PocketSphinx was pre-populated with only 121 food items from the menus of Dunkin Donuts and McDonalds, two fastfood restaurants. After rebuilding the recognizer's corpus, a subject read out various orders from each of these menus. Figure 2 shows the recognition rate for various text lengths and environmental noise levels (in decibels). Clearly, limiting the recognizer's range significantly improved its accuracy.

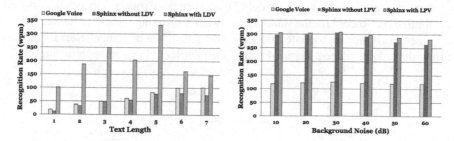

Fig. 2. Speech recognition speeds of CMU Sphinx vs Google Voice for different text lengths (left) and background noise (right)

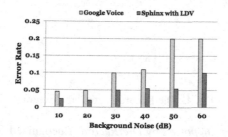

Fig. 3. Error rates of Sphinx with Location-Dependent Vocabularies (LDV) vs Google Voice, different background noise

The error rate was calculated as the number of errors in recognized words divided by the total number of words spoken. Figure 3 shows that Pocketsphinx with the limited recognition corpus has a lower error rate than Google Voice.

(2) *Personalization based on Speaker Identification:* CMU Sphinx has several high-quality acoustic models we used to adapt to the user's speaking style. To train the acoustic models, we generated an adaptation corpus by recording the smartphone owner speaking menu items. This adaption data consisted of a list of order sentences, a dictionary describing the pronunciation of all words in that list of sentences, and a recording of users speaking each of those sentences.

4   The DietRecord Restaurant Order Recognition App

Overview: Based on our findings, we created the DietRecord Android app that auto-matically recognizes and records food orders spoken by a smartphone user. DietRecord detects the user's arrival at a restaurant and retrieves the menus of nearby restaurants using the Foursquare API. These menu items are used as a corpus into DietRecord's PocketSphinx-based speech recognition module. Distances to all restaurants in the user's vicinity are computed and the user is assumed to be in the restaurant that is closest to their current location. An acoustic model of the smartphone owner's speech is also used to customize DietRecord for the smartphone owner's speaking style. DietRecord inserts recognized foods into appropriate categories (breakfast, lunch, dinner, snack), based on the time the order is placed. Figure 4 shows the DietRecord system architecture.

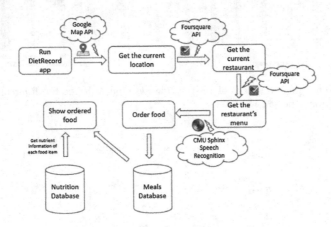

Fig. 4. DietRecord system architecture

User Interaction Modes Supported by DietRecord: Recognized food orders are stored in a database on the smartphone. Over time, meal entries become a diet diary, which also includes nutrition information such as calories, carbohydrates, protein. Users may interact with DietRecord either by speaking their food orders or using DietRecord's interfaces to browse their order history.

Nearby Restaurant Detection: The Google Map API was used to detect the user's current location (longitude and latitude), which is used by the Foursquare API to obtain a list of restaurants within 500 m and their menus. Figure 5 shows (a) DietRecord's restaurant detection screen. Figure 5(b) shows some recognized foods.

Extraction of Nutrition Information of Ordered Food: DietRecord presents users with nutrition information of their recorded diet (See Fig. 5(c)), which was retrieved from the USDA national nutrition database.

DietRecord Implementation: DietRecord is implemented in the Android operating system. DietRecord's interfaces were created by extending Android's activity class. A Service class detected the user's location and performed background processing such

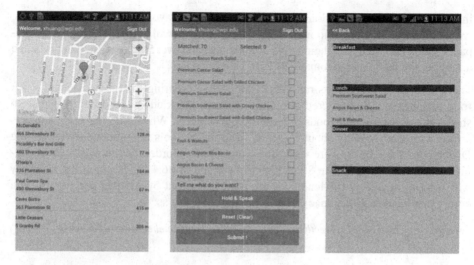

Fig. 5. Screens (a) Restaurant detection (b) Recognized foods (c) Nutrition information.

as running the PocketSphinx speech recognition engine. Content Providers were used to store data in DietRecord. An intent was used to start an activity, service or broadcast from another activity. The diet data was stored in SQLite, a lightweight database.

5 DietRecord Evaluation

Study 1: We recruited 23 Worcester Polytechnic Institute students aged 23 to 29 (15 male, 8 female). Participants were given a questionnaire to gauge their general interest

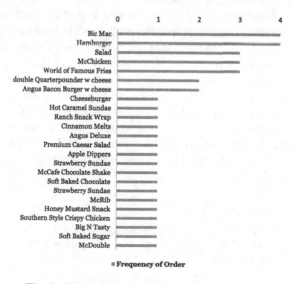

Fig. 6. Distribution of foods ordered by subjects.

in a diet recording application such as DietRecord. To avoid biasing their responses, we did not present this group with DietRecord or any actual app. Over 82 % of participants were concerned with their daily calorie intake and over 50 % of participants wanted a mobile app that could automatically track their meals.

Study 2: Four other subjects ran DietRecord while ordering food at McDonald's fast food restaurants. They ordered a total of 40 items (26 kinds of food items). Figure 6 shows the distribution of foods ordered by the subjects. When ordering food, subjects spoke with their mouths about 5 inches from the phone's microphone. After testing DietRecord, the subjects were asked questions. For food orders of 1–6 words, the recognition accuracy ranged from 80 to 93.3 % (average of 86.4 %). Recognition accuracy was not influenced by the length of the food name, but by whether the word was a compound word (e.g. Big mac). We computed accuracy as:

$$Accuracy = Number\ of\ correctly\ recognized\ words\ /\ Total\ number\ of\ words\ in\ a\ dish \qquad (1)$$

6   Related Work

Other mobile speech entry applications include Parakeet [7], a continuous speech recognition system for mobile touch-screen devices. Users entered text by speaking into their phones. However, Parakeet was less accurate than desk tops and users experienced delays as long as 1 min for some words. Commercial diet tracking apps such as MyFitnessPal have also been proposed but require manual input.

7   Conclusion and Future Work

In this paper, we investigated using speech recognition to record foods ordered by smartphone users at restaurants. We demonstrated higher recognition accuracy and speed by building location-dependent speech vocabularies to limit the recognition range and an acoustic model to adapt to the smartphone owner's speaking style. We proposed DietRecord, a smartphone app that can automatically record users' restaurant orders. Participants in our user studies found DietRecord convenient and useful.

However, DietRecord has some limitations. The Foursquare API we used for retrieving a list of nearby restaurants has some missing food items. The DietRecord app also requires GPS to detect the user's current location, which drains the smartphone's battery. Making DietRecord energy efficient is future work. Finally, the subjects in our user study were mostly from China. In future we will diversify our participants.

References

1. National Center for Health Statistics. http://www.cdc.gov/nchs/
2. Kong, F., Tan, J.: DietCam: regular shape food recognition with a camera phone. In: Proceedings of the BSN. IEEE (2011)

3. Food Research and Action Center (FRAC), Overweight and Obesity in the US. http://frac.org/initiatives/hunger-and-obesity/obesity-in-the-us/

4. Rozzi, W.A., Stern, R.M.: Speaker adaptation in cont. speech recognition via estimation of correlated mean vectors. In: IEEE Proceedings of the ICASSP 1991 (1991)

5. Jyothi, P., et al.: Distributed discriminative language models for Google voice-search. In: Proceedings of the ICASSP. IEEE (2012)

6. Huggins-Daines, D., et al.: Pocketsphinx: a free, real- time cont. speech recognition system for hand-held devices. In: Proceedings of the IEEE ICASSP (2006)

7. Vertanen, K., Kristenssen, P.: Parakeet: a cont. speech recognition system for mobile touch-screen devices. In: Proceedings of the ACM IUI 2009 (2009)

8. Andrew, A.H., Boriello, G., Fogarty, J.: Simplifying mobile phone food diaries. In: Proceedings of the Pervasive Health 2013 (2013)

9. Hsu, H.H., Min-Ho, C., Neil, Y.Y.: A health man- agement application with QR-code input and rule inference. In: Proceedings of the ISIC. IEEE (2012)

10. Ohbuchi, E., Hiroshi, H., Lim, A.H.: Barcode readers using the camera device in mobile phones. In: Proceedings of the International Conference Cyberwords (2004)

DRSTI: A Workbench for Querying Retinal Image Data of Age-Related Macular Degeneration Patients

Abhinav Parakh, Parvathi Chundi$^{(\boxtimes)}$, and Mahadevan Subramaniam

Computer Science Department, University of Nebraska-Omaha,
Omaha, NE 68182, USA
{abhinavparakh,pchundi,msubramaniam}@unomaha.edu

Abstract. Age-related macular degeneration (AMD) affects the vision of millions of people around the world. Currently there are a few treatment options to treat and/or arrest the visual distortions in AMD patients; however, they are not uniformly effective. Retinal health of AMD patients is monitored using imaging of the retina using optical coherence tomography, fluorescein agiography, etc. The visual distortions experienced by the patients are monitored using *Amsler* grids. All these different types of image data can be used to study the retinal health of patients and develop correlations among data collected from different images, particularly from the Amsler grids annotated by AMD patients. This paper proposes a conceptual and logical data model that combines all of the image data from AMD patients and describes a query model for accessing the data for a single as well as across multiple patients. All retinal images are processed to construct a **retinal map** for each eye of a patient. The rich retinal map data is then stored in a relational database for further querying.

Keywords: Age-related macular degeneration · Distortions · Retinal map · Relational data model

1 Introduction

Age-related macular degeneration (AMD) is a leading cause of low vision in the developed world. The National Eye Institute estimates that around 2 million people in the U.S. currently suffer from AMD and this number is projected to double by 2030, and almost triple by 2050 [12].

Computational methods to analyze the images of the retinas of AMD patients have played a crucial role in assessing the extent of the disease and devise appropriate treatments. The advent of sophisticated imaging techniques has made it possible to obtain a diverse set of images (see Fig. 1) concerning the function, morphology, and the pathology of the retina of an AMD patient. Amsler grids [13], displayed in Fig. 1(a)

Research Supported by Faculty Innovation Research Enterprise Grant from University of Nebraska-Omaha.

X. Zheng et al. (Eds.): ICSH 2015, LNCS 9545, pp. 340–349, 2016.
DOI: 10.1007/978-3-319-29175-8_32

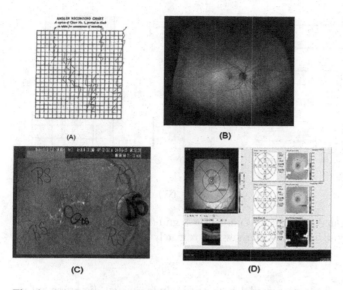

Fig. 1. (A) An Amsler grid annotated by a patient (B) FA image (C) SLO image (D) OCT image

are used by physicians to diagnose and monitor the severity visual distortions in AMD pateints. Flourescein Angiography (FA) images, Fig. 1(b), provide information about leakages, (SLO) images, Fig. 1(c), provide information about relative and dense scotomas, areas where visual function is lost, and OCT images, Fig. 1(d), provide information about areas of retinal thickening or thinning due to AMD.

With the availability of these diverse images, there is an increased interest in correlating these images to provide a more detailed view of AMD to aid physicians. Recently, multi-modal correlations [11] of OCT and FA images of a single retina have been used to provide physicians with more accurate information regarding the affected macular regions, their shapes, and their sizes. OCT images of one eye have been correlated to those of the other eye [1] of a patient to aid physicians to predict disease progress in the second eye and perform early intervention.

While achieving impressive successes, most of these studies are restricted to analyzing one or two types of retinal images of a single patient, trying to find correlations among function, morphology, and pathology. In order to provide a compre-hensive view of the status of the retinal health of an AMD patient it is necessary to seamlessly represent and manipulate heterogeneous retinal image data about an AMD patient. The target representation should not only support easy update, and maintenance of the heterogeneous image data over the course of treatment but also be amenable to cor-relation analyses across several AMD patient discover common health profiles. This is the main objective of this paper.

Towards this goal, in this paper, we propose a data representation for a variety of retinal image data including FA, OCT, SLO, and Amsler grid images that is amenable for querying and correlating data of a single patient to both eyes of multiple patients across all these image types. We propose the notion of a *retinal map,* an $n \times n$ spatial grid to summarize the crucial health information obtained from the FA, OCT, SLO, and Amsler grid images. We first describe a conceptual model of the data captured by the retinal map. We then obtain a relational schema from the conceptual model, which can then be used to query the retinal map data to find possible correlations among different types of retinal images.

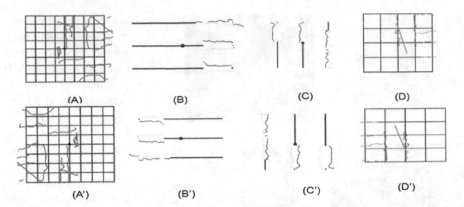

Fig. 2. Distortions seen by an AMD patient (A) in an 8×8 grid (B) in horizontal lines (C) in vertical lines (D) in a 4×4 grid. Images A'– D' show approximately how these images fall on the patient's retina.

An important feature of our data model is that it includes visual distortion information of AMD patients in addition to that obtained by the FA, OCT, and SLO images. Explaining visual distortions based on retinal images does not seem to have received much attention earlier. It is nontrivial to quantify distortions seen and annotated by a patient on a paper-based Amsler grid. In order to study the visual distortion problem, we have used an Amsler grid image displayed on an Android-tablet to elicit the types of distortions seen by a patient. The patient shown an image on a tablet and is then asked to trace the distortions using the touch interface. The resulting grid annotated by a patient can then be analyzed to gather quantitative information about the shape, magnitude, and location of distortions. See Fig. 2(A)–(D). Retinal maps that incorporate data from the retinal images as well as distortions on a single cohesive spatial grid are likely to provide a unique opportunity for a systematic study and tracking of the AMD visual distortions and ultimately, their corrections.

The rest of the paper is organized as follows. Section 2 discusses the notion of a retinal map. Section 3 discusses the conceptual data model, a sample set of relations and SQL queries. Section 4 describes the implementation of the conceptual data model using the OCT image data of about 10 patients. We built a query interface using which the OCT data can be queried and the result can be analyzed. Processing and storing the other types of retinal image data is ongoing.

2 Retinal Maps

Computational methods for processing retinal images is an active area of research [4, 8]. We employed simple image processing techniques such as image segmentation and edge and contour detection [14] to process retinal images to obtain relevant information from each image. The information is transferred from each retinal image to a retinal map after super-imposing an $n \times n$ grid on each of the images and marking each grid cell with the information obtained from the image. We use only the average retinal thickness map (the top-left corner of the OCT image) of the OCT image. Each retinal map cell spans a part of the retinal image and represent the health of the retina covered by the grid cell. For example, consider the FA image and a retinal map cell *(x, y)*. If *(x, y)* overlaps with the lesion part of the image, then our algorithm will mark its numeric value as 0. If the grid cell *(x, y)* is outside or on the boundary of the lesion, then we will set its numeric value as the difference between the average RGB value of *(x, y)* and the average RGB value of all pixels in the lesion area. Our intuition here is that, if a grid cell has a very small numeric value corresponding to the FA image, then it is likely to be unhealthy.

After the processing of each of the images, we associate each retinal map cell (x, y) with a 4-tuple <v1; v2; v3; v4>. Value v1 is obtained from an SLO image and specifies if (x, y) is a part of relative scotoma, a dense scotoma, a preferred retinal locus, or empty. Value v2 is obtained from the FA image and specifies whether or not (x, y) is a part of the lesion. Value v3 is obtained from the OCT average retinal thickness map and specifies the thickness, volume values of that part of the retina, and the ETDRS map region[1]. To transfer the information from Amsler grid images to the retinal map, we process each grid image (Figs. 1(A) and 2(A)–(D)) by computing the amount of distortion marked in each retinal map. We use the following heuristic to orient the position of an Amsler grid image on the retina. When an image is viewed by a patient (using only one eye at a time), the image formed by eyes lens system is smaller than the object viewed, inverted (upside-down) and reversed (right-left). We map the center of the Amsler grid to the center of the retinal map and use the above guidelines to position the Amsler grid image on the retinal map. Then, we compute a distortion value for each retinal value cell as a numeric value that specifies the amount of distortion in the Amsler grid underlying the retinal map cell (x, y).

3 Conceptual Data Model

Figure 3 shows an Entity-Relationship model of the retinal health information of a patient[2]. The patient demographic information, the information from the retinal tests – OCT, FA, and SLO, are represented as entities. The attributes of the patient entity are – patient_id, age, sex, visual acuity values for both right and left eyes. The OCT entity's attributes are – which eye (OS/OD), retinal map column number, retinal map row number, thickness and volume values for that retinal map grid cell, the macular region the cell falls in, the average RGB value of the retina map grid cell, the and the date of the test. The attributes for the SLO and FA entities are mostly similar.

The distortion data of each patient is stored in a Is-A hierarchy [10]. The general entity *Distortion* is used to capture the fact that the information gathered from any Amsler grid image annotated by the patient is the same. Each grid type used to record the distortions seen by a patient is captured as a specialization of the Distortion entity. The attributes of the Distortion entity are the same as those of other entities such as the

---

[1] The 9 macular regions as defined by the Early Treatment Diabetic Retinopathy Study (ETDRS).

[2] Figure 3 lists only a few of the attributes for each entity due to lack of space.

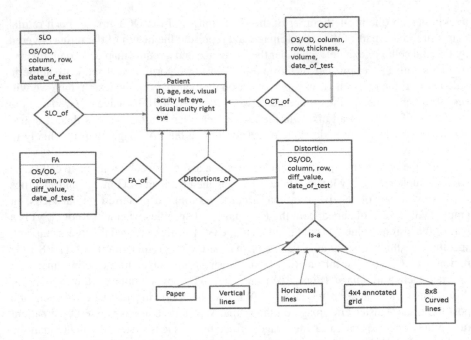

Fig. 3. An entity-relationship model for the retinal map data

SLO entity. There is a one-to-many relationship between the patient entity and the OCT entity. For each patient in the patient entity set, there could be zero or more OCT entities mapped to it in the relationship. But for any one entity in the OCT entity set, there must be only one patient in the relationship set. This constraint is captured by the total participation of the OCT entity in the relationship set OCT_Of. The same is true for entity sets FA, SLO, and Distortion entity sets.

The relational schema obtained by the above E-R model is given below. The relational model is developed with the types of queries to be processed over the data. In this case, the central part of the data model is the $n \times n$ retinal map data collected from the retinal images of each patient's eye. The data model must support queries to access the retinal map data of a single patient for a specific location (a single retinal map cell or a collection of cells) or that of multiple patients across different locations and types.

The logical (relational) data model contains the patient relation to store the demographic information, with ID as the primary key. Then there is one relation for each of the OCT, SLO, and FA entities. Each of these relations will include the ID of the patient as one of the columns in addition to its attributes. There are different options for storing the distortion data of a patient. One option is to store the data collected from different distortion images 8×8, 4×4, etc., in the same table, with the type of the grid as an additional column. Another option is to create a separate a table for each distortion type. The latter option is better for clarity of the relational data model and hence, that option is chosen. The relational data model is shown below. The underlined attribute(s) in each relation definition constitutes the primary key of that relation (Fig 4).

Patient (patient_id, age, sex, OS, OD)
SLOData (patient_id, OS/OD, column, row, status, date_of_test)
FAData (patient_id, OS/OD, column, row, diff_value, date_of_test)
OCTData (patient_id, OS/OD, column, row, thickness, volume, macular region,
RGB color, date_of_test)
PaperAmsler (patient_id, OS/OD, column, row, distortion_value, date_of_test)
VerticalLines (patient_id, OS/OD, column, row, distortion_value, date_of_test)
HorizantalLines (patient_id, OS/OD, column, row, distortion_value, date_of_test)
FourByFour (patient_id, OS/OD, column, row, distortion_value, date_of_test)
EightByEight (patient_id, OS/OD, column, row, distortion_value, date_of_test)

	1	2	3	4
1	OCT (257, 1.36) FA(0.1) SLO(RS) Distortion(<8x8, 0.5>, <4x4, 0.2> <horizontal, 0.2>, <vertical, 0.01>)	OCT(279, 1.48) FA(0.08) SLO(Normal) Distortion(<8x8, 0.2>, <4x4, 0.1>, <horizontal, 0.2>)	OCT (282, 1.52) FA(0.08) SLO(RS) Distortion(<8x8, 0.2>, <4x4, 0.1>, <horizontal, 0.2>)	OCT(293, 1.55) FA(0.1) SLO(RS) Distortion(<vertical, 0.2>)
2	OCT (257, 1.36) FA(0.07) SLO(RS) Distortion(<8x8, 0.6>, <4x4, 0.4> , <horizontal, 0.2>, <vertical, 0.1>)	OCT(304, 0.48) FA(0.05) SLO(DS) Distortion(<8x8, 0.6>, <4x4, 0.4> <horizontal, 0.2> ,<vertical, 0.01>)	OCT(305, 0.48) FA(0.02) SLO(DS) Distortion(<8x8, 0.6>, <4x4, 0.4> <horizontal, 0.2> ,<vertical, 0.4>)	OCT(293, 1.55) FA(0.07) SLO(RS) Distortion(<vertical, 0.2>)
3	OCT (259, 1.38) FA(0.1) SLO(Normal) Distortion(<8x8, 0.6>, <4x4, 0.4> <horizontal, 0.2>, <vertical, 0.01>)	OCT(242, 0.19) FA(0.07) SLO(RS) Distortion(<8x8, 0.6>, <4x4, 0.2> <horizontal, 0.2>, <vertical, 0.4>)	OCT(307, 0.48) FA(0.02) SLO(RS) Distortion(<8x8, 0.6>, <4x4, 0.4> <horizontal, 0.2>, <vertical, 0.01>)	OCT(272, 1.48) FA(0.08) SLO(RS) Distortion(<vertical, 0.2>)
4	OCT (263, 1.40) FA(0.1) SLO(RS) Distortion(<8x8, 0.5>, <4x4, 0.2>, <horizontal, 0.2>, <vertical, 0.4>)	OCT(263, 1.40) FA(0.09) SLO(Normal) Distortion(<8x8, 0.5>, <4x4, 0.2> <horizontal, 0.2>, <vertical, 0.4>)	OCT(299, 0.65) FA(0.1) SLO(RS) Distortion(<vertical, 0.2>)	OCT(263, 1.40) FA(0.1) SLO(RS) Distortion(<vertical, 0.2>)

Fig. 4. A sample retinal map

We show above a sample retinal map for an eye of a patient. A 4 × 4 retinal map was superimposed on each of the images collected for monitoring of the left eye of a patient and the image segment underlying each retinal map cell *(i, j)* was processed to compute the values from different images and stored in the map. Some sample data for a few tables based on the concept of retinal maps is shown below. We list a few records for each table.

Patient(1, 82, F, 20/40, 20/40) Patient(2, 65, M, 20/200, 20/200)
SLOData(1, OS, 1, 1, RS, 01/11/2014) SLOData(1, OS, 1, 2, RS, 01/11/2014)
OCTData(1, OS, 1, 1, 257, 1.36, fovea, dccdc, 01/11/2014)
EightByEight(1, OS, 1, 1, 0.5, 01/11/2014) VerticalLines(1, OS, 1, 1, 0.01, 01/11/2014)

Using these relations, we can extract information pertaining to multiple tests of a single patient. As an example, consider the following query to extract the FA diff_value for patient ID 1 for all the retinal map cells where the SLO status is "DS" (dense scotoma).

select FAData.diff_value from FAData natural join SLOData where FAData,patient_id = 1 and SLOData.status = "DS".

4   DRSTI Workbench for OCT Average Thickness Map Images

The proposed conceptual data model was implemented using the EasyPHP MySQL™ server. The database currently stores the patient demographic information of about 10 patients, and the average retinal thickness map data collected from the OCT images of their left and right eyes. The retinal thickness map was divided into 9 regions – fovea, upper focal, lower focal, nasal focal, temporal focal, upper periphery, lower periphery, nasal periphery, and temporal periphery using MATLAB subroutines. Each macular segment was identified by using an appropriate mask to remove the unwanted part of the thickness map. Each thickness map was processed with a set of 9 masks, for each macular segment.

The size of the retinal map was set to the width and length of the OCT average thickness map image, 400 × 400. Each retinal cell was stored as a row in the OCT table. For each pixel in the thickness map, the RGB value and the macular region value were stored in the table. Additionally, the average thickness and volume values were collected manually from the numeric values provided in the OCT test image and stored.

After the average thickness maps of both eyes of the patients are processed and stored in the data form, users can retrieve interesting information by writing SQL queries. A query form is developed and displayed so that users can conveniently use it to specify their queries. A query form, shown in Fig. 5 on the left side, is displayed to the user to select attributes to query on, the constraints on values of these attributes, and the attributes to be returned in the query result. After consulting with the physicians, we decided to include the following information on a query form that a user can choose to include or not in a query – Patient IDs, dates when the OCT image as taken, macular regions of the OCT image, color, thickness, and volume attributes. It was suggested by physicians that red and blue color on a thickness map indicated unhealthy regions. So, we decided to allow a user to query the RGB color attributes of an image. A user can also specify the macular regions he/she interested in. This will allow physicians to retrieve patients with abnormalities in specific regions of the retina. For convenience sake, the default is set to select all regions. By selecting a region, the user is deselecting other regions.

In this query form, the user has selected to access the macular regions of all patients where the average red color in the average thickness map is between 50 to 100 % (high or unhealthy). The right side of Fig. 5 shows the result of this query. There are two patients that satisfy the constraint. For each of the average thickness maps that satisfy the query constraints, the result displays the thickness map itself, with the macular regions that meet the query constraints, and the regions that do not, and a histogram of RGB values, one for each macular region in the query result, and the average thickness and volume values for each region.

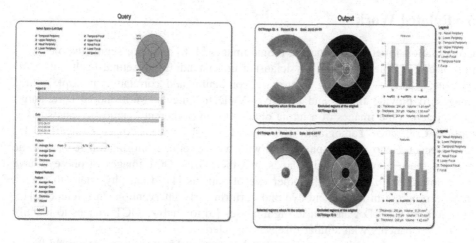

Fig. 5. Query 1 and results

Figure 6 shows a query (form is displayed on the left side of the figure) where the user selected 5 specific macular regions and set a constraint that these macular regions must be healthy in each of the thickness maps in the result. The result of this query contains a single user whose thickness map is shown in the right side of the figure. As can be seen from the color histogram in the result, the red color pixels are low in number in this thickness map which indicates that the retina is relatively healthy.

The design of the query and result forms is ongoing. We consult with the physicians frequently to evaluate the efficacy of these forms.

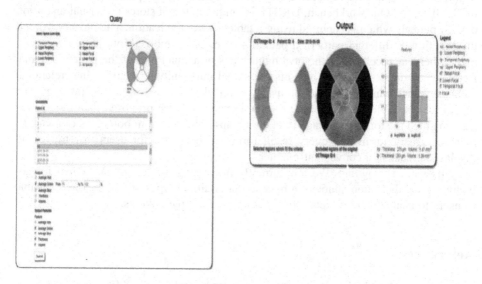

Fig. 6. Query 2 and result

5 Related Work

Computational methods to analyze retinal images [4, 8] and their segmentations [2, 7] play a crucial role in aiding physicians in understanding the retinal health of AMD patients. There is increasing interest in combining and correlating multiple retinal images to provide timely and effective AMD treatments. Multi-modal correlations [3, 11] across the images of a retina obtained using different diagnostic tests such as Optical Coherence Tomography (OCT) and the Fluorescein Angiography (FA) [5] have been used to provide physicians with more accurate information regarding the affected macular regions, their shapes, and their sizes. OCT images of one eye have been correlated to those of the other eye of patients [1] to aid physicians to predict disease progress in the second eye and perform early intervention. In references [15, 16], authors use LDA and clustering analyses [6] to analyze OCT images to identify clusters of patients with similar disease characteristics.

The conceptual and relational data models proposed in this paper are quite different from the previous works on retinal image processing. The proposed work combines the power of relational data model with a simple and novel notion of a retinal map, which is similar to the image data model proposed in [9]. We anticipate that the DRSTI workbench, when completed, will provide a flexible and convenient environment for AMD researchers to study and correlate visual distortions to retinal health attributes.

6 Conclusion and Future Work

In this paper we describe a conceptual and relational data model to capture the retinal health of AMD patients, represented by different imaging equipments such as the FA, OCT, SLO, etc. Our workbench, DRSTI, is unique in that it stores the visual distortion data of patients which is captured using a tablet based application. The physiology and the function of different parts of a patient's retina are combined into an $n \times n$ *retinal map,* where each cell stores the health attributes of a small part of the patient's retina. Retinal map data of multiple patients are stored into multiple relations in a relational database which can then be queried using powerful SQL. The paper illustrates the data model and possible queries through several examples. The proposed data model was implemented to store the average thickness maps collected from both eyes of about 10 patients. Query forms and query result forms were created for users to retrieve and display the data in a convenient manner.

This work is ongoing. We are currently processing the rest of the retinal images including the distortion annotation data so that multiple types of features are available to users to analyze and correlate features across multiple patients.

References

1. Amissah-Arthur, K.N., Panneerselvam, S., Narendran, N., Yang, Y.C.: Optical coherence tomography changes before the development of choroidal neovascularization in second eyes of patients with bilateral wet macular degeneration. Eye **26**, 394–399 (2012)

2. Chiu, S.J., Lokhnygina, Y., Dubis, A.M., Dubra, A., Carroll, J., Izatt, J.A., Farsiu, S.: Automatic cone photoreceptor segmentation using graph theory and dynamic programming. Biomed. Opt. Expr. **4**(6), 924–937 (2013)

3. Chundi, P., Subramaniam, M., Margalit, E.: Discovering themes from AMD retinal maps using topic models. In: IEEE Engineering in Medicine and Biology Society Conference (2014)

4. DeBuc, D.C.: A review of algorithms for segmentation of retinal image data using optical coherence tomography. In: Ho, P. (ed.) Image Segmentation (2011). ISBN: 978-953-307-228-9

5. Malamos, P., Sacu, S., Georgopoulos, M., Kriss, C., Pruente, C., Schmidt-Erfurth, U.: Correlation of high-definition optical coherence tomography and fluorescein angiography imaging in neovascular macular degeneration. Invest. Opthamology Cis Sci. **50**(10), 4926–4933 (2009)

6. Mardia, K., et al.: Multivariate Analysis. Academic Press, New York (1979)

7. Niemeijer, M., Staal, J.: Comparative study of retinal vessel segmentation methods on a new publicly available database. In: Proceedings of SPIE Conference on Medical Imaging (2004)

8. Pattona, N., Aslamc, T.M., MacGillivray, T., Dearye, I.J., Dhillon, B., Eikelboom, R.H., Yogesana, K., Constable, I.J.: Retinal image analysis: concepts, applications and potential. Prog. Retinal Eye Res. **25**(1), 99–127 (2006)

9. Grosky, W.I., Stanchev, P.L.: An image data model. In: Laurini, R. (ed.) VISUAL 2000. LNCS, vol. 1929, pp. 14–25. Springer, Heidelberg (2000)

10. Silberschatz, A., Korth, H.F., Sudarshan, S.: Database System Concepts. McGraw Hill Higher Education, New York (2009)

11. Taibl, J.N., Sayegh, S.I.: Multimodality imaging in clinical diagnosis and treatment of macular disease. In: Proceedings of the SPIE 8567, Ophthalmic Technologies, XXIII (2013)

12. http://www.nei.nih.gov/eyedata/

13. Amsler, M.: Earliest symptoms of diseases of the macula. Br. J. Ophthalmol. **37**, 521 (1953)

14. Parker, J.R.: Algorithms for Image Processing and Computer Vision. Wiley, New York (2011)

15. Go, S., Chundi, P., Subramaniam, M.: Analyzing OCT images of age-related macular degeneration patients to identify spatial health correlations. In: IEEE Conference on Engineering in Medicine and Biology (2015)

16. Subramaniam, M., Chundi, P., Margalit, E.: Discovering themes from AMD retinal maps using topic models. In: IEEE Conference on Engineering in Medicine and Biology (2014)

Proposal to Handle the Interoperability of Clinical Information Systems Across Different Stakeholders

Alexandra López[1], Brayan S. Reyes Daza[2],
and Octavio J. Salcedo Parra[2,3]

[1] Secretaria Distrital de Salud, Bogotá, Colombia
alopez@saludcapital.gov.co
[2] Internet Inteligente Research Group Universidad Distrital Francisco José de
Caldas, Bogotá, Colombia
bsreyesd@correo.udistrital.edu.co
osalcedo@udistrital.edu.co
[3] Universidad Nacional de Colombia, Bogotá D.C., Colombia

Abstract. This paper presents the results of a technological proposal for the implementation of health standards that permit interoperability in industry without throw away the efforts jointly by the governing body of the health sector for the Capital District and by the entities health providers of Network Attached via a service-oriented architecture that provides the ability to integrate all efforts previously made and provides the evolutionary capacity of the HCEU platform.

Keywords: CDA · HL7 · HCEU · XDS

1 Introduction

The technological framework of the health sector is complex and problematic because every institution providing health services, funding, insurance and regulatory as well as various governments agencies, universities and other actors in the health system, have created islands of information in themselves, where the exchange of information with other parties is the exception (Acevedo-Bernal, 2011). In this scenario the efforts are not coordinated, processes are duplicated, yield is lost and increase costs. Then, regulators entities and government have a partial and belated vision what happens in institutions, unable to evaluate the implementation and impact of the projects. Finally, this makes the planning of new health policies and adds noise to the decision-taking at the level of the regulator sector.

2 Research Methodology

Based on the proposed objectives as a result of the operation model for the system of Electronic Health Record Unified (HCEU) it must be determined at the application level the overall architecture of the system, to determine this architecture is used the

© Springer International Publishing Switzerland 2016
X. Zheng et al. (Eds.): ICSH 2015, LNCS 9545, pp. 351–352, 2016.
DOI: 10.1007/978-3-319-29175-8

projective research methodology to guide the process of developing of the architectural system proposal. In this methodological process by reviewing reports on states of management of clinical information about patients of the health system of the Capital District previously developed by the Ministry of Health, existing the problematic of the impossibility of sharing by a timely way the clinical information regarding the medical history of the patients given the high degree of heterogeneity and various states of development or absence of the information systems of the Provider Entities Health Network Attached Capital District (University District, 2012). The standard selected for the system because its different advantages and great adaptability was HL7, with the implementation of IHE profiles for application and review of architectural styles was selected because the service-oriented architecture advantages. How is applied the service-oriented architecture using HL7 is the result of this research.

3   Research Results: General Architecture of the HCEU System

The design of the architecture supports the integration of existing applications on each attached network entity, created to support the mission of the District Health System, by building a technological solution based on interoperability, and fully available, which has a lower impact in each one of the consumers applications of the HCEU services.

Additionally, it is important the HCEU positioning as a resource of the District Health System, which from the beginning is projected to extend its capabilities, and its use and re-use in changing processes and evolutionary focusing on providing a health service highest quality to each of the beneficiaries.

4   Conclusions

Using HL7 allows the District and SDS supported by integrated services architecture integrate on a scalable form the various entities that make up the framework of the Capital District Health, and even the extension of the national model by integrating health networks substantially improve the nation's health.

The resulting health model of the Capital District supported by HL7 standards group, IHE profiles and service-oriented architectural style is a viable, scalable and evolutionary model that allows the determination of health sector policies that facilitate the promotion and prevention management of the morbidity - mortality due to the availability of information for episodes of care of patients in the sector.

References

1. Health Level Seven International. Introduction to hl7 standards, 2014. http://www.hl7.org/implement/standards/index.cfm?ref=nav
2. Universidad Distrital SDS. Modelo de Operación HCEU. Universidad Distrital, Reading, MA, 2012
3. Dirección General de Información en Salud. Norma Oficial Mexicana NOM-024-SSA3-2012, 2012. http://www.dgis.salud.gob.mx/intercambio/nom024.html

Author Index

Printed in the United States
By Bookmasters